Paula

Evidence-Based Rehabilitation

A Guide to Practice

SECOND EDITION

EDITED BY

MARY LAW, PHD, OTREG(ONT), FCAOT

SCHOOL OF REHABILITATION SCIENCE

MCMASTER UNIVERSITY

HAMILTON, ONTARIO, CANADA

JOY MACDERMID, PT, PHD

SCHOOL OF REHABILITATION SCIENCE

MCMASTER UNIVERSITY

HAMILTON, ONTARIO, CANADA

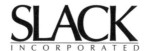

Delivering the best in health care information and education worldwide

www.slackbooks.com

ISBN: 978-1-55642-768-8

Copyright © 2008 by SLACK Incorporated

Evidence-Based Rehabilitation: A Guide to Practice, Second Edition Instructor's Manual
is also available from SLACK Incorporated. Don't miss this important companion to
Evidence-Based Rehabilitation: A Guide to Practice, Second Edition.
To obtain the Instructor's Manual, please visit http://www.efacultylounge.com.

Cover illustration by Doris M. Law and kindly used with permission.

SLACK Incorporated uses a review process to evaluate submitted material. Prior to publication, educators or clinicians
provide important feedback on the content that we publish. We welcome feedback on this work.

Published by: SLACK Incorporated
                       6900 Grove Road
                       Thorofare, NJ 08086 USA
                       Telephone: 856-848-1000
                       Fax: 856-853-5991
                       www.slackbooks.com

Library of Congress Cataloging-in-Publication Data

Evidence-based rehabilitation : a guide to practice / edited by Mary Law, Joy MacDermid. -- 2nd ed.
   p. ; cm.
Includes bibliographical references and index.
ISBN 978-1-55642-768-8 (alk. paper)
1. Medical rehabilitation. 2. Evidence-based medicine. 3. Occupational therapy. I. Law, Mary C. II. MacDermid, Joy.
  [DNLM: 1. Rehabilitation--methods. 2. Evidence-Based Medicine--methods. 3. Treatment Outcome. WB 320 E93
2008]

RM930.E934 2008
617'.03--dc22
                                                                                                2007039244

For permission to reprint material in another publication, contact SLACK Incorporated. Authorization to photocopy
items for internal, personal, or academic use is granted by SLACK Incorporated provided that the appropriate fee is paid
directly to Copyright Clearance Center. Prior to photocopying items, please contact the Copyright Clearance Center
at 222 Rosewood Drive, Danvers, MA 01923 USA; phone: 978-750-8400; website: www.copyright.com; email: info@
copyright.com

Printed in the United States of America.

Last digit is print number: 10 9 8 7 6 5 4

CONTENTS

Evidence-Based Rehabilitation: A Guide to Practice, Second Edition Instructor's Manual
is also available from SLACK Incorporated. Don't miss this important companion to
Evidence-Based Rehabilitation: A Guide to Practice, Second Edition.
To obtain the Instructor's Manual, please visit http://www.efacultylounge.com.

ACKNOWLEDGMENTS

We have been very fortunate to be supported in this book by excellent authors who have willingly shared their knowledge to writing chapters of this book. We thank to each of them for their thoughtful and comprehensive contributions. Our work in evidence-based rehabilitation has been stimulated and supported by colleagues and students at McMaster University, Canada. We are grateful to work in an environment where new ideas are explored, challenged, and developed.

ABOUT THE EDITORS

Mary Law, PHD, OTReg(Ont), FCAOT, FCAHS is a Professor and Associate Dean (Health Sciences) Rehabilitation Science and associate member of the Department of Clinical Epidemiology and Biostatistics at McMaster University. She holds the John and Margaret Lillie Chair in Childhood Disability Research. Mary, an occupational therapist by training, is Co-Founder of CanChild Centre for Childhood Disability Research, a multidisciplinary research center at McMaster University. Mary's research centers on the development and validation of client-centered outcome measures, evaluation of occupational therapy interventions with children, the effect of environmental factors on the participation of children with disabilities in day to day activities, and transfer of research knowledge into practice. In her educational activities, Mary is involved in teaching the theoretical basis of occupational therapy practice and evidence-based occupational therapy practice in the occupational therapy program, as well as supervising graduate students. Mary is the lead author of the Canadian Occupational Performance Measure, a client-centered outcome measure for occupational therapy, and has written books on client-centered occupational therapy and measurement of occupational performance.

Joy MacDermid, PT, PhD, is an Associate Professor in Rehabilitation Science at McMaster University (Hamilton, ON), and is the Co-director of Clinical Research at the Hand and Upper Limb Centre (London, ON). She is funded as a (physical therapist/epidemiologist) scientist by the Canadian Institutes of Health (CIHR New Investigator). She has published more than 100 articles including systematic reviews, development/evaluation of outcomes measures, clinical trials, knowledge transfer, clinical practice guidelines, and identification of clinical predictors. Her clinical interests are in musculoskeletal pain and disability resulting from upper quadrant disorders and the impact of these disorders on work and subsequent health and quality of life. Joy teaches courses in upper extremity musculoskeletal clinical skills, evidence-based practice, work disability, quality of life, and knowledge exchange and transfer. She is the Vice-President of the American Society of Hand Therapists (ASHT); has twice won its best scientific paper award; and was awarded the Natalie Barr Lecture in 2006, the Philadelphia Hand Meeting Honored Professorship in 2006, and the CIHR Quality of Life Award in 2007. She is an associate editor for *The Journal of Hand Therapy* and *The Journal of Orthopaedic and Sports Physical Therapy* and is the editor for the ASHT Clinical Outcome Assessment Recommendations for the Wrist/Hand.

Contributing Authors

Jill Ball, BP, BHScOT
Occupational Therapist
Renfrew Educational Services
Calgary, Alberta, Canada

Laura Bradley, MSc OT, OTReg(Ont)
Clinician
Early Childhood Program
Ottawa Children's Treatment Center
Ottawa, Ontario, Canada

Winnie Dunn, PhD, OTR, FAOTA
Professor and Chair
Department of Occupational Therapy Education
University of Kansas Medical Center
Kansas City, KS

Paola Durando, BA, MLS
Public Services Librarian
Bracken Health Sciences Library
Queen's University
Kingston, Ontario, Canada

Robin Gaines, PhD, SLP(C), CASLPO, CCC-SLP
Clinical Researcher
Children's Hospital of Eastern Ontario Research Institute,
Adjunct Professor
School of Rehabilitation Sciences
University of Ottawa
Ontario, Canada

Sally Home, BAppSc(OT) Hons, GradCert(Mgt)
CRS Australia
Nowra, New South Wales, Australia

Emma Housser, BSc
Division of Community Health & Humanities
Memorial University, St. John's
Newfoundland and Labrador, Canada

Jennie Q. Lou, MD, MSc, OTR
Director, Master of Science in Biomedical Informatics Program
Professor of Public Health & Internal Medicine
College of Osteopathic Medicine
Nova Southeastern University
Ft. Lauderdale, FL

Maria Mathews, PhD, MHSA, BA, BSc
Division of Community Health & Humanities
Memorial University, St. John's
Newfoundland and Labrador, Canada

Annie McCluskey, PhD, MA, DipCOT
Faculty of Health Sciences
The University of Sydney
Sydney, Australia

Susan Michlovitz, PT, PhD, CHT
Ithaca, NY
Adjunct Associate Professor, Rehabilitation Medicine
Program in Physical Therapy
Columbia University
New York, NY

Cheryl Missiuna, PhD, OTReg(Ont)
Associate Professor
School of Rehabilitation Science
Director
CanChild, Centre for Childhood Disability Research
McMaster University
Hamilton, Ontario, Canada

Nancy Pollock, MSc, OTReg(Ont)
Associate Clinical Professor
School of Rehabilitation Science
Co-Investigator
CanChild, Centre for Childhood Disability Research
McMaster University
Hamilton, Ontario, Canada

Jessica Telford, BA
Assistant/Coordinator
School of Rehabilitation Science
McMaster University
Hamilton Ontario, Canada

Lauren Thompson, BAppSc(OT) Hons
Port Kembla Hospital
Wollongong, New South Wales, Australia

Linda Tickle-Degnen, PhD, OTR/L, FAOTA
Professor and Chair
Department of Occupational Therapy
Director
Health Quality of Life Lab
Tufts University
Medford, MA

Diane Watson, PhD, MBA, BScOT
Faculty, Centre for Health Services and Policy Research
University of British Columbia
Director of Research and Analyses
Health Council of Canada

PREFACE

Science is not formal logic... it needs the free play of the mind in as great a degree as any other creative art. It is true that this is a gift which can hardly be taught, but its growth can be encouraged in those who already posses it.

Max Born (1882 1970)

Evidence-based practice continues to be one of the most discussed and debated topics in health care over the past decade. Initially described and developed in an area of medicine, evidence-based practice is now part of every health care discipline and professional education program. While everyone agrees that it is important to use evidence in practice, the challenges of finding, evaluating, and using evidence are substantial. For rehabilitation, our evidence base is growing rapidly but moving these findings into practice remains a substantial challenge. Integrating research findings with clinical wisdom and clients' preferences and values is the goal of evidence-based rehabilitation. Our aim in editing this text is to provide information to students and practitioners in rehabilitation to aid in the development and use of evidence-based practice.

The book is designed to outline the concepts, methods, and strategies underpinning evidence-based rehabilitation. There are four sections within the text. Section I, Introduction to Evidence-Based Practice, describes the basic concepts of evidence-based rehabilitation and discusses how knowledge is developed within a discipline. The role of reflective practice in supporting evidence-based practice is outlined. Section II, Finding the Evidence, centers on outcomes in evidence-based rehabilitation and methods to search for evidence. Evaluation, critical appraisal, and systematic review of evidence are highlighted in Section III, Assessing the Evidence. An example of a completed systematic review of evidence in area of rehabilitation practice illustrates these methods. Finally, Section IV, Using the Evidence, discusses strategies to build evidence in practice and communicate evidence to clients, managers, funders, and practitioners. The relationship between practice guidelines and evidence-based practice is described in the chapter outlining the use of guidelines. Information about knowledge exchange and transfer is discussed. An example of a coordinated approach to knowledge development and transfer in an area of rehabilitation services is provided to stimulate discussion and learning regarding the transfer of knowledge into practice and policy.

We have benefited greatly from feedback about the first edition of this book. We hope that rehabilitation students, practitioners, and educators will explore the issues and methods in this book and find it useful to build professional knowledge. We welcome your thoughts and comments about the book's content.

Mary Law and Joy MacDermid
Hamilton, Ontario, Canada
October 29, 2007

SECTION I:

INTRODUCTION TO EVIDENCE-BASED PRACTICE

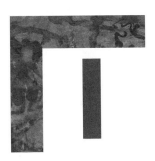

Introduction to Evidence-Based Practice

Mary Law, PhD, OTReg(Ont), FCAOT and Joy MacDermid, PT, PhD

LEARNING OBJECTIVES

After reading this chapter, the student/practitioner will be able to:

- Understand the origins and definitions of evidence-based practice (EBP) and recognize the key elements.
- Critically discuss the concepts and misconceptions surrounding EBP.
- Recognize the nature of EBP in rehabilitation.
- Understand and explain the key characteristics of evidence-based rehabilitation (EBR), including awareness, consultation, judgment, and creativity.

"I have used this intervention for many years, and now researchers have shown that it is not effective. How do I know whether I should believe them and stop using this approach?"

"The program in which I work is starting a new service designed to improve the work tolerance and function of injured workers. We will need to demonstrate that the outcomes of this new program are excellent. How do I identify assessment tools to evaluate client outcomes after receiving the program?"

"Several studies have shown that a short, intensive therapy intervention may be more effective than therapy for a longer period of time. What are the cost implications of this type of service delivery?"

EVIDENCE-BASED REHABILITATION

Any rehabilitation practitioner could ask these questions. Occupational therapists, physical therapists, speech pathologists, and other rehabilitation health professionals, need high-quality information on which to base clinical and managerial decisions. These issues point to the need for practice based on available evidence. EBP in rehabilitation has emerged as one of the most influential concepts in the past decade.

The very mention of EBP brings out different reactions from rehabilitation practitioners. The concept of such practice may seem daunting to the beginner—finding applicable evidence, evaluating it, and putting its recommendations into practice is no small feat! However, if done correctly, EBP is not a burden but a very powerful tool that helps practitioners provide higher quality services for their clients and families.

EBP is often perceived as an "all-or-nothing" approach but, in reality, it can be put into practice in stages through setting priorities for action. Learning about and implementing EBP is best done one step at a time. The fears that surround EBP are largely unfounded and based on a misunderstanding of the concept. Indeed, EBP is probably one of the most misunderstood concepts in health care today because of its newness and the degree to which it breaks from traditional practice. This chapter aims to provide a number of working definitions of EBP and to debunk the myths surrounding it.

The Origins of Evidence-Based Practice

EBP emerged in medicine based on a clear need for a better way to make clinical decisions and fueled by developments in the field of clinical epidemiology. Although a number of scientists were active in moving the emerging field of clinical epidemiology forward at different institutions in Canada and in Europe, McMaster University, Hamilton, ON, Canada has been recognized as the birthplace of evidence-based medicine (EBM). This credit is largely attributable to the original work of David Sackett who worked with colleagues in the new and innovative "problem-based" medical program established at McMaster University in 1970. The first textbook on clinical epidemiology (Sackett, Haynes, & Tugwell, 1985), which was published with Sackett's colleagues in the Department of Clinical Epidemiology at McMaster University contained many of the core concepts of EBM. Colleagues like Bryan Haynes and Gord Guyatt continued to develop and disseminate the key principles and methods of EBM, the latter often credited with coining the term evidence-based medicine. Despite the concept's relative youth, it has infiltrated many different disciplines and is now recognized worldwide. In fact, it was recently named one of the top ten developments in medicine (Dickersin, Straus, & Bero, 2007). Concepts can be adapted for greater impact as they dissipate, but they can also be misused and misunderstood so it is important to retain the key principles.

DEFINING EVIDENCE-BASED PRACTICE

"What does the evidence say?"

"Have you looked at the evidence?"

"Based on the evidence, I recommend..."

Sound familiar? The term *evidence-based practice* is appearing more and more frequently in the literature, educational programs, client groups, and job descriptions in health care. Numerous attempts have been made to conclusively define EBP, and these variants reflect the necessary process of adapting and refining the classic definition to different environments. EBM and EBP are often used interchangeably to mean the same thing. Technically, EBM refers only to the "medical" field, whereas EBP encompasses more aspects of health care, including rehabilitation.

As EBP has developed, a number of variant definitions have been proposed. EBM, as first described by researchers and practitioners at McMaster University, was described as "a new paradigm for medical practice" (Evidence-Based Medicine Working Group, 1992, p. 2420). In this first article outlining EBM, Guyatt and colleagues wrote about the need for physicians to develop skills in critical appraisal and the application of evidence guidelines to the provision of care. In that paper, EBM was not given a formal definition. A later paper defined EBM as the "conscientious, explicit and judicious use of current best evidence in making decisions about the care of individual patients/clients" (Sackett, Rosenberg, Gray, Haynes, & Richardson, 1996, p. 71). The practice of EBM means integrating individual clinical expertise with the best available external clinical evidence from systematic research. This definition has been carefully worded to strike a fine balance between "clinical expertise" and "external clinical evidence."

One of the greatest obstacles to the spread of EBP is that some established practitioners are opposed to it on ideological grounds. They object to EBP on the grounds that it pays no heed to the experience and expertise that professionals have been developing throughout entire careers. This is one of the main misconceptions about EBP; it does not ignore clinical skill; in fact, it welcomes it. EBP tries to root out assessment procedures and interventions that have worked their way into accepted practice but which may not be the most beneficial for the client.

The argument for EBP is simple: If there is a better way to practice, therapists should find it. This means critically evaluating what has already been done to see if it could be improved, making EBP a heavily client-centered approach to providing care. However, EBP in no way advocates ignoring the clinical experience of established practitioners. If anything, that experience is more important, for knowledgeable practitioners are the ones who will know how best to implement EBP's findings. EBP's central message here is one of flexibility and of being able to blend the old ways with the fruits of research and new knowledge. As Sackett et al. (1996) say, "By individual clinical expertise we mean the proficiency and judgment that individual clinicians acquire through clinical experience and clinical practice."

As the idea of EBP unfolded, the definition began to expand and to include components other than current literature. Soon, EBP was seen as an approach to decision making that used the best evidence available in conjunction with client choices to decide upon an option that suits the client best (Muir Gray, 1997). Initially, EBP reduced the emphasis on clinical judgment, instead favoring research studies. Now there is seen to be more of a balance between research and clinical judgment, recognizing that the clinicians and their colleagues bring valuable information to client choices (Guyatt, 2004).

EBP is seen as a process, beginning with clinical questions, appraisal of the evidence, application of the evidence (considering the clients wishes and needs), and finishing with an evaluation of the clinical outcomes (Haynes, 2002). The Canadian Health Services Research Foundation (CHSRF) (2004) adds that evidence-based practitioners combine not only research evidence, but also political and organizational evidence to arrive at clinical decisions. EBP has also been described as a total process beginning with knowing what clinical questions to ask, how to find best practice, and how to appraise evidence for validity and applicability to a particular care situation. The best evidence then must be applied by a practitioner with expertise in considering the patient's unique values and needs. The final aspect of this process is the evaluation of the effectiveness of care and the continual improvement of this process (DePalma, 2000).

During the past few years, research evidence has also played a larger role in informing policy initiatives. For policy, the use of evidence has been termed *evidence-informed practice*, in light of the fact that policy decisions are influenced by other factors besides research evidence (e.g., budgets, political decisions) (CHSRF, 2005).

In essence, EBP is based on a self-directed learning model, whereby practitioners must not only continue learning but also continue evaluating their techniques and practice in light of this learning to see what can be improved. This is—in the truest sense of the form—the ability to critically examine, evaluate, and apply knowledge and then assess one's own findings. Strange as it may sound, practitioners must maintain a humble attitude about their own practice patterns to excel at EBP. The ability to admit one's own errors and oversights and to critically assess one's own prior work is crucial because knowing one's own limitations (and when to look for help) is the basis of EBP. If you maintain this attitude, EBP's use of the "best external evidence" allows you to tap into the work of thousands of professionals around the world in order to find the best possible interventions for your clients. As Sackett et al. (1996) say, "By best available external clinical evidence we mean clinically relevant research, often from the basic sciences of medicine, but especially from patient-centered clinical research..."

Thus the definition offered by Sackett et al. (1996) is an acknowledgment that health care is an imperfect science that requires both overarching clinical guidelines and individual judgment in equal parts. EBP works with the interplay of these two factors, making it a powerful tool that practitioners can use to guide their clinical decisions. EBP uses research evidence but not in isolation.

Another useful definition of EBP comes from another expert in the field, Dr. Trisha Greenhalgh. She offers a simple definition of EBP: "Evidence-based medicine requires you to read the right papers at the right time and then to alter your behavior (and, what is often more difficult, the behavior of other people) in light of what you have found" (Greenhalgh, 1997, p. 2). A more detailed definition comes from Rosenberg and Donald (1995) in their paper, "Evidence-based medicine: An approach to clinical problem solving." They write that EBM/practice is "the process of systematically finding, appraising, and using contemporaneous research findings as the basis for clinical decisions. EBM asks questions, finds and appraises the relevant data, and harnesses that information for everyday clinical practice" (p. 1122).

The definition offered by Rosenberg and Donald (1995) outlines EBP and also provides a step-by-step method of going about it. The four steps are questioning, searching, evaluating, and implementing and should be a constant cycle for the dedicated practitioner of EBP. At any moment, practitioners will likely be faced with a number of problems to which they must apply EBP, and they will be at various stages of the process at different times.

Recent literature has emphasized an expanded definition and scope for EBP. Haynes (2004, p. 2) states, "EBM advocates want patients, practitioners, health care managers and policy makers to pay attention to the best findings from health care research that meet the dual requirements of being both scientifically valid and ready for clinical application." The goal of EBP is to create strategies and tools for practitioners to access, understand, and use the latest research knowledge to improve services for clients. Much work has been done to increase the accessibility of research knowledge through the development of critical review guides, systematic reviews, and easy-to-understand knowledge transfer materials.

There is now a recognition among EBP proponents that research knowledge is only one of several factors that is considered in clinical decision-making (Haynes, 2002; Law, Pollock, & Stewart, 2004).

As Law et al. (2004, p. 14) state:

> *In fact, EBP can be considered to be a combination of information from what we know from research, what we have learned from clinical wisdom, and what we learned from information from the client and their family. This combination of information enables us to work together with clients and families to make the best use of knowledge.*

Despite the different word choices in the many definitions of EBP, therapists use a combination of many facets of current literature, client choice, expertise, and clinical judgment to best serve the clients in their practice.

CONTROVERSY IN EVIDENCE-BASED REHABILITATION

Knowing that EBR is the standard practitioners must reach is not enough. How then do we become evidence-based practitioners? On the outset, this seems a simple process. Discover the client's wishes, research different alternatives, appraise the evidence available, confer with colleagues, weigh the pros and cons of each option, and come to a choice. In practice, some feel that this is not as easy as it appears. Clinicians report several challenges associated with becoming and remaining evidence-based practitioners.

There is a heavy cost associated with generating high-level, good-quality studies. As researchers may be financially limited in what they can produce, consumers of research may be left with fewer choices of evidence. There may be relatively few high-level quality studies available on a given topic, but more research being done at lower, less expensive levels. This will leave clinicians at a loss to find large banks of high-level evidence to support or refute a treatment option (Guyatt, 2004).

Evidence of all qualities is being generated and indexed in the databases at an astounding rate. Many practitioners feel that this is simply too much to contend with and are not able to effectively create summaries that are current. Because of the influx of information, past systematic reviews are often not updated, leaving clinicians with "older" evidence (Guyatt, 2004).

Practitioners incorporating research into current clinical practice can run into problems due to the design of studies. Evidence-based practitioners must incorporate research into their current therapies to ensure best practice. However, methodological differences in current studies may affect the clinician's ability to use them. For example, randomized control trials (RCTs) and meta-analyses are considered the highest level of quantitative evidence, but many of them cannot be generalized due to subgroup make up, clinical size of effect, or quality of outcome measures used. This will limit the practitioner's ability to use the conclusions clinically (Grimmer, 2004).

Presentation of evidence can also impede the ability of clinicians to incorporate it into practice. Research is often presented in a language that clinicians have difficulty understanding with the implications to current practice not always outlined. Without someone to help "translate" the findings into a format that clinicians can understand and apply, the research does not reach its intended audience and clients are not able to benefit from it (Sudsawad, 2005).

Finally, clinicians feel that there is often a lack of time and resources preventing them from becoming effective evidence-based practitioners (Curtin & Jaramazovic, 2001). Many feel they are not skilled in effectively searching the evidence, and when they do, the studies they wish to access are not available (Bennett et al., 2003; Curtin & Jaramazovic, 2001).

Despite these concerns, rehabilitation clinicians are positive about using evidence in their practice (Curtin & Jaramazovic, 2001), and a recent Australian survey suggests that 96% of practitioners say EBP is important to therapists (Bennett et al., 2003). With this in mind, how can we become (and remain) effective evidence-based practitioners?

If client values and therapist values are not the same, we can research all options and present graded recommendations based on all available options (Guyatt, 2004). Researchers can liaise with clinicians to ensure that clinically relevant information is being presented in a way that practitioners can understand (Grimmer, 2004). Companies and hospitals can offer practical incentives of time to therapists, as well as targeted educational initiatives around search strategies to assist the implementation of research into current practice (Bennett et al., 2003; Curtin & Jaramazovic, 2001).

Table 1-1	
MYTHS OF EVIDENCE-BASED PRACTICE	
Myth	*Reality*
• Evidence-based practice already exists	• Many practitioners take little or no time to review current medical findings
• Evidence-based practice is impossible to put into place	• Even extremely busy practitioners can initiate evidence-based practice through little work
• Evidence-based practice is cookie-cutter medicine	• Evidence-based practice requires extensive clinical expertise
• Evidence-based practice is a cost-cutting mechanism	• Evidence-based practice emphasizes the best available clinical evidence for each client's situation

MYTHS SURROUNDING EVIDENCE-BASED PRACTICE

Despite attempts to publicize the realities surrounding EBP, there continue to be some "myths" surrounding it (Table 1-1), which Sackett et al. (1996) and Haynes (2002) discuss in their articles. The misconception that EBP is either "already in place" or "impossible to practice" is their first target. Addressing the first point, Sackett et al. point out that while completely keeping up with the health research literature is impossible for any person, many practitioners take little or no time in their weekly routine to examine journals and publications, preferring instead to rely completely on their initial training to guide their practice (Sackett et al., 1996)

EBP does not mean that every clinical situation will send a practitioner slavishly running to the library, but it does mean that when a new situation presents itself, a clinician should employ research skills to find an answer and pass this information on to colleagues. Unfortunately, this is not always the case; many clinicians rely solely on the expertise of others, which, while it can be helpful, is inherently based on the quirks of individual experience. As previously stated, a balance between the two sources of information can hardly hurt practitioners in making more accurate and more insightful diagnoses.

This argument also meshes with Sackett et al.'s (1996) further point that EBP is not impossible to put into place. In fact, they specifically state that "studies show that busy clinicians who devote their scarce reading time to selective, efficient, client-driven searching, appraisal and incorporation of the best available evidence can practice evidence-based medicine." Practicing EBP is not a matter of inundating one's self with evidence—it is a matter of deftly locating and using the evidence from the ever-growing pile of research and rehabilitation knowledge. This practice becomes easier as systems are developed to filter or evaluate the wealth of published studies.

Another criticism of EBP is that it is "cookie-cutter" medicine or devoid of the need for individual clinical judgment. This criticism returns to the earlier fears of EBP making clinicians' expertise irrelevant, and Sackett et al. (1996) again attempt to clarify the goals of EBP. As they state, "external clinical evidence can inform, but can never replace, individual clinical expertise; this expertise will assist the practitioner in deciding whether the external evidence applies to the individual client at all and, if so, how it should be integrated into a clinical decision." No supporter of EBP has argued for the removal of regular training for practitioners; they have merely suggested that the training include information on how EBP fits into the clinical equation.

Table 1-2

IMPORTANT CONCEPTS IN EVIDENCE-BASED REHABILITATION

- Awareness
- Creativity

- Judgment
- Consultation

Lastly, Sackett et al. (1996) debunk the concept that EBP is merely a malicious tool of health-policy makers—either introduced to cut costs or insisting that each clinical intervention be backed by a RCT. Both issues miss the point of EBP—to bring the best available clinical evidence to each client's situation. Using the best available evidence does not reduce the need for costly interventions; it simply attempts to ensure that each client gets the treatment appropriate for his or her condition. Furthermore, EBP insists that each case is treated with the best available evidence and is not so haughty that it rejects anything that is not a RCT outright. Because of the strength of EBP, it can be applied now in all forms of health care. This fact is discussed by

While the health care climate may create a situation in which some policy makers misuse the core concepts of EBP, it is clear that EBP definitions do not encourage suspending treatments if there are no RCTs available to support them; they merely suggest that the best available evidence inform the choice.

EVIDENCE-BASED REHABILITATION

One goal of this book is to assist students in becoming better practitioners and caregivers through using evidence-based strategies and tools. The previous discussion of EBP provides a theoretical understanding of the concept. The remainder of the chapter focuses on a discussion of EBR, which students may find more applicable and more relevant to their future work. EBR is a subset of evidence-based clinical practice, which has been discussed at length. Let us look at some ideas that will help us to ascertain the key skills that assist clinicians practice EBR (Table 1-2).

Awareness

The first definition is from the Health Informatics Research Unit (HIRU) at McMaster University, which states, "Evidence-based clinical practice (EBCP) is an approach to health care practice in which the clinician is aware of the evidence that bears on her clinical practice, and the strength of that evidence" (HIRU, 2002). The HIRU makes an important point—the clinician must be aware of the evidence related to his or her practice. This does not mean that he or she must read every new journal that comes out cover-to-cover, but he or she should find ways of staying up-to-date with what new research is happening in his or her field. There are many ways to do this, from journals that specifically summarize research advances to Web sites that bring information together to online discussion groups and chat forums in which practitioners can interact. Instead of awareness of everything without comprehension, the goal is focused awareness, or knowledge, of where to look. Each practitioner must find his or her own natural way to stay up-to-date. This is important because striving for excellence means giving the best to each client and his or her family.

Consultation

A second definition comes from J. A. Muir Gray's (1997) book on evidence-based health care, in which he points out, "Evidence-based clinical practice is an approach to decision making in which the clinician uses the best evidence available, in consultation with the patient, to decide upon the option which suits that patient best." Muir Gray's definition is a reminder of one of the most important aspects of health care—transparency. Practitioners have a specialized set of skills and knowledge, and an essential part of their job has always been to be good communicators. Their role is to work together with the client to ascertain the problem(s) and how it can be resolved in the easiest possible terms. With the advent of EBR, that job remains the same, albeit somewhat more complex. EBP is a method for distilling information from the findings of others and, equally, a vehicle for educating the client. Practitioners who are able to adeptly explain the practice of EBR to their clients, how they have found the clinical data they are using, and what they are doing with it will be the most successful. This opens the process up to the client, so he or she can see what the practitioner is doing. EBP turns the focus toward the community, with the practitioner working as an educator as well as a service provider.

Judgment

Although EBP and EBR represent a major advance in the field of rehabilitation, they should not be embraced blindly. At the 60th Annual Assembly of the American Academy of Physical Medicine and Rehabilitation, keynote speaker Dr. Joel DeLisa (1999) made these remarks about EBP and rehabilitation, "However, there are problems in the 'evidence' of evidence-based medicine... the laudable goal of making clinical decisions based on evidence can be impaired by the restricted quality and scope of what is collected as 'best available evidence'" (p. 7).

The problems or limits to the evidence in EBP cannot and should not be ignored. As DeLisa (1999, p. 7) points out:

> Derived almost exclusively from randomized trials and meta-analysis... the results [of EBP work in rehabilitation] show comparative efficacy of treatment for an "average" randomized patient and are not for pertinent subgroups formed by cogent clinical features such as severity of symptoms, illness, comorbidity, and other clinical nuances.

Practitioners must possess good clinical judgment to differentiate how to apply the recommendations of EBP and how they must be tailored to the specifics of each client's situation.

Creativity

A final definition of evidence-based health care, which lends itself to EBR, comes from an article in the *Journal of the American Medical Association*, which summarizes a discussion on the practice of EBM. The definition that comes from this round table is that evidence-based health care is "a conscientious, explicit, and judicious use of the current best evidence to make a decision about the care of patients" (Marwick, 1997). Using the best effort in a "conscientious, explicit, and judicious" way will not always be straightforward, and practitioners will have to use their creative skills to meet the challenges of real life. Learning EBP is both a science and an art and, as such, must be melded to the already existing body of skills that a practitioner has in his or her repertoire. EBR may sound like "cookie-cutter" practice but, in actuality, it requires a great deal of creativity and insight to work correctly. Ultimately, EBP allows practitioners to "write their own textbook," so to speak, and teach themselves what they need to do. This makes creativity essential.

Conclusion

EBR is an important part of current practice. Practicing confident, resourceful, and creative rehabilitation is an art and must be developed over time. It is hoped that this book will serve to speed that process for many practitioners as they formulate their own definition of EBR.

Evidence-Based Practice

- There are misunderstandings of EBP because of the way in which it breaks with traditional practice; it can be seen as a powerful tool, not a burden.
- EBP maintains a fine balance between clinical expertise and external clinical evidence.
- EBP is based on an ongoing and self-directed learning model.
- EBP can support a strongly client-centered approach to rehabilitation.
- Clinical experience remains crucial because knowledgeable practitioners will best implement their findings based on evidence.
- EBP makes use of the current best methods of treatment.

Evidence-Based Rehabilitation

- EBR is an adaptation of the concepts of EBP to rehabilitation practice and necessitates specific skills that allow clinicians to use evidence within the complex decision making required for rehabilitation practice.
- Awareness: The clinician must be aware of the evidence that has to do with practice and maintain focused awareness.
- Consultation: The practitioner must have a specialized set of skills and knowledge to be a good communicator; the practitioner works as an educator/service provider.
- Judgment: The practitioner differentiates between cases about how to apply recommendations of EBP; tailored to specifics of each client's situation.
- Creativity: EBR requires creativity and insight as the practice and application of the best available evidence is not always straightforward.

Web Links

- *Definitions of Evidence-Based Practice*
  www.shef.ac.uk/~scharr/ir/def.html
  This site has an extensive selection of definitions for EBP, including many found in this chapter. It also has links to other resources for learning more about the essential aspects of EBP.
- *Evidence-Based Medicine Learning Resources*
  www.herts.ac.uk/lis/subjects/health/ebm.htm
  This site features a large section of definitions of EBP and a list of links to centers and institutes that work with EBP, giving an overview of the work being done in the field.
- *Centre for Health Evidence*
  www.cche.net
  This site has many measures to help practitioners with evidence-based practice.

- *Evidence-Based Occupational Therapy web portal*
  www.otevidence.info
  This site is an internationally developed and supported portal for information on evidence-based occupational therapy. The site development was funded through the Canadian Association of Occupational Therapists and McMaster University School of Rehabilitation Science and is endorsed by the World Federation of Occupational Therapists.
- *Alberta Evidence-Based Medicine Toolkit*
  www.ebm.med.ualberta.ca
  This site has tools for identifying and appraising evidence.
- *OTseeker: Occupational Therapy Systematic Evaluation of Evidence*
  www.otseeker.com/default.htm
  OTSeeker, developed in Australia, is a database containing abstracts of systematic reviews and RCTs relevant to occupational therapy. All trials cited have been critically appraised and rated regarding their validity.
- *PEDro*
  www.pedro.fhs.usyd.edu.au/index.html
  PEDro, developed in Australia, is a database of abstracts of systematic reviews, RCTs, systematic reviews, and practice guidelines in physiotherapy. All citations have been critically appraised and rated regarding their validity.
- *Resource Guide for Evidence-Based Rehabilitation Practice*
  www.library.ualberta.ca/subject/evidencerehab/guide/index.cfm#sources
  This site provides information and links to resources pertaining to EBP in rehabilitation

TAKE HOME MESSAGES

Evidence-Based Practice (EBP)

✔ There are misunderstandings of EBP because of the ways in which it breaks with traditional practice; it can be seen as a powerful tool, not a burden.

✔ EBP maintains a fine balance between clinical expertise, external clinical evidence and client values and needs.

✔ EBP is based on a self-directed learning model.

✔ EBP can support a strongly client-centred approach to rehabilitation.

✔ Clinical experience remains crucial because knowledgeable practitioners will best implement their findings based on evidence.

✔ EBP makes use of the current best methods of treatment.

Evidence-Based Rehabilitation (EBR)

✔ EBR is a subset of the clinical practice of EBP.

✔ Awareness: clinician must be aware of the evidence which has to do with practice; maintain focused awareness.

✔ Consultation: specialized set of skills and knowledge to be a good communicator; the practitioner works as an educator/service provider.

✔ Judgment: practitioner differentiates between cases about how to apply recommendations of EBP; tailored to specifics of each client's situation.

✔ Creativity: EBR requires creativity and insight as the practice and application of the best available evidence is not always straightforward.

LEARNING AND EXPLORATION ACTIVITIES

The purpose of this segment is to introduce the concept of EBP through the exploration of key definitions found in the literature. The following exercises guide the student through a process of thinking critically about the definition of EBP and applying this knowledge to possible clinical scenarios. The work done in these exercises should be saved by the students as a good reference during their study of EBP.

1. Defining Evidence-Based Practice

a. What is your conception of EBP? What was your conception before you read this chapter? Make a chart and list both side by side, then attempt to locate where the gaps were in your knowledge. Then address the follow-up questions by thinking on a wider scale. How could misinformation about EBP be misleading other practitioners? What could be done about it?

b. Build upon the ideas uncovered in the previous step by writing your own definition of EBP. You can incorporate parts of the definitions given above if you would like, but make sure that the definition is meaningful and makes sense for you. Keep this definition written down somewhere, and look at it again once you have finished working through this book. Has your definition changed? Why?

c. In small groups, write out a definition of EBP, listing the most crucial aspects. Prepare a short (5 minute) presentation about your definition, and present it to the rest of the class. This can include debate or creative elements (dramatic, artistic, etc.). Your goal is to get the message across and make it stick in the minds of your audience.

d. Myths surrounding EBP are presented in this chapter, along with the responses from Sackett et al. (1996). What are your assumptions about EBR? Write these down. How do you propose that these myths can be addressed?

2. Best Practice

a. What is your definition of "best practice"? How does that definition compare to your thoughts before and after reading this chapter? How does the concept of best practice fit into EBP? Are they components of one another, or different concepts?

3. Evidence-Based Rehabilitation

a. The four principles of EBR outlined in the chapter—Awareness, Consultation, Judgment, and Creativity—serve as good guideposts for practitioners implementing EBR, but they are not perfect. Can you think of any other guideposts for yourself? If not, can you further define what is meant from each of the original guideposts?

b. List briefly the differences and similarities between how EBM and EBR might be practiced. What are the key dissimilarities? How are EBM and EBR the most different? How are they the most similar? Why?

REFERENCES

Bennett, S., Tooth, L., McKenna, K., Rodger, S., Strong, J., Ziviani, J., et al. (2003). Perceptions of evidence-based practice: A survey of Australian occupational therapists. *Australian Occupational Therapy Journal, 50*(1), 13-22.

Canadian Health Services Research Foundation. (2004). What counts? Interpreting evidence-based decision-making for management and policy. 6th CHSRF annual workshop. Retrieved August 1, 2006, from http://www.chsrf.ca/knowledge_transfer/pdf/2004_workshop_report_e.pdf

Canadian Health Services Research Foundation. (2005). Conceptualizing and combining evidence for health system guidance. Retrieved August 1, 2006, from http://www.chsrf.ca/other_documents/evidence_e.php

Curtin, M., & Jaramazovic, E. (2001). Occupational therapists' views and perceptions of evidence-based practice. *British Journal of Occupational Therapy, 64*(5), 214-222.

DeLisa, J. A. (1999). Issues and challenges for psychiatry in the coming decade. *Archives Physical Medicine & Rehabilitation, 80*, 1-12.

DePalma, J. A. (2000). Evidence-based clinical practice guidelines. *Seminars in Perioperative Nursing, 9*(3),115-120.

Dickersin, K., Straus, S. E., & Bero, L.A. (2007). Evidence-based medicine: increasing, not dictating, choice. *British Medical Journal, 334*(Suppl. 1), 10.

Duncan, P. W. (1997). Evidence-based medicine. *Physiotherapy Research International, 2*, 271-272.

Evidence-Based Medicine Working Group. (1992). Evidence-based medicine. A new approach to teaching the practice of medicine." *Journal of the American Medical Association, 268*, 2420-2425.

Greenhalgh, T. (1997). *How to read a paper: The basics of evidence-based medicine*. London: BMJ Press.

Grimmer, K. (2004). Implementing evidence in clinical practice: the 'therapies' dilemma. *Physiotherapy, 90*(4), 189-194.

Guyatt, G. (2004). Evidence-based medicine has come a long way. *British Medical Journal, 329*, 990-996.

Haynes, B. (2002). What kind of evidence is it that evidence-based medicine advocates want health care providers and consumers to pay attention to? *BMC Health Services Research, 2*, 1-7.

Haynes, R. B. (2004). What kind of evidence is it that evidence-based Medicine advocates want health care providers and consumers to pay attention to? *BMC Health Services Research, 2*, 3.

Health Information Research Unit. (2002). How to teach evidence-based clinical practice 2002. Retrieved February 14, 2002, from http://hiru.mcmaster.ca.

Law, M., Pollock, N., & Stewart, D. (2004). Evidence-Based occupational therapy: concepts and strategies. *New Zealand Journal of Occupational Therapy, 51*(1), 14-22.

Marwick, C. (1997). Proponents gather to discuss practicing evidence-based medicine. *Journal of the American Medical Association, 278*(7), 531-532.

Muir Gray, J. A. (1997). *Evidence-Based health care: How to make health policy and management decisions*. London: Churchill Livingstone.

Rosenberg, W., & Donald, A. (1995). Evidence-based medicine: An approach to clinical problem solving. *British Medical Journal, 310*(6987), 1122-1126.

Sackett, D. L., Haynes, R. B., & Tugwell, P. (1985). *Clinical epidemiology: A basic science for clinical medicine*. London: Little Brown.

Sackett, D. L., Rosenberg, W. M., Gray, J. A., Haynes, R. B., & Richardson, W. S. (1996). Evidence-based medicine: What it is and what it isn't. *British Medical Journal, 312*(7023), 71-72.

Sudsawad, P. (2005). A conceptual framework to increase usability of outcome research for evidence-based practice. *American Journal of Occupational Therapy, 59*(3), 351-355.

2

Development of Evidence-Based Knowledge

Winnie Dunn, PhD, OTR, FAOTA and Jill Ball, BP, BHScOT

LEARNING OBJECTIVES

After reading this chapter, the student/practitioner will be able to:

- Recognize and understand the multiple levels at which knowledge develops within a discipline.
- Define the different periods of development for the practitioner and explain the corresponding relationship with the development of knowledge.
- Understand the subsequent responsibilities and challenges of the practitioner as an individual, a member of a discipline, and a representative of a discipline.
- Understand the challenges in developing evidence in rehabilitation.

INTRODUCTION

It is easy to believe that the knowledge of a particular discipline has been there for all time, was established quickly by experts who were defining the discipline, and was carried forth by all subsequent generations as stable and clear factors that characterize the discipline's perspectives and work. With this belief, persons would only have to acquire the knowledge, skills, and viewpoints of the discipline so they can use the information and then pass it along with little need for ongoing re-evaluation. Therapists have long recognized the need for ongoing development of knowledge, skill, and the associated clinical reasoning. For example, high participation rates in continuing education and peer consultation are most commonly used by rehabilitation therapists as a means of gathering and implementing new knowledge (Rappolt & Tassone, 2002).

In fact, knowledge develops at many levels within one's own discipline and in concert with other disciplines that are interested in similar ideas. Additionally, as each new insight emerges, people have the opportunity to understand their profession in a new way and to consider what new dilemmas this insight reveals. There are many issues that people cannot even conceive are present until certain other knowledge becomes clear to them.

Knowledge is a collection of ideas and facts about a topic. People tend to say they have knowledge when information and ideas have stood the test of time and experience. Evidence is information that makes a conclusion apparent, and it is the accumulation of these conclusions that leads to new insights. The accumulation of evidence typically advances knowledge in a particular area, and knowledge, in turn, introduces other possibilities for gathering evidence. Although people generally refer to formal research as evidence for professional practice, in actuality, each professional act provides evidence that accumulates into that professional's knowledge base.

An Example

It was standard practice in the United States during the early 1900s to institutionalize persons with disabilities (i.e., people with disabilities were housed in large government-funded facilities and provided basic care for their survival). This practice was based on the belief that persons who were mentally or physically deficient could not contribute to and could not care for themselves; therefore, they need to be isolated from society and cared for.

People then began to demonstrate that individuals with disabilities could learn. This insight led people to question their beliefs about individuals with disabilities: Could these individuals take care of themselves and contribute to society? People began to consider what the possibilities were for persons who could learn; they had to reconsider the standard practice of institutionalization, which by its very nature kept people with disabilities from participating in certain activities, including contributing to society and learning to care for themselves. Some members of society began to press for persons with disabilities to be moved out of institutions so they could become members of communities and realize their potential (i.e., the deinstitutionalization movement).

Deinstitutionalization operationalized the knowledge about persons with disabilities having the potential to learn and, therefore, the possibility to contribute to society. When communities began to move people out of institutions, everyone realized that the communities did not have the infrastructure in place to support these new community members. Communities needed housing for all these persons; this issue had been irrelevant when people with disabilities were housed in large institutions. The community members who had worked in the institutions were now displaced from their work, creating an economic shift in the community. Communities were certainly able to tackle these challenges, but prior to deinstitutionalization there was no opportunity to see these issues; therefore, there was no opportunity to develop knowledge. As each insight occurred, other opportunities for insight presented themselves.

A century later, it can be seen that those who had the courage to challenge institutionalization beliefs and practices began a process of changing services for persons with disabilities forever. Those who provided institutional care could not have conceived of some of our current practices (e.g., buildings that are accessible to everyone) because these innovations were too divergent from their beliefs and practices.

Evidence-based knowledge serves a generative function in the evolution of information for practice. It invites us to simultaneously gain insight to solve a current problem and see the dilemmas that are only visible from the next vantage point.

PURPOSE

The purpose of this chapter is to introduce the ways that evidence-based knowledge develops within a discipline. Primarily, there are three vantage points for knowledge development. First, the individual professional travels through a developmental process beginning with preservice educational preparation and continuing through the "expert" phase of the professional career path. Second, professionals develop and share information with each other within their own disciplines. Finally, professionals develop and share information across disciplines to inform a wider circle of thinkers. We will discuss each of these in turn and consider what our responsibilities are in the development of evidence-based knowledge.

THE INDIVIDUAL PROFESSIONAL

Responsibilities

Individual professionals are responsible for facilitating knowledge development as insights emerge in daily practice. In order to accomplish this, professionals must first develop awareness of their own beliefs. It is essential to recognize that knowledge is not a prerequisite for a belief (Quine & Ullian, 1978). Beliefs emerge from experiences, viewpoints of those we trust, and sociocultural influences. Awareness of individual beliefs is important because beliefs form a filter through which professionals view and, therefore, interpret events and information. When beliefs are undefined, professionals are unaware of the reasons for their choices in practice (i.e., they act on interpretations that are guided surreptitiously by their beliefs), masking alternative interpretations.

For example, therapists may believe in the benefits of a therapeutic modality based on practice experience and a mentor's fervor for the method, while scientific knowledge of how the modality works may be scarce. Conductive education techniques are an example of this. Conductive education has been used with children who have cerebral palsy, although there is little evidence to support its efficacy (Bairstow, Cochrane, & Rusk, 1991; Bochner, Center, Chapparo, & Donelly, 1999; Darrah, Watkins, Chen, & Bonin, 2004; Lonton & Russell, 1989; Reddihough, King, Coleman, & Catanese, 1998). Similarly, manual therapy is an area of physical therapy practice in which practitioners have strong beliefs in hands-on techniques that are commonly passed on by "gurus," frequently before adequate evidence is in place to support their use. Therapists have a belief in the power of movement, hands-on treatment, and therapeutic interaction and have experienced changes in their patients with these types of interventions. Therefore, they have a predisposition toward believing that these techniques are effective, even when research is sparse and varied. Reddihough et al. (1998) studied 34 children with cerebral palsy and found that those receiving conductive education made similar progress to children in alternative intervention groups. Bochner et al. (1999) reported that results of conductive education were quite variable with children who have motor disabilities, with some children showing no changes and others learning specific motor skills; however, they also cited lack of generalization of skills as a problem. Systematic reviews on the use of manual therapy for neck pain indicate manual therapy is less effective when used alone as compared to exercise which has the larger impact (Gross et al., 2002)

The example of conductive education and other therapies that have been embraced within rehabilitation without adequate supporting evidence illustrates what Quine and Ullian (1978) describe: "the intensity of a belief cannot be counted on to reflect its supporting evidence" (p. 7). When developing EBP, professionals must remain aware of the power of personal beliefs, be open to identifying the source and nature of the beliefs, and be willing to search for evidence-based knowledge to inform their practice techniques separate from their beliefs. Many professional practices begin with an experienced professional acting out a hunch; this willingness to discover new possibilities is appropriate as long as we take the next steps to evaluate effectiveness.

Evaluating effectiveness is the second responsibility for professionals (Feyerbend, 1993). The ability to continually question current information and seek new answers is often described as lifelong learning for the individual; this process forms the basis of EBP for the profession. Developing knowledge about how to search for and critically appraise research studies is an important skill for all rehabilitation practitioners. In the absence of such knowledge, evaluating the outcomes of intervention for each person receiving services is vital. This idea is discussed in more detail later in this section.

The third responsibility is a willingness to use information to abandon ineffective methods and/or erroneous ideas and beliefs in favor of more effective options. This responsibility is challenging to fulfill because it requires professionals to entertain the possibility that their particular framework for thinking and problem solving needs adjustment. Beliefs and conceptual frameworks are interwoven; if one's framework does not change, the beliefs within that framework will be difficult to alter (Kuhn, 1996).

For example, rehabilitation professionals educated within a medically based framework may have difficulty abandoning the belief that *doing something to or for the patient is best* as part of the "professional as expert" conceptual framework. A client-centered framework suggests that professionals collaborate with the client and family, and it has been shown to be an effective approach (Dunst, Deal, & Trivette, 1996; Rosenbaum, King, Law, King, & Evans, 1998). However, it requires professionals to reconstruct their beliefs to acknowledge the client and family as active participants in planning.

To meet the responsibility of knowledge development for EBP, professionals must also share their emerging insights and broader beliefs with others. Open dialogue and the ability to request feedback in practice encourages the development of efficacious practices. It enables professionals to remain flexible in their approach to practice challenges and facilitates ongoing improvements in practices (Feyerbend, 1993).

Finally, professionals must participate in activities that are effective in their practices. In order to implement effective practices, professionals must conduct critical reviews of the literature, participate in quality reviews, and/or participate in formal data collection activities. Vigilance in collecting data enables patterns to emerge, hypotheses to be tested, and decisions to be made based on information actually available within the practice. There is potential to gather evidence-based data for a variety of audiences (e.g., for the professional's own practice, for the discipline, for the consumer, for the payer). With each audience, the evidence is gathered as a means of convincing the professionals that interventions are effective, providing support for the viability of the discipline, demonstrating changes to consumers, and/or convincing payers that they are using their resources to purchase valuable services.

In summary, several personal responsibilities that facilitate professional knowledge development have been highlighted, including awareness of personal beliefs, evaluating the effectiveness of current practices, maintaining open dialogue and feedback regarding current practices, and participating in activities that will enhance current practice. Although several personal responsibilities exist, it is important to acknowledge that professionals do not practice in isolation. Responsibilities also exist beyond the individual to include the health care profession, the organization or institution, and the interdisciplinary team to support the acquisition and implementation of knowledge development within the health care system (Hannes et al., 2005; Ketefian, 2001; Reimer, Sawka, & James, 2005). These influences will be explored further when we examine the challenges in developing evidence in practice.

Phases of Professional Development

Professionals do not leave their educational preparation and enter work fully equipped to meet all of the responsibilities of serving as evidence-based professionals. The course of one's career affords different possibilities (Table 2-1).

Table 2-1

PROFESSIONAL KNOWLEDGE DEVELOPMENT

Preservice Experience
- Becomes aware of own beliefs and learns initial strategies for questioning beliefs

Novice Professional Period
- Begins to generalize ideas, determines effective and ineffective methods for practice, and tests knowledge and beliefs

Experienced Professional Period
- Establishes methods for evaluating effectiveness, hypothesizes successful therapeutic techniques, and shares with colleagues

Expert Professional Period
- Participates in formal methods of collecting data and evaluating interventions, shares knowledge more globally, and critiques work of others

Preservice Experiences

Through preservice experiences, students learn the knowledge base of the discipline and are exposed to the available evidence for current interventions. In this initial stage, the professional learns how to use the available evidence to construct preliminary clinical reasoning strategies and decision-making guides. The knowledge development for preservice students occurs within the current thought paradigms of the discipline, thereby focusing their learning to include current knowledge and evidence (Kuhn, 1996; Schell, 1998). Preservice professionals meet the first and second responsibilities of becoming evidence-based professionals (i.e., they become aware of their beliefs and learn initial strategies for questioning those beliefs in the interest of effectiveness).

Novice Professional Period

In the novice period, professionals learn how others apply knowledge and evaluate evidence. Novice professionals try ideas and evaluate their effectiveness in individual situations. It is during this period of development that professionals begin to generalize ideas across peoples and settings, determining effective and ineffective methods for practice, thus building a resource of professional experiences that guides future decisions. The novice professional period provides opportunities to test the knowledge and beliefs that professionals have acquired through educational preparation, increasing clarity and generalizability of knowledge for practice. This period provides an opportunity for professional socialization and organizational socialization in which the novice professional experiences the attitudes, values, and beliefs of the profession and the organization in which they work (Miller, Solomon, Giacomini, & Abelson, 2005; Solomon & Miller, 2005). This period forms the foundation for understanding how clinical reasoning occurs within the broader context of the professional and work environments. Therefore, the novice professional period forms the foundation for clinical reasoning as knowledge and personal beliefs, now grounded in experience, begin to merge.

Experienced Professional Period

With further experience, professionals begin to create a personal "database" from all their professional experiences and learning. The experienced professional period enables the individual to establish methods for evaluating the effectiveness of selected interventions based on their personal database (Feyerbend, 1993). Professionals working within particular settings will be able to evaluate the effectiveness of therapeutic interventions on functional outcomes achieved by clients in that setting. The experienced professional is better able to hypothesize those therapeutic techniques that will be most successful for clients admitted with particular functional concerns due to the breadth and depth of the professional practice to inform these decisions. They are able to make evidence-based clinical decisions by weighing multiple factors, including their practice context, their clinical expertise, the knowledge of expert colleagues, and their client's preferences (Wilkins, Jung, Wishart, Edwards, & Gamble-Norton, 2003). As professionals generate evidence in practice, they also begin to share their personal "evidence" with other professionals; sharing facilitates development of collective knowledge about effective practices. This collective knowledge can be shared in team meetings, focus groups, and professional conference presentations for specific areas of practice.

Expert Professional Period

In the expert professional period, professionals participate in more formal methods of collecting data and evaluating effectiveness of interventions. Professionals may solicit funding to conduct research within their service setting or population. For example, professionals may participate in a RCT to try to determine which of two intervention methods is most effective, or they may publish a case study to illustrate a client's experience with a particular disability. The knowledge gained through this research allows professionals to make findings more globally available to other professionals. When expert professionals share in more public forums, they can impact EBP knowledge development by inviting less advanced colleagues to benefit from the expert's insights. This period also includes critiquing the works and insights of others to advance knowledge for the discipline (Feyerbend, 1993; Quine & Ullian, 1978).

PROFESSIONALS WITHIN A DISCIPLINE

Just as in individual development, professionals within a discipline have collective responsibilities to contribute to evidence-based knowledge. These include challenging current beliefs, sharing information with colleagues, introducing new ideas, and formally testing hypotheses for their new ideas.

The growth of knowledge in a discipline is possible only when the members and interested others challenge current beliefs and theories. By challenging current theory, a discipline ensures thoroughness and refinement and fosters further development of knowledge. Knowledge development within a professional community requires its members to constantly push the limits imposed by current working paradigms. By encouraging professionals to participate in dialogues about knowledge development and understanding, both the discipline and the individual professionals evolve (Feyerbend, 1993), creating a generative cycle.

Individuals within a discipline relate their practice knowledge base to theories of the profession. Theories within the profession guide practice decisions and practice experiences, in turn informing the theory. It is valuable to recognize the challenge that members have in introducing new ideas to a professional group with established theories that form the basis for current research and communication within the profession. One may expect new ideas to be encouraged because new ideas serve to further develop professional knowledge. However, new ideas also challenge the foundation of current activities, which can be threatening to the stability of professional beliefs (Feyerbend, 1993).

Professionals within a discipline are responsible for designing and implementing formal methods for testing hypotheses that grow out of the cycle of practice-construct dialogue. Professionals need to have current beliefs to begin, but these ideas need to be challenged in some way in order to advance current forms of professional practice and, ultimately, refine the constructs and beliefs. Thus, tension between research and practice is inevitable and a necessary struggle for the advancement of knowledge (Quine & Ullian, 1978). For researchers to understand how to propose change, they must understand that issues arise in practice that seem contradictory to currently held beliefs. Schachter and Cohen (2005) suggest several factors that enhance the potential of a professional community to adopt a change in practice based on new evidence, including "an onsite champion, staff buy-in, a willingness to see systems change, and the availability of additional resources"(p. 1). New data can be generated to inform more advanced thinking, thus advancing the discipline's body of knowledge. How a professional community adopts or rejects innovative or controversial information determines its evolution and viability (Chinn & Brewer, 1993).

PROFESSIONALS ACROSS DISCIPLINES

Evidence-based knowledge development must also occur in collaboration with other disciplines that are interested in similar ideas. There are many professional practice problems that simply cannot be solved with a single discipline's perspective. When the knowledge of a variety of disciplines is shared, there emerges many more possibilities for knowledge development. To enable the sharing of knowledge across disciplines, members of professional communities have several responsibilities.

First, professionals must remain open to other points of view. Collaboration among professionals requires teamwork with a desire to share and receive new ideas. Second, it is important to remain aware of how decisions made by a variety of disciplines may impact families and individuals being served. The paradigm of family-centered care provides a good example of this need for collaboration. Professionals employing this paradigm encourage and support family involvement regardless of the expertise of any particular discipline. For family-centered care to be effective, professionals then need to identify the unique and complementary knowledge that will enable a family to act on their goals without creating undue burden on the family (e.g., an undue burden would be each discipline designing its own intervention plans, expecting the family to carry all of them out).

The third responsibility professionals have is to recognize and facilitate awareness about the similarities and differences in approaches to problem solving and knowledge development for each discipline. Clear communication between professionals about investigation approaches and methods is necessary to ensure effective collaboration across disciplines. Awareness about similarities and differences may be enhanced through interdisciplinary training (Clark, 2004; Fertman, Dotson, Mazzocco, & Reitz, 2005; Rodehorst, Wilhelm, & Jensen, 2005) and collaborative learning facilities (Moore, Vaughan, Hayes, & McLendon, 2005).

The fourth responsibility in advancing collective evidence-based knowledge among disciplines is to collaboratively conduct research. Professionals can work together to design and implement formal methods for testing hypotheses that grow out of the interdisciplinary dialogue. Research can focus on problems that are best tested from an interdisciplinary perspective, which draws upon a range of theoretical frameworks thereby resulting in a comprehensive perspective (Barbour & Barbour, 2003).

For example, several disciplines contribute to knowledge about barrier-free design (sometimes called universal design or universal access). Individuals with backgrounds in occupational therapy, physiotherapy, architecture, interior design, environmental psychology, human ecology, and urban and regional planning all have knowledge and skills related to barrier-free design. The collective knowledge of these professionals expands the possible solutions for designing a barrier-free environment (Cooper, Cohen, & Hasselkus, 1991; Steinfeld & Shea, 1993).

Finally, professionals from across disciplines must recognize uncomfortable places as opportunities for knowledge development. It is naturally difficult for individuals with different theoretical paradigms to collaborate with each other; however, each discipline evolves from the reflection of colleagues from other disciplines. The product of interdisciplinary collaboration can advance knowledge for each discipline and for collective knowledge in an area of interest.

CHALLENGES IN DEVELOPING EVIDENCE FOR PRACTICE

There are several different challenges in developing evidence for practice:

- Producing generalizable evidence
- Disseminating this evidence in an accessible and relevant format
- Implementing evidence into practice

First, evidence needs to be generalizable to the professional's current practice environment. Consideration should be given to contextual factors, including policy guidelines and the client's circumstance (Glasgow, Magid, Beck, Ritzwoller, & Estabrooks, 2005; Nananda, 2005). Second, disseminating evidence to maximize uptake by professionals requires that the evidence is accessible and relevant. Remaining current with EBR research requires constant effort by clinicians to seek out evidence (Stegink-Jansen, 2002). Barriers to accessing evidence may include lack of time, lack of access to resources, or a lack of desire to enhance current knowledge and skills (Hannes et al., 2005). Therefore, evidence should be presented in a format that is efficient for the professional to digest and applicable to current practice.

Third, implementing evidence into current practice or "closing the gap between what is known and what is practiced" (Weaver, Warren, & Delaney, 2005) is a challenge faced across health care disciplines. This challenge exists within the larger context of the practice environment and includes the health care profession, the organization or institution, and the interdisciplinary team. Implementing evidence into practice requires the support of the practice environment (Hannes et al., 2005; Ketefian, 2001; Reimer et al., 2005) to seek out information and a willingness to change current practice if evidence supports this change. Rogers (1995) proposes that professionals need to identify the key players in contexts that are both early adopters of innovation and are well respected by the constituent groups in order to get groups to adopt new ideas. This means that professionals need to identify key leadership that has influence for both administrative and staff changes to adopt new ideas.

AN EXAMPLE ILLUSTRATING THE CONTRIBUTION OF RESEARCH AND EVIDENCE TO DEVELOPING EVIDENCE-BASED KNOWLEDGE FOR PRACTICE AND KNOWLEDGE DEVELOPMENT

All of the ideas presented in this chapter and throughout this book are platitudes if there is no evidence that knowledge development and evolution actually occur in these ways. Those of us who are further along on our professional journeys have a sense of knowledge development from our own lived experiences, but it is inefficient for a discipline to rely on "living it" to see the power of the knowledge development. As disciplines mature, we must be willing to conduct formal analyses of knowledge development; this not only includes the facts and data from studies, but also the evolution of insights at each new point in the knowledge development process. Without scholars willing to wonder, muse, and hypothesize about the meaning of information, all the data in the world would not advance knowledge. Additionally, we need practitioners who are open to new ideas and who question current practice so that hypotheses can be tested and refined.

We will highlight these principles using a powerful example from the occupational therapy (and related disciplines) literature: the development of knowledge about sensory integration. This area of knowledge development illustrates all levels of evolution: individual scholars moving from novice to expert, the discipline increasingly incorporating advancing knowledge into the collective thinking, and the impact of occupational therapy's work on other disciplines' knowledge development.

Early Developments and Insights

Occupational and physical therapy have a long history of relying on the neuroscience literature to guide thinking about assessment and intervention. Many early theorists have discussed the importance of nervous system operations for the production of adaptive human behaviors (Ayres, 1955; Blashy & Fuchs, 1959; Bobath & Bobath, 1955; Cruickshank, Bice, & Wallen, 1957; Fay, 1948; Rood, 1952). These scholars were peers in the 1950s so much of their work was interdependent. For this discussion, we shall focus specifically on the evolution of sensory integration knowledge, which we primarily attribute to Dr. A. Jean Ayres.

Dr. Ayres' was an occupational therapist and licensed clinical psychologist whose early thinking arose from her study of neuroscience during her doctoral and postdoctoral work (Sieg, 1988). She had experience working with children and adults with various central nervous system conditions (Cruickshank, 1974). Therefore, from an individual perspective, we would say Dr. Ayres was in her experienced professional period (see Table 2-1). As you recall from earlier in the chapter, this means she would have created a personal database for decision making and would be sharing her perspectives with others. She was also seeking formal doctoral and postdoctoral education at this time, foreshadowing her intent to enter the expert professional period.

Dr. Ayres was fascinated by what she observed in children with cerebral palsy and learning disabilities. She began to hypothesize about the nature of these children's performance difficulties based on her studies and her professional experiences. She emphasized visual motor functions and perceptual and proprioceptive facilitation to improve upper extremity function (Henderson, Llorens, Gilfoyle, Myers, & Prevel, 1974). She wrote several articles to share her ideas with others (Ayres, 1954, 1958, 1960, 1963), as do most people in the experienced professional period.

At the discipline level, Dr. Ayres was generating an impact in two ways. First, she was beginning to change the course of occupational therapy thinking. Second, those in related disciplines who also had an interest in children's perceptual motor skills considered Dr. Ayres a visionary scholar. Dr. William Cruickshank (1974), a noted scholar of education and psychology and one of Dr. Ayres' peers, stated in reviewing Dr. Ayres early work, "…the writings of Jean Ayres… have been instrumental in setting new directions for a total discipline, or at least have directed the profession of occupational therapy in two areas that are historically and functionally different… prior to 1955" (p. viii).

Testing Hypotheses to Gain New Perspectives

After publishing her ideas and insights on children's perceptual motor skills and completing her postdoctoral education, Dr. Ayres began to test her theoretical ideas with larger samples and sound measurement methods.

These actions represent the expert professional period of her individual career path. She was quite prolific in writing during this period, reporting on her findings, interpreting the results in light of her own and the work of other scholars, and making more refined hypotheses for subsequent research.

In order to test some of the theoretical constructs, Dr. Ayres identified available methods and constructed some of her own methods of measuring children's sensory, perceptual, motor, and praxis abilities. In her 1965 article, "Patterns of Perceptual Motor Dysfunction in Children," she reported on the first of several factor analytic studies, a creative and insightful work for the time. Using data from 100 children with perceptual deficits and 50 typically developing children, Dr. Ayres hypothesized that there were five syndromes representing dysfunction, including apraxia, tactile and visual perception, tactile defensiveness, bilateral integration, and poor figure ground perception.

With this study and subsequent work to refine these patterns, Dr. Ayres began to validate theoretical constructs that would provide a specific focus for occupational therapy research for the next four decades and beyond. Simultaneously, this work has influenced work in related disciplines by informing them of occupational therapy's significant and unique contributions and advancing knowledge to their work as well.

Dr. Ayres continued to elucidate perceptual motor and sensory integrative constructs in a series of factor analytic studies (Ayres, 1965, 1966a, 1966b, 1969a, 1969b, 1971, 1972a, 1972b). She and colleagues standardized the Southern California Sensory Integrative Tests, which enabled professionals to identify specific types of sensory integrative performance problems.

By 1972, Dr. Ayres had identified five types of sensory integrative dysfunction:

1. Visual/tactile/kinesthetic form and space perception

2. Motor planning and tactile perception

3. Tactile perception, hyperactivity, distractibility, and tactile defensiveness

4. Postural and ocular muscle control

5. Auditory language functions

She increasingly refined her measures in her studies, so that she could illustrate these categories of performance problems with more clarity. Because she had demonstrated the presence of several of these factors across study populations, she spoke with more confidence about their integrity and applicability to assessment and intervention planning in practice situations. Dr. Ayres also conducted other studies to examine the effectiveness of interventions based on her hypotheses (Ayres, 1972a, 1976). These intervention studies informed therapists how they might apply her ideas in their practice.

The Second Generation Develops Insights

As Dr. Ayres traversed through her expert professional period, she was influencing many younger therapists with her ideas. The knowledge that Dr. Ayres developed and validated through her research moved into occupational therapy curricula as core knowledge, and sensory integration theory and practice began to be inherent in service planning for children. As these "second generation" colleagues moved from their novice periods into their experienced professional periods, they began making and testing hypotheses of their own.

Armed with the tools that Dr. Ayres provided (i.e., the data, the tests, new knowledge, expert insights), occupational therapists serving children began to emphasize sensory integration factors when evaluating and designing intervention programs. Occupational therapy graduate students and scholars who were studying Dr. Ayres' work began to design and implement intervention studies to evaluate the effectiveness of a sensory integrative approach in therapy. (Note: Since our purpose here is to examine the knowledge development process and not provide a comprehensive review of this literature, please review Fisher, Murray, & Bundy [1991] for an in-depth reporting of the work during this period.)

This was a prolific period for testing hypotheses and generating insights about the role of sensory integration in persons' performance. Dr. Ayres had provided such a rich foundation of ideas that what began as a few musings and insights had now become a whole body of ideas to consider. Because Dr. Ayres was so vigilant at disseminating her ideas in writing and in presentations, the possibility of advancing knowledge multiplied geometrically with this new cohort of novices emerging to experienced professionals. For example, Ottenbacher (1982) found 49 articles reporting on research about sensory integrative interventions. His meta-analysis revealed a positive effect for sensory integrative interventions, but only eight of the articles met his criteria for inclusion in the review process. Other studies reported more equivocal results (Feagans, 1983; Ferry, 1981; Ottenbacher & Short-DeGraff, 1985), suggesting that further work still needed to be done to demonstrate the appropriate application of sensory integrative constructs for EBP.

Another important event in knowledge development at the discipline level occurred during this time. Because there was more information available about the constructs and application (both effective and ineffective) of sensory integration, scholars from other disciplines began to consume this knowledge, with mixed results. For example, Arendt, MacLean, and Baumeister (1988) published a critique of sensory integration therapy as it might be applied to persons with mental retardation and reported that it would be inappropriate to apply these methods based on the available evidence. The editor recognized the provocative nature of this topic and invited five scholars in occupational therapy to respond to this article. The entire series of articles is published in one volume, providing an excellent example of scholarly discourse. From a knowledge-development perspective, critiques such as these are not possible until knowledge has developed to the point that others can study it and consider their perspectives on the ideas.

It was also during this period that scholars conducted clinical trials of sensory integration interventions (Humphries, Snider, & McDougall, 1993; Humphries, Wright, McDougall, & Vertes, 1990; Humphries, Wright, Snider, & McDougall, 1992; Kaplan, Polatajko, Wilson, & Faris, 1993; Polatajko, Kaplan, & Wilson, 1992; Polatajko, Law, Miller, Schaffer, & Macnab, 1991; Wilson & Kaplan, 1994; Wilson, Kaplan, Fellowes, Gruchy, & Faris, 1992). These research teams reported similar results (i.e., that sensory integration therapy was equally effective as other interventions [e.g., perceptual motor, tutoring, traditional interventions], not more effective at affecting sensorimotor outcomes and that results on the impact of sensory integration on academic performance were equivocal).

These studies reflect the maturation of therapists' thinking about sensory integration and its increasing visibility in the larger professional arenas. There was more interest and pressure to demonstrate the usefulness of these "new" ideas. Those outside the "web of belief" were appropriately asking questions about the claims of effectiveness. It was time for researchers to study the nature and scope of sensory integration practices and for those in practice to understand when sensory integration interventions would be the appropriate or inappropriate choice to make. This process of refinement had an important impact on knowledge generation in that it illuminated the possible limitations of this knowledge for particular intervention practices. It is critical that both effective and ineffective methods become clear in the research; this establishes the parameters for proper use of knowledge and invites scholars to reconceptualize the nature and meaning of their constructs for use in practice and in subsequent research.

The "Renaissance Period"

So here we are more than a decade later from all this activity. We have another cohort of occupational therapy professionals who are in their experienced professional period, only this time they have been able to study not only the knowledge that Dr. Ayres provided but also all the knowledge that the first cohort provided (who are now in their expert professional periods). This breadth of information and distance from the original seeds of knowledge provide a new vantage point for considering the ideas. Additionally, the culture of scholarly endeavors has matured as well, affording new tools and strategies for testing the fidelity of knowledge and the effectiveness of its application in practice.

Great things are happening, as they do when knowledge has the time to settle in, and scholars can take a fresh look with new tools. Occupational therapy scholars have been studying neuroscience and sensory integration knowledge and are adding clarity to some of Dr. Ayres' original ideas, as well as proposing new ideas for consideration. As an indicator of the available accumulating knowledge, Miller and Lane (2000) produced a three-part series of articles that provided a taxonomy of definitions related to sensory integration and sensory processing, inviting scholars to use consistent terms for this burgeoning body of knowledge.

As one example of knowledge being reformulated, Dr. Ayres discussed tactile defensiveness and gravitational insecurity as conditions in which the person was unable to tolerate touch and movement input, respectively (Ayres, 1972b). Researchers of today are revisiting one's inability to process sensory input as part of modulating the amount and type of information a person might need for creating adaptive responses. They are using the knowledge developed thus far and applying contemporary methods of research to characterize sensory modulation as a range of responses to sensory events (Baranek, Foster, & Berkson, 1997; Dunn, 2000), thus broadening original ideas and observations. We have also broadened ideas about the domain of study.

In the early years, sensory integration concepts and treatment methods were the focus of the research but, in more recent years, scholars have identified constructs that are more properly classified in the larger context of sensory processing. While sensory integration is a component of sensory processing (i.e., the nervous system's capacity to process sensory input [Miller & Lane, 2000, p. 2]), the term *sensory processing* encompasses the application of broader neuroscience constructs to the human experience (i.e., the way the nervous system receives, modulates, integrates, and organizes incoming sensory information [Miller & Lane, 2000]). Studies of children with poor coping skills (Williamson & Szczepanski, 1999), poor regulatory abilities (DeGangi, 2000), autism (Baranek et al., 1997; Kientz & Dunn, 1997), and fragile X syndrome (Belser & Sudhalter, 1995) provided evidence that a broader consideration was appropriate. Additionally, studies of intervention in natural settings (Case-Smith & Bryan, 1999; Kemmis & Dunn, 1996) have suggested that some of the findings of ineffectiveness of sensory integration interventions may be related to a too-narrow perspective.

With a broader perspective, it becomes imperative for scholars to conduct studies with scholars from other disciplines. Furthermore, scholars from other disciplines are finding sensory processing knowledge from the literature themselves and using knowledge from occupational therapy to inform their research programs.

For example, DeGangi, Sickel, Wiener, and Kaplan (1996) studied fussy babies by combining occupational therapy methods and psychophysiological methods and found that there are distinct patterns of performance, indicating hyper-responsivity to stimuli. Baranek et al. (1997) conducted a factor analysis of behaviors of children and adults with developmental disabilities and found two factors that both supported the idea of sensitivities to sensory input. Miller and colleagues (MacIntosh, Miller, Shyu, & Hagerman, 1999; Miller et al., 1998) have reported behavioral and psychophysiological data indicating poor sensory modulation in children with fragile X syndrome and identified a distinct pattern of performance they call sensory modulation disorder. Dunn and colleagues (Dunn, 1994; Dunn & Brown, 1997; Dunn & Westman, 1997; Ermer & Dunn, 1998; Kientz & Dunn, 1997) have reported on distinct patterns of children's responses to sensory events in daily life based on disabilities such as autism and attention deficit hyperactivity disorder (ADHD). Belser and Sudhalter (1995) found distinct arousal difficulties in children with fragile X syndrome when compared to children with autism and ADHD, and they hypothesized about their ability to modulate input for responding.

Personal Reflection—by Winnie Dunn

My professional development has occurred during the periods I have briefly described. As a novice in 1972, I had the advantage of Dr. Ayres' work from the onset of my studies to be an occupational therapist. Looking back, I certainly had no idea that I, as a novice, was part of this new direction (as Dr. Cruickshank called it). I just thought of sensory integration as part of occupational therapy knowledge. At that time, the role of researcher was a distant and disconnected one from practice. I certainly began to realize the power of this knowledge evolution as I attended workshops and studied. If someone had told me then that I would be contributing to this body of knowledge, I would have laughed and dismissed the comment. That is the way of novices—we do not have insight about the impact we have on others and ourselves; nevertheless the impact occurs.

For me, it was the plague of a practice dilemma for which I could not find an answer in my books and references. I was completely focused on solving my dilemma without any awareness that *this* was the beginning of my research career. It was many years later that I was able to identify the beginning of my "researcher self."

In the last few years, as I have studied sensory processing and developed the sensory profile tools for research and practice, I came upon some of my work pages from my novice period. I found a diagram I had been trying to formulate that contained the same constructs that I reported in an article in 1997 (Dunn, 1997). What strikes me is that it took me more than 20 years to achieve clarity about these ideas; yet, it also strikes me that I had these ideas more than 20 years ago!

I relay this experience because many novices feel discouraged, feeling that they will never learn and know what their mentors do. I invite you to be aware of the raw material ideas you produce during your novice period; perhaps we need to plant those seeds early so that we can release them to the public at a later date. Pay attention to your own development and how it affects you, the persons you serve, and your profession. Yes, *you* affect knowledge development with every action you take. Experts are sometimes encumbered by their own history, making it difficult to see knowledge in a new way—in the role of the novice entering the world of knowledge development.

CONCLUSION

In this chapter, we considered how knowledge develops. There are simultaneous activities occurring that enable knowledge to emerge and evolve. Professionals develop along their respective career paths, profiting from the work that has come before them and gathering their own information and insights along the way. As individuals in a profession gather and discuss their ideas, collective insights form as hypotheses that can be formulated and tested. As data become available, professionals reformulate their hypotheses and gain new insights. Interdisciplinary discourse also advances knowledge by adding perspectives to evolving ideas. These are the processes that occur to produce evidence for practice.

There is still much to discover about the nature of rehabilitation interventions and their appropriate application in practice. With the wealth of colleagues attending to this body of knowledge, there is no doubt that this journey will continue and be a fruitful source of knowledge development. It is through the persistent processes of professionals moving from novice to expert and disciplines evolving that this will occur.

TAKE HOME MESSAGES

✔ Knowledge develops at many different levels—simultaneously within a discipline and in collaboration with other disciplines.

✔ The tension between practice and knowledge is inevitable and acts in a positive way as the source for the advancement of knowledge.

✔ The role of the individual professional within a discipline area passes through four distinct stages: preservice experience, novice professional period, experienced professional period, and expert professional period. Knowledge, skill, and clinical reasoning evolve through these stages.

✔ An understanding of how knowledge develops must include a recognition of the three different vantage points for knowledge (individual professional, professional within a discipline, professionals across disciplines).

✔ Novices can enact a positive influence on knowledge development by becoming aware of their research self, choosing a methodical and critical approach to finding and implementing new knowledge, and encouraging new ideas.

✔ There are different responsibilities for the practitioner in each of the three different vantage points for the development of knowledge:

Individual Professional

- Remaining aware of influence of own personal beliefs/biases
- Evaluating effectiveness through questioning current information and seeking answers
- Willing to use this information to abandon ineffective practices

Professional Within a Discipline

- Challenging current beliefs and sharing information with colleagues
- Introducing new ideas and formally testing hypotheses

Professionals Across Disciplines

- Conducting research collaboratively and being open to other points of view
- Remaining aware of how decisions are being made by a variety of disciplines may impact families
- Facilitating awareness of various approaches to problem solving between disciplines
- There are several challenges in developing evidence in rehabilitation: producing generalizable evidence, evidence dissemination, and the implementation of evidence into practice

LEARNING AND EXPLORATION ACTIVITIES

The purpose of this chapter is to introduce the different vantage points at which knowledge develops and to demonstrate how these levels interact in practice.

1. Select one of the following topics of rehabilitation practice that interests you:

   a. Treatment of acute low back pain

   b. Outcomes of medical versus stroke units for person experiencing a stroke

   c. Home-based treatment for persons with arthritis

   d. School-based treatment for children with cerebral palsy

   e. Community reintegration for persons with schizophrenia

   Complete the following activities for the topic you have selected:

   a. Using your current knowledge and a literature search, construct a preliminary clinical reasoning strategy to guide treatment and practice for this topic area. Focus on what you know as a student and the elements of practice that should be put into place based on the evidence that you find.

   b. Interview a practitioner in the same topic area. Ask him or her to tell you about his or her clinical reasoning strategy to guide practice.

   c. Compare the results of what you found and what you discussed with the practitioner. Are the two approaches congruent? If not, what are the differences? Why might these differences occur, and how do they relate to the development of knowledge in rehabilitation practice?

2. Three arms of knowledge development within professions contribute to EBP: the individual professional's path, intradisciplinary development, and interdisciplinary development. Think of an example in current clinical practice. How will each of these arms address the issue in order to contribute to EBP?

3. Think of a population with which you have already worked or a population that you are interested in working with in the future (e.g., children with cerebral palsy, older adults with dementia, teenagers with eating disorders). List any assumptions or personal beliefs you carry about that population. How will these beliefs affect your use of the evidence surrounding this population? How may they affect intradisciplinary development? Interdisciplinary development?

REFERENCES

Arendt, R., MacLean, W., & Baumeister, A. (1988). Critique of sensory integration therapy and its application in mental retardation. *American Journal on Mental Retardation, 92*, 401-411.

Ayres, A. J. (1954). Ontogenetic principles in the development of arm and hand functions. *American Journal of Occupational Therapy, 8*(3), 95-99, 121.

Ayres, A. J. (1955). Proprioceptive facilitation elicited through the upper extremities: Part 3: Special applications to occupational therapy. *American Journal of Occupational Therapy, 9*(3), 121-126.

Ayres, A. J. (1958). The visual motor function. *American Journal of Occupational Therapy, 12*(3), 130-138.

Ayres, A. J. (1960). Occupational therapy for motor disorders resulting from impairment of the central nervous system. *Rehabilitation Literature, 21*, 302-310.

Ayres, A. J. (1963). The development of perceptual motor abilities: A theoretical basis for treatment of dysfunction. *American Journal of Occupational Therapy, 17*(6), 221-225.

Ayres, A. J. (1965). Patterns of perceptual motor dysfunction in children. *Perception and Motor Skills, 20*, 335-368.

Ayres, A. J. (1966a). Interrelations among perceptual motor abilities in a group of normal children. *American Journal of Occupational Therapy, 20*(6), 288-292.

Ayres, A. J. (1966b). Interrelationships among perceptual motor functions in children. *American Journal of Occupational Therapy, 20*(2), 68-71.

Ayres, A. J. (1969a). Relation between Gesell development quotients and later perceptual motor performance. *American Journal of Occupational Therapy, 23*(1), 11-17.

Ayres, A. J. (1969b). Deficits in sensory integration in educationally handicapped children. *Journal of Learning Disabilities, 2*, 160-168.

Ayres, A. J. (1971). Characteristics of types of sensory integrative dysfunction. *American Journal of Occupational Therapy, 25*(7), 329-334.

Ayres, A. J. (1972a). Improving academic scores through sensory integration. *Journal of Learning Disabilities, 5*, 338-343.

Ayres, A. J. (1972b). Types of sensory integrative dysfunction among disabled learners. *American Journal of Occupational Therapy, 26*(1), 13-18.

Ayres, A. J. (1976). *The effect of sensory integrative therapy on learning disabled children: The final report of a research project.* Los Angeles, CA: University of Southern California.

Bairstow, P., Cochrane, R., & Rusk, I. (1991). Selection of children with cerebral palsy for conductive education and the characteristics of children judged suitable and unsuitable. *Developmental Medicine & Child Neurology, 33*(11), 941-942.

Baranek, G., Foster, L., & Berkson, G. (1997). Sensory defensiveness in persons with developmental disabilities. *Occupational Therapy Journal of Research, 17*(3), 173-185.

Barbour, R. S., & Barbour, M. (2003). Evaluating and synthesizing qualitative research: the need to develop a distinctive approach. *Journal of Evaluation in Clinical Practice, 9*(2), 179-186.

Belser, R., & Sudhalter, V. (1995). Arousal difficulties in males with fragile X syndrome: A preliminary report. *Developmental Brain Dysfunction, 8*, 270-279.

Blashy, M., & Fuchs, R. (1959). Orthokinetics: A new receptor facilitation method. *American Journal of Occupational Therapy, 13*(5), 226-234.

Bobath, K., & Bobath, B. (1955). Tonic reflexes and righting reflexes in the diagnosis and assessment of cerebral palsy. *Cerebral Palsy Review, 16*(5), 4-10.

Bochner, S., Center, Y., Chapparo, C., & Donelly, M. (1999). How effective are programs based on conductive education? A report of two studies. *Journal of Intellectual and Developmental Disability, 24*(3), 227-242.

Case-Smith, J., & Bryan, T. (1999). The effects of occupational therapy with sensory integration emphasis on preschool-age children with autism. *American Journal of Occupational Therapy, 53*(5), 489-497.

Chinn, C., & Brewer, W. (1993). The role of anomalous data in knowledge acquisition: A theoretical framework and implications for science instruction. *Review of Educational Research, 63*(1), 1-49.

Clark, P. G. (2004). Institutionalizing interdisciplinary health professions programs in higher education: The implications of one story and two laws. *Journal of Interprofessional Care, 18*(3), 251-261.

Cooper, B. A., Cohen, U., & Hasselkus, B. R. (1991). Barrier-free design: A review and critique of the occupational therapy perspective. *American Journal of Occupational Therapy, 45*(4), 344-350.

Cruickshank, W. (1974). Foreword. In A. Henderson, L. Llorens, E. Gilfoyle, C. Myers, & S. Prevel (Eds.), *The development of sensory integrative theory and practice: A collection of the works of A. Jean Ayres.* Dubuque, IA: Kendall/Hunt Publishing.

Cruickshank, W., Bice, H., & Wallen, N. (1957). *Perception and cerebral palsy.* Syracuse, NY: Syracuse University Press.

Darrah, J., Watkins, B., Chen, L., & Bonin, C. (2004). Conductive education intervention for children with cerebral palsy: an AACPDM evidence report. *Developmental Medicine and Child Neurology, 46*(3), 187-203.

DeGangi, G. (2000). *Pediatric disorders of regulation in affect and behavior: A therapist's guide to assessment and treatment.* San Diego, CA: Academic Press.

DeGangi, G., Sickel, R., Wiener, A., & Kaplan, E. (1996). Fussy babies: To treat or not to treat? *British Journal of Occupational Therapy, 59*(10), 457-464.

Dunn, W. (1994). Performance of typical children on the sensory profile: An item analysis. *American Journal of Occupational Therapy, 48*(11), 967-974.

Dunn, W. (1997). A conceptual model for considering the impact of sensory processing abilities on the daily lives of young children and their families. *Infants and Young Children, 9*(4), 23-35.

Dunn, W. (2000). The sensations of everyday life: Empirical, theoretical, and pragmatic considerations. *American Journal of Occupational Therapy, 55*(6), 608-620.

Dunn, W., & Brown, C. (1997). Factor analysis on the sensory profile from a national sample of children without disabilities. *American Journal of Occupational Therapy, 51*, 490-495.

Dunn, W., & Westman, K. (1997). The Sensory Profile: The performance of a national sample of children without disabilities. *American Journal of Occupational Therapy, 51*, 25-34.

Dunst, C. J., Deal, A. G., & Trivette, C. M. (1996). *Supporting & strengthening families: Methods, strategies and practices, Volume 1.* Cambridge, MA: Brookline Books, Inc.

Ermer, J., & Dunn, W. (1998). The Sensory Profile: A discriminant analysis of children with and without disabilities. *American Journal of Occupational Therapy, 52*(4), 283-290.

Fay, T. (1948). The neurophysical aspects of therapy in cerebral palsy. *Archives of Physical Medicine, 29*(6), 327-334.

Feagans, L. (1983). A current view of learning disabilities. *Journal of Pediatrics, 102*(4), 487-493.

Ferry, P. C. (1981). On growing new neurons: Are early intervention programs effective? *Pediatrics, 67*(1), 38-41.

Fertman, C. I., Dotson, S., Mazzocco, G. O., & Reitz, S. M. (2005). Challenges of preparing allied health professionals for interdisciplinary practice in rural areas. *Journal of Allied Health, 34*(3), 163-168.

Feyerbend, P. (1993). *Against method* (3rd ed.). London, England: Verso.

Fisher, A. G., Murray, E. A., & Bundy, A. C. (1991). *Sensory integration theory and practice.* Philadelphia, PA: F. A. Davis Company.

Glasgow, R. E., Magid, D. J., Beck, A., Ritzwoller, D., & Estabrooks, P. A. (2005). Practical clinical trials for translating research to practice: design and measurement recommendations. *Medical Care, 43*(6), 551-557.

Gross, A. R., Kay, T. M, Kennedy, C., Gasner, D., Hurley, L., Yardley, K., et al. (2002). Clinical Practice guidelines on the use of manipulation or mobilization in the treatment of adults with mechanical neck disorders. *Manual Therapy, 7*(4), 193-205.

Hannes, K., Leys, M., Vermeire, E., Aertgeerts, B., Buntinx, F., Depoorter, A. M. (2005) Implementing evidence-based medicine in general practice: a focus group based study. *BMC Family Practice, 9*, 6-37.

Henderson, A., Llorens, L., Gilfoyle, E., Myers, C., & Prevel, S. (1974). *The development of sensory integrative theory and practice: A collection of the works of A. Jean Ayres.* Dubuque, IA: Kendall/Hunt Publishing.

Humphries, T., Snider, L., & McDougall, B. (1993). Clinical evaluation of the effectiveness of sensory integrative and perceptual motor therapy in improving sensory integrative function in children with learning disabilities. *Occupational Therapy Journal of Research, 13*(3), 163-182.

Humphries, T., Wright, M., McDougall, B., & Vertes, J. (1990). The efficacy of sensory integration therapy for children with learning disability. *Physical and Occupational Therapy in Pediatrics, 10*(3), 1-17.

Humphries, T., Wright, M., Snider, L., & McDougall, B. (1992). A comparison of the effectiveness of sensory integrative therapy and perceptual-motor training in treating children with learning disabilities. *Journal of Developmental Behavior and Pediatrics, 13*(1), 31-40.

Kaplan, B. J., Polatajko, H. J., Wilson, B. N., & Faris, P. D. (1993). Reexamination of sensory integration treatment: A combination of two efficacy studies. *Journal of Learning Disabilities, 26*(5), 342-347.

Kemmis, B., & Dunn, W. (1996). Collaborative consultation: The efficacy of remedial and compensatory interventions in school contexts. *American Journal of Occupational Therapy, 50*(9), 709-717.

Ketefian, S. (2001). Issues in the application of research to practice. *Rev Latino-am Enfermagen, 9*(5), 7-12.

Kientz, M., & Dunn, W. (1997). A comparison of the performance of children with and without autism on the Sensory Profile. *American Journal of Occupational Therapy, 51*(7), 530-537.

Kuhn, T. (1996). *The structure of scientific revolutions* (3rd ed.). Chicago, IL: University of Chicago Press.

Lonton, A. P., & Russell, A. (1989). Conductive education—magic or myth? *Z-Kinderchir, 44*(Suppl 1), 21-23.

MacIntosh, D., Miller, L., Shyu, V., & Hagerman, R. (1999). Sensory modulation disruption, electrodermal responses, and functional behaviors. *Developmental Medicine & Child Neurology, 41*, 608-615.

Miller, L., & Lane, S. (2000). Toward a consensus in terminology in sensory integration theory and practice, part 1: Taxonomy of neurophysiological processes. *Sensory Integration Special Interest Section Quarterly, 23*(1), 1-4.

Miller, L., McIntosh, D., McGrath, J., Shyu, V., Lampe, M., Taylor, A., et al. (1998). Electrodermal responses to sensory stimuli in individuals with fragile X syndrome: A preliminary report. *American Journal of Medical Genetics, 83*, 268-279.

Miller, P. A., Solomon, P., Giacomini, M., & Abelson, J. (2005). Experiences of novice physiotherapists adapting to their role in acute hospitals. *Physiotherapy Canada, 57*(2), 145-153.

Moore, M. E., Vaughan, K. T. L., Hayes, B. E., & McLendon, W. (2005). Developing an interdisciplinary collaboration center in an academic health sciences library. *Medical References Services Quarterly, 24*(4), 99-107.

Nananda, F. (2005). Challenges in translating research into practice. *Journal of Women's Health, 14*(1), 87-95.

Ottenbacher, K. (1982). Sensory integration therapy: Affect or effect? *American Journal of Occupational Therapy, 36*, 571-578.

Ottenbacher, K., & Short-DeGraff, M. (1985). *Vestibular processing dysfunction in children.* Binghamton, NY: Haworth Press, Inc.

Polatajko, H., Kaplan, B., & Wilson, B. (1992). Sensory integration treatment for children with learning disabilities: Its status 20 years later. *Occupational Therapy Journal of Research, 12*(6), 323-341.

Polatajko, H., Law, M., Miller, J., Schaffer, R., & Macnab, J. (1991). The effect of a sensory integration program on academic achievement, motor performance, and self-esteem in children identified as learning disabled: Results of a clinical trial. *Occupational Therapy Journal of Research, 11*(3), 155-174.

Quine, W., & Ullian, J. (1978). *The web of belief* (2nd ed., pp. 9-34). New York, NY: McGraw-Hill.

Rappolt, S., & Tassone, M. (2002). How rehabilitation therapists gather, evaluate, and implement new knowledge. *The Journal of Continuing Education in the Health Professions, 22*, 170-180.

Reddihough, D. S., King, J., Coleman, G., & Catanese, T. (1998). Efficacy of programmes based on conductive education for young children with cerebral palsy. *Developmental Medicine & Child Neurology, 40*(11), 763-770.

Reimer, B., Sawka, E., & James, D. (2005). Improving research in the addictions field: a perspective from Canada. *Substance Use & Misuse, 40*, 1707-1720.

Rodehorst, T. K., Wilhelm, S. L., & Jensen, L. (2005) Use of interdisciplinary simulation to understand perceptions of team members' roles. *Journal of Professional Nursing, 21*(3), 159-166.

Rogers, E. (1995). *Diffusion of Innovations* (4th ed.). New York: The Free Press.

Rood, M. (1952). Neurophysiological mechanisms utilized in the treatment of neuromuscular dysfunction. *American Journal of Occupational Therapy, 10*(4), 220-225.

Rosenbaum, P., King, S., Law, M., King, G., & Evans, J. (1998). Family-centred service: A conceptual framework and research review. *Physical and Occupational Therapy in Pediatrics, 18*(1), 1-20.

Schachter, K. A., & Cohen, S. J. (2005). From research to practice: Challenges to implementing national diabetes guidelines with five community health centers on the U.S.-Mexico border. *Preventing Chronic Disease, 2*(1), 1-6.

Schell, B. (1998). Clinical reasoning: The basis of practice. In M. Neistadt & E. Crepeau (Eds.), *Willard and Spackman's occupational therapy* (9th ed.). Philadelphia, PA: Lippincott, Williams & Wilkins.

Sieg, K. (1988). A. Jean Ayres. In B. Miller, K. Sieg, F. Ludwig, S. Shortridge, & J. Van Deusen (Eds.), *Six perspectives on theory for practice of occupational therapy* (pp. 95-142). Rockville, MD: Aspen Publishers.

Solomon, P., & Miller, P.A. (2005). Qualitative study of novice physical therapists' experiences in private practice. *Physiotherapy Canada, 57*(3), 190-198.

Stegink-Jansen, C.W. (2002). Outcomes, treatment effectiveness, efficacy, and evidence-based practice: Examples from the world of splinting. *Journal of Hand Therapy, 15*(2), 136-143.

Steinfeld, E., & Shea, S. (1993). Enabling home environments. Identifying barriers to independence. *Technology and Disability, 2*(4), 69-79.

Weaver, C. A., Warren, J. J., & Delaney, C. (2005). Bedside, classroom and bench: collaborative strategies to generate evidence-based knowledge for nursing practice. *International Journal of Medical Informatics, 74*, 989-999.

Wilkins, S., Jung, B., Wishart, L., Edwards, M., & Gamble-Norton, S. (2003). The effectiveness of community-based occupational therapy education and functional training programs for older adults: A critical literature review. *Canadian Journal of Occupational Therapy, 4*(70), 214-225.

Williamson, G., & Szczepanski, M. (1999). Coping frame of reference. In P. Kramer & J. Hinojosa (Eds.), *Frames of reference for pediatric occupational therapy* (pp. 431-468). Philadelphia, PA: Lippincott, Williams & Wilkins.

Wilson, B. N., & Kaplan, B. J. (1994). Follow-up assessment of children receiving sensory integration treatment. *Occupational Therapy Journal of Research, 14*(4), 244-266.

Wilson, B. N., Kaplan, B. J., Fellowes, S., Gruchy, C., & Faris, P. (1992). The efficacy of sensory integration treatment compared to tutoring. *Physical and Occupational Therapy in Pediatrics, 12*(1), 1-36.

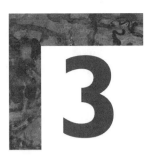

3

Becoming an Evidence-Based Practitioner

Annie McCluskey, PhD, MA, DipCOT; Sally Home, BAppSc(OT) Hons, GradCert(Mgt); and Lauren Thompson, BAppSc(OT) Hons

LEARNING OBJECTIVES

After reading this chapter, the student/practitioner will be able to:

- Reflect on his or her own stage of development as an evidence-based practitioner.
- Recognize the different levels of engagement with EBP that practitioners may display.
- Describe the skills, knowledge, attitudes, and behaviors that may be required to become an evidence-based practitioner.
- Identify characteristics of their own organization that may influence the progress of EBP.
- List strategies that can be used to facilitate EBP.

INTRODUCTION

The specific process of "doing" EBP will be described later in this book. In preparation for this chapter, think about the general process of applying evidence to practice. The first step in the EBP process is to write a focused clinical question to guide database searching. Next, conduct searches in an organized manner, and select the best research to answer your question. Third, read and critically appraise this research. If the research is robust enough, decide if changes to practice are needed, disseminate and implement findings, and in due course, evaluate health outcomes for individual clients.

The process of becoming an evidence-based practitioner appears relatively simple at first glance. In our experience, learning to write focused questions and search more effectively are the easier skills to learn, although both require practice. Learning to critically appraise research is more challenging, as we will discuss in this chapter, partly because of a need to interpret statistics and understand a range of research designs. Then there is the matter of using these skills to inform practice, which more difficult than it first appears. And finally, changing practice in line with new evidence is one of the most challenging aspects of becoming an evidence-based practitioner.

This chapter describes the process of becoming an evidence-based practitioner and was informed by a study involving Australian occupational therapists. This mixed methods study followed a group of practitioners for several months after they had attended a workshop on EBP. First, the study methods and key findings will be presented. Second, a typology of practitioners will be described. Third, strategies that practitioners used postworkshop to become more evidence based are described, along with factors that helped them during the change process. Finally, key messages and implications for individual rehabilitation practitioners, managers, educators, and researchers are discussed.

THE RESEARCH PROJECT

In late 2002, 114 Australian occupational therapists were recruited to a study using a before-and-after design (McCluskey, 2004). Participants were offered a 2-day, low-cost workshop on EBP and follow-up support for 8 months (the intervention). In exchange, they were asked to do three things. First, they would complete a survey and knowledge test three times (before and immediately after the workshop, and 8 months later). Second, they were asked to complete a critically appraised topic (or CAT [see Chapter 10 for more information on CATs]), in pairs or alone. Finally, participants were asked to keep a diary, before and for 8 months postworkshop, and record any searching, reading, and appraisal activities. The intention was that the CAT assignment would encourage therapists to use their skills and knowledge, thereby increasing the frequency of their search and appraisal activities.

Measurable Outcomes

Key findings were that skills and knowledge improved markedly but behavior changed little, based on the frequency of searching and appraisal activities (see McCluskey & Lovarini, 2005). Preworkshop, 6% engaged in critical appraisal increasing to 18% in the 2 months postworkshop and 18% at the 8-months follow-up. Nearly two thirds (60%) were not reading any research, let alone appraising it, at follow-up. Twenty-three participants (20%) completed their CAT assignment within 12 months (available free of charge at www.otcats.com).

While disappointing, these findings are consistent with other research focused on knowledge transfer involving general health physicians in Norway (Forsetlund et al., 2003). We know that workshops help practitioners to learn search and appraisal skills, which many did not acquire as students. However, workshops do not guarantee that skills and knowledge will be used, practiced, shared with colleagues, or applied for the benefit of clients. Behavior change is difficult, and most practitioners will require self-reflection and other assistance to change their practice.

Qualitative Data From Participant Interviews

After 18 months, 10 of the most active and "successful" Australian practitioners were purposely selected for interview. The aim was to choose people who had shown a measurable change in their skills and knowledge based on knowledge test results and diary activities. We also selected people who we knew, from personal contact, had championed EBP at work. Our aim was to explore occupational therapists' experience of a social process. Therefore, a specific population that had experienced change was required.

Practitioners were asked two key questions. First, they were asked to describe what they had done upon return to work after the 2-day workshop ("*Last year you attended a 2-day workshop on evidence-base practice. What happened between then and now?*"). Second, they were asked to talk about factors that had helped or hindered them during this time ("*Tell me about any*

Table 3-1

CHARACTERISTICS OF THE INTERVIEW SAMPLE (N = 10)

Characteristic	n (%)
Level of Initial Occupational Therapy Qualification	
Diploma	2 (20%)
Undergraduate degree	8 (80%)
Time Since Graduation	
<5 years	2 (20%)
≥5 but <10 years	1 (10%)
≥10 years by <20 years	5 (50%)
≥10 years	2 (20%)
Postgraduate Qualification	
No	5 (50%)
Yes	5 (50%)
Enrolled in Postgraduate Study	
Yes	0 (0%)
No	10 (100%)
Employment Status	
Full-time	8 (80%)
Part-time (25 hours per week or less)	2 (20%)
Geographical Work Location	
Metropolitan	4 (40%)
Regional or rural	6 (60%)

Adapted with permission from McCluskey, A. (2004). *Increasing the use of research evidence by occupational therapists [Final report]*. Penrith South, Australia: School of Exercise and Health Sciences, University of Western Sydney.

factors that you think might have helped or hindered your ability to put ideas into practice at work following the workshop").

Data were analyzed independently by the authors using grounded theory methods (Glaser & Strauss, 1967; Schreiber, 2001; Strauss & Corbin, 1998). Constant comparative techniques were used in which we looked for similarities and differences across participants. For example, what was similar and different about the language used or the workplace of participants who were more or less active and engaged in the process postworkshop? How were these subgroups similar or different? We also examined their stories for process, strategies, conditions, and consequences (Fagerhaugh, 1986; Glaser, 1996). For example, what steps did participants follow when proceeding with their CAT? What strategies did they use to make time for this additional work? All three researchers met frequently to discuss the categories and subcategories.

The Sample

Demographic characteristics of the interview sample are summarized in Table 3-1. Most of the participants had been working as an occupational therapy practitioner for more than

Figure 3-1. Typology of practitioners according to their engagement in evidence-based practice. (Adapted from McCluskey, A. [2004]. *Increasing the use of research evidence by occupational therapists* [Final Research Report]. Penrith South, Sydney: University of Western Sydney and Thompson, L. [2003]. *Becoming an evidence-based occupational therapist.* [Unpublished undergraduate honours thesis]. Campbelltown, New South Wales: School of Exercise & Health Sciences, University of Western Sydney. Model adapted from Bonner, A. [2001]. *Producing the magnum opus: The acquisition and exercise of nephrology nursing expertise.* Unpublished doctoral dissertation, University of Western Sydney, Australia.)

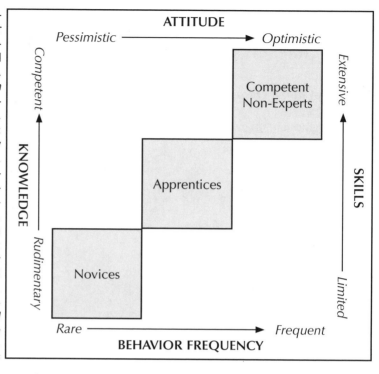

10 years (70%) and worked full-time (80%). Half of the participants had postgraduate qualifications (increasing the likelihood that they already knew how to search for articles and use electronic databases preworkshop).

First, a typology of practitioners will be described. Characteristics that defined each type or category of practitioner will be presented, including the skill, knowledge, behavior, and attitudes observed. Strategies used during the change process to become an evidence-based practitioner will then be explored along with factors that influenced change.

KEY FINDINGS FROM THE QUALITATIVE STUDY

A Typology of Evidence-Based Practitioners

There were three distinct categories of participants according to their level of engagement with EBP. These categories were labeled *Novices, Apprentices,* and *Competent Non-Experts.* It was difficult to choose an appropriate label to represent the latter group because even after 18 months, none could be classified as experts in EBP. Instead, the term *Competent Non-Expert* was chosen to reflect their enhanced skills and knowledge and increased proficiency at activities such as searching and critical appraisal. The three categories existed on a continuum, ranging from those who mostly operated as experience-based practitioners (*Novices*), to those who were more evidence-based in the way they thought and worked (*Competent Non-Experts*) (Figure 3-1).

Practitioners in each category displayed different levels of skill and knowledge (Table 3-2). The frequency of behaviors such as searching and appraisal also varied across the three categories of practitioner, as did their attitudes to EBP. Each category of practitioner was defined

Table 3-2

CATEGORIES AND CHARACTERISTICS OF PRACTITIONERS

		Categories	
Characteristic	**Novices**	**Apprentices**	**Competent Non-Experts**
Skills	Rudimentary	Developing	Competent
Knowledge	Limited	Developing	Extensive
Behavior	Rare	Irregular	Regular
Attitude	Pessimistic	More optimistic	Optimistic

(Adapted with permission from McCluskey, A. [2004]. *Increasing the use of research evidence by occupational therapists* [Final Research Report]. Penrith South, Sydney: University of Western Sydney and with permission from Thompson, L. [2003]. *Becoming an evidence-based occupational therapist.* [Unpublished undergraduate honours thesis]. Campbelltown, New South Wales: School of Exercise & Health Sciences, University of Western Sydney. Model adapted from Bonner, A. [2001]. *Producing the magnum opus: The acquisition and exercise of nephrology nursing expertise.* Unpublished doctoral dissertation, University of Western Sydney, Australia.)

according to the presence or absence of these characteristics and the use or nonuse of certain strategies.

Novices possessed basic skills, limited knowledge, rarely engaged in search and appraisal activities, and displayed a somewhat negative, pessimistic attitude to EBP. Conversely, *Competent Non-Experts* had achieved skill competency, possessed extensive knowledge, engaged in search and appraisal activities regularly, and displayed a positive, optimistic attitude to EBP. *Apprentices* were somewhere in between these two categories.

Skills were the practical abilities that individuals needed to possess in order to use evidence. An example of a skill was the ability to construct a search strategy. Skills were influenced by knowledge and the practitioner's attitude toward EBP. The level of skill also affected behavior. Those with a higher level of skill tended to apply the process of EBP more often. Skills were initially acquired as a consequence of attending the workshop on EBP and developed through continued practice. Skill levels ranged from rudimentary to advanced. *Novices* were still developing skills for finding and using evidence. The more *Competent Non-Experts* could manage basic as well as more complex skills, such as applying evidence in practice.

Knowledge involved knowing facts and procedures related to the "doing" of EBP (i.e., what databases were available, how to access them on the Internet, and knowing the levels of evidence). Skills and knowledge were interrelated. Participants had to possess knowledge of the concepts involved to develop and apply skills. Participants' knowledge ranged from limited to extensive. *Novices* possessed only limited knowledge. They were still developing an understanding of EBP, including related terminology and available databases. *Apprentices* had developed their knowledge further, while the *Competent Non-Experts* possessed extensive knowledge of most EBP concepts.

Behavior referred to the application of skills and knowledge. In our study, frequency of behavior referred to how regularly participants engaged in the process of searching for, appraising, and implementing research evidence into practice. Participants' behavior ranged from infrequent use of skills and knowledge, to regular engagement in EBP.

Attitude was defined as the mental view, disposition, or opinion of the occupational therapist with regard to EBP. Attitudes were closely linked to motivation and eagerness to become more evidence based. For example, some occupational therapists placed great importance on using research evidence. Others were negative and felt that EBP was unnecessary. Attitudes ranged from being pessimistic and focusing on barriers to being optimistic and committed to overcoming barriers. Attitudes were also closely linked to behaviors. The *Competent Non-Experts,* who were generally positive and optimistic about EBP, tended to apply their skills and knowledge more frequently than the *Novices*, who were generally more negative and pessimistic.

The Novices

Two of the 10 occupational therapists in our study were classified as *Novices.* They were still at the beginning of their journey along the path to becoming evidence based. Although 18 months had passed since they attended the initial workshop on EBP, they were not proficient at using their skills and knowledge. Becoming evidence based required a significant change in their skills and knowledge, as well as a change in behavior and attitudes.

Rudimentary Skills

Novices did not have the skills to appraise or implement evidence. They wrote clinical questions and searched the databases for evidence. However, even when working through these processes, the *Novices* encountered many difficulties and needed help:

> *… having a better knowledge of looking at how to put together a clinical question… I'm still not all that practised and skilled at doing it (OT5)*

> *I then did try to do a search relating to a client and wasn't able—wasn't successful in the search (OT8)*

Novices reported limited Internet and computer skills prior to joining the project. This lack of skills became a barrier to progress when they wanted to search for evidence. For example, when one *Novice* was asked about barriers encountered, this was her response:

> *…a lack of practical understanding on how to access databases and search techniques and computer use generally. Frustration when my first search was unsuccessful… that was a real big turn-off (OT8)*

Limited Knowledge

Novices had limited knowledge of the range of databases available and appropriate search terms to use when seeking information to answer their question. Further, they had limited knowledge of EBP jargon. For example, they did not use technical language, misused terminology, or were unable to remember appropriate terms. In place of using technical terms, these occupational therapists used words like "stuff" and "things." For example:

> *I didn't have enough computer skills… to know anything about search engines or how to go about finding stuff (OT5)*

Another participant referred to "random control trials" rather than "randomized controlled trials." At times, they were at a loss for the appropriate term to use, such as systematic reviews, which they had not heard of before the workshop.

Infrequent Behavior

Due to the difficulties that *Novices* faced when trying to search, they did not apply the process of EBP often. They did not appear able to appraise or implement evidence and rarely wrote questions or searched for literature:

> *I don't necessarily use specific clinical questions I suppose, I kind of try and look at target words I guess... [but] it's not day-to-day (OT5)*

A behavioral indicator of *Novices* was that they searched for, collected, and sometimes read journal articles but did not engage in appraisal:

> *I read it... that's it (OT5)*

> *I still don't... necessarily... critique a journal article. I know I should but I don't (OT8)*

Pessimistic Attitude

Novices were more pessimistic about achieving EBP than other categories of occupational therapists. Although they reported a prior interest in further education and keeping up-to-date, they tended to focus on barriers rather than on how to overcome them. For example, when lack of time was identified as a barrier, *Novices* did not look at ways to make time but instead determined that it was not possible for them to fit searching and appraisal into their day. *Novices* were also flippant about the importance and validity of using evidence in practice. They used phrases such as *"playing around," "to-ing and fro-ing,"* and *"trying,"* which implied less commitment to EBP than that displayed by the *Apprentices* and *Competent Non-Experts.*

Another defining attitudinal characteristic of *Novices* was low internal motivation. They needed external prompting from their project "buddy" or the outreach support person employed on the project to pursue EBP. *Novices* became frustrated when they had difficulty or hit a barrier. This frustration affected their confidence and led them to give up altogether when faced with difficulties.

The Apprentices

The *Apprentices* existed between the *Novices* and *Competent Non-Experts* on a continuum ranging from experience-based to evidence-based practitioners. Five of the 10 study participants were classified as *Apprentices*. They had a sound understanding of the process of EBP and the activities they should be undertaking. However, they were still developing and refining their skills. *Apprentices* were able to write clinical questions and search for information with little difficulty. They were also beginning to use available resources to appraise the evidence located.

Generally, *Apprentices* had a fragmented experience of working through the process of EBP. When they hit a barrier, they tended to "shelve" that task for a while. However, they would always return to and master the task. Their level of enthusiasm and confidence varied according to the degree of difficulty experienced. When things went according to plan, they were excited and motivated. When tasks became difficult or could not be completed without help, they lost confidence. All of the *Apprentices* displayed similar behaviors, skills, knowledge, and attitudes.

Developing Skills

The *Apprentices* were still learning, refining, and developing their skills. They had moved beyond writing a clinical question, searching for information, and reading the articles found. They possessed the skills to comfortably write clinical questions and were confident that they could design searches that would locate available evidence:

I have the skills now to look something up... it feels good to be able to just type some-thing in and "right, great, I've got what I need" and I know how to get what I need (OT2)

Although the *Apprentices* were critically appraising evidence, this was not without difficulty. All reported difficulty analyzing and understanding statistical information:

I started a new question... did all the searches... got all the articles... read them all... started the summary and then got stuck on the stats... I've done the summary of what they actually did, but it's come down to actually analyzing the stats and trying to com-pare all the different results that they got. And that's the bit I got stuck on (OT1)

Apprentices were learning to manage such difficulties with analysis by identifying and using resources available to them. These resources included statistical texts and the research project officer/outreach support person employed on the project. However, *Apprentices* were not implementing evidence in practice. They knew they should be implementing research and some were trying to. The *Apprentices* recognized, however, that they were not yet comfortable with implementing evidence and needed further practice:

...The final stages of the process... implementing change... I'm not very good at it, I know that much (OT1)

Developing Knowledge

The *Apprentices* were still developing their knowledge. They had a clear understanding of the process of EBP and knew they should be doing more than just reading articles. They were appraising studies but not without difficulty. Most did not fully understand statistical concepts required to appraise research articles. The *Apprentices* were actively using their skills and knowl-edge but were not yet proficient. They had a thorough knowledge of available databases and search engines and how to access and use these. The *Apprentices* had a greater knowledge of technical language and terminology related to EBP than the *Novices*. They were beginning to use terms such as levels of evidence, clinically effective, randomized trials, and critical appraisal.

Irregular Behavior

The main behavioral indicator of the *Apprentices* was that they had moved beyond search-ing and reading. They were now critically appraising articles. Because they were able to move further through the process of EBP than the *Novices*, they were using their skills and knowledge more often. Occupational therapists at this stage were also beginning to plan for the future and thinking about other clinical questions they might investigate. Some had begun to formulate new questions and conduct searches. Such behavior suggested that the *Apprentices* were thinking about the place of evidence in their practice more often than *Novices* but were still not using evidence regularly.

More Optimistic Attitude

Apprentices were more positive about using evidence in practice. Like the *Novices*, they were keen to keep learning and stay up-to-date. All of the *Apprentices* were aware of, and mentioned the importance of using, research evidence in practice. However, they acknowledged that they were not basing their practice on evidence as much as they should be:

I'm... aware that I really should take the time and look this up... not that I actually have the time to do that (OT2)

In general, the *Apprentices'* motivation and enthusiasm varied in accordance with their fragmented engagement. They were more motivated when they were achieving results but less so when they had put tasks aside due to lack of time or difficulty. Because the *Apprentices* were still mastering skills, they confronted many challenges. When they came across a challenging task, they tended to put the project aside for a while and book over their allocated time. The evidence-based summary (a CAT) that they were producing for the research project was not always a priority. *Apprentices* were beginning to address barriers faced. They were not always successful, but they still had greater optimism about EBP than the *Novices*.

Competent Non-Experts

Three of the 10 study participants were classified as *Competent Non-Experts*. They possessed extensive knowledge, advanced skills, and were very active in using these frequently. They used jargon related to EBP appropriately and comfortably. *Competent Non-Experts* also had a positive attitude toward EBP. They mentioned barriers less frequently than the *Novices* and *Apprentices* and were putting strategies in place to overcome barriers.

These participants were committed to the process of EBP. They were active in their departments and encouraged other occupational therapists to increase their use of evidence. *Competent Non-Experts* took on the roles of educator and leader. As with the other two categories, *Competent Non-Experts* were characterized by the skills they possessed, their EBP knowledge, the frequency of their behavior, and the attitude toward EBP.

Competent Skills

The *Competent Non-Experts* had moved beyond appraising and were thinking about how to use findings. They felt competent writing clinical questions and searching for and appraising literature. They had the skills to complete these three steps with little difficulty. They were also beginning to develop skills for using evidence in practice.

Extensive Knowledge

The *Competent Non-Experts* knew a great deal about EBP. They were able to work through most of the stages of the EBP process. They were proficient in using databases and the Internet to locate articles. *Competent Non-Experts* had extensive knowledge of evidence-based terminology. They used jargon appropriately and talked comfortably during the interview about "systematic reviews," "levels of evidence," and "confidence intervals." Use of such terms suggested a higher level of understanding of concepts than that demonstrated by *Apprentices* and *Novices*.

Frequent Behavior

The key behavioral indicator of *Competent Non-Experts* was that they regularly used the EBP process. They were planning for a future that included EBP and had written new questions they hoped to answer. Although changing practice was not easy, they were thinking and talking about it routinely:

> *I now use the McMaster appraisal tool... and... make a recommendation to the organization whether or not we take on board anything about new practice, depending on the level of evidence provided (OT7) (See Appendices A to D for McMaster tools)*

Competent Non-Experts were also active within their departments, encouraging peers to use the EBP process. They were involved in changing and writing departmental policies and procedures. Most had started a journal club. One participant had developed a business plan that included EBP. They taught other health professionals about EBP and encouraged the use of evidence among their peers:

I did a series of in-services. I tried to use some of the structure that had been applied in the workshop where we looked at how to write a clinical question first and did the in-services on that. Then looked at databases and what are around and some sessions on how to search databases and that sort of thing. And then we did a series of in-services as well on how to critically appraise... (OT9)

I came back and within 6 weeks... did a presentation to them about the workshop and what was involved with the workshop, and then from that we started to formulate how, as a group, we could be more evidence-based in what we did...from that we started a group where we meet once a month now and work through... appraising some articles together...using a McMaster form (OT3)

Optimistic Attitude

Another defining characteristic of *Competent Non-Experts* was their positive attitude to EBP. They embraced the concept and were optimistic about being able to achieve EBP. They were not so concerned about problems and barriers, which they felt they could overcome. Most had been interested in EBP for some time and had volunteered to participate in the research project to enhance their learning:

I was really keen to look at EBP and how it could be incorporated (OT3)

When I saw it advertised [the EBP project]... given the interest I had in EBP, and feeling that it was very much a thing of the future...that I needed to know more about, I put my hand up for it then (OT7)

STRATEGIES USED AND CONDITIONS NECESSARY FOR BECOMING AN EVIDENCE-BASED PRACTITIONER

Three key strategies were used, more often and more consistently by *Competent Non-Experts* than by other participants. These strategies were labeled *Finding Time for EBP, Developing Skills and Knowledge,* and *Staying Focused* (Table 3-3). Participants used these strategies to overcome barriers such as lack of time, and limited skills and knowledge.

There were also certain conditions or factors that facilitated the move to an evidence-based approach, or conversely that limited their progress toward this goal. These conditions were readiness for change, personal and organizational expectations, the presence of deadlines, and the availability of support (Table 3-4). If these conditions were present and positive, these practitioners were more likely to progress. If these conditions were absent or negative, progress was hindered.

The consequence of not adopting these strategies, and not having certain conditions present, was that participants appeared to remain more experienced based in the way they thought and practiced. The categories of practitioner (or the typology), strategies, and conditions form a provisional model or theory of change from non-EBP to EBP. This provisional grounded theory will require further testing and development. The following section provides examples of the strategies, conditions, and consequences identified through analysis of the 10 interview transcripts.

Table 3-3

STRATEGIES USED TO BECOME AN EVIDENCE-BASED PRACTITIONER

Strategies	*Subcategories*
Finding time for EBP	• Prioritizing activities • Planning ahead
Developing skills and knowledge	• Using evidence • Teaching others • Seeking help
Staying focused	• Making a commitment • Being persistent • Being motivated

Adapted with permission from McCluskey, A. (2004). Increasing the use of research evidence by occupational therapists [Final report]. Penrith South, Australia: School of Exercise and Health Sciences, University of Western Sydney. Adapted with permission from Home, S. (2003). *Finding time to become an evidence-based practitioner.* [Unpublished undergraduate honours thesis]. Campbelltown, New South Wales: School of Exercise & Health Sciences, University of Western Sydney.

Table 3-4

CONDITIONS THAT INFLUENCED CHANGE AND THE UPTAKE OF EVIDENCE-BASED PRACTICE

Conditions	*Definition*
Readiness for change	Time ready, intellectually ready, resource ready, or skill ready. Readiness to change work habits and allocate time to EBP-related activities
Personal and organizational expectations	Personal expectations of achievement Use of evidence encouraged and expected by individuals and their organization Managers and supervisors were enquiring and interested and expected new knowledge to be applied and shared with others in the organization
Presence of deadlines	Intrinsic or extrinsic, negotiable or non-negotiable, urgent or nonurgent The presence of deadlines helped initiate and stimulate further activity levels and provided direction and focus for participants
Availability of support	Encouragement, physical resources (Internet, journals, computer, databases), financial assistance, and work concessions Support from managers, organizations, buddies, and peers

Adapted with permission from McCluskey, A. (2004). Increasing the use of research evidence by occupational therapists [Final report]. Penrith South, Australia: School of Exercise and Health Sciences, University of Western Sydney. Adapted with permission from Home, S. (2003). *Finding time to become an evidence-based practitioner.* [Unpublished undergraduate honours thesis]. Campbelltown, New South Wales: School of Exercise & Health Sciences, University of Western Sydney.

Finding Time for Evidence-Based Practice

This strategy involved *prioritizing* activities and *planning* ahead. Time was in short supply and was the major barrier to engaging in EBP for all participants, as indicated by the following quote:

> *There are always loads of additional projects that we're working on, meetings and supervision. So, definitely it is very difficult to find the time (OT9)*

In order to find time, *Competent Non-Experts* made research utilization a priority. They negotiated time and set time aside in and out of work hours for EBP-related activities. Conversely, *Novices* complained about lack of time and did not implement these strategies. A few *Novices* tried to set aside time but were not persistent in maintaining this commitment, partly because they and their organization did not place a high value on activities associated with EBP:

> *… if it doesn't get… a little old lady… back home, well then [it's not considered important] (OT6)*

> *We had talked about getting Internet access at work but the management felt that that would take away from time spent seeing clients so it was better [for the Internet] not to be there… [which] made it impossible to do any of the searching or the analysis within the work place (OT3)*

Searching, reading, and critical appraising were not necessarily considered essential parts of the day-to-day work of an occupational therapist by *Novices* or their organizations. Nor were these activities valued in comparison to "hands-on" clinical work. As a consequence, participants often felt guilty when they engaged in EBP-related activities at work:

> *…every month I… had to book over that time for clinical appointments to meet the caseload demands…so that was interesting in itself….rather then protecting that time and doing evidence-based work, I kept putting it off (OT4)*

Private practitioners were concerned about their "billable time" and the cost and time effectiveness of using evidence—particularly if they could not charge clients for their time. They prioritized billable work hours ahead of searching or appraising and completed EBP activities outside of work hours:

> *There was billable work to be done and income to be generated. I couldn't afford to say "Oh this 2 weeks of work time, I'll set aside"…so it was [done] on top of the [other] work (OT10)*

Several participants recognized that EBP *had* to become part of their routine work for it to be sustainable, with a certain number of hours being allocated per week or month:

> *We've got to change our cultures and job descriptions… to include the time… rather than it being something you can tack on when you've got a free moment (OT4).*

Planning ahead was how they managed. They scheduled time for EBP activities. Scheduling time in a diary acknowledged the importance of this work. *Competent Non-Experts* planned their workload by breaking work toward their CAT into smaller parts, so that the task did not seem so overwhelming. They were more likely than *Novices* to set time aside and stick to this commitment:

> *Seeing this whole project stretching out in front of me in its enormity (completion of the CAT), and wondering how I was ever going to find my way to the end… step goals …was the way I managed (OT7)*

> *I see it (the CAT assignment) as a giant iceberg and [I'm] just slowly chipping away at bits and pieces (OT3)*

Novices did set aside time, but often it was not enough or they failed to use the time efficiently: *I just ran out of time basically and I didn't go very far with it.* They also wasted more time on unproductive searching. Lack of success sometimes caused them to give up entirely.

In summary, *Finding Time for EBP* was difficult for all participants. Lack of time was the major barrier to adopting EBP. While *Novices* struggled to prioritize and plan, *Competent Non-Experts* managed their time by prioritizing EBP activities ahead of other work and scheduling time in advance in their diary. Thus, effective time management appeared to be an important and defining characteristic of an evidence-based practitioner.

Developing Skills and Knowledge

The second strategy used by participants on their journey to becoming evidence-based practitioners was developing their skills and knowledge. They managed this by *using evidence, teaching EBP to others*, and *seeking help* when faced with difficulties.

Using evidence involved the application of skills and knowledge acquired during the 2-day workshop (e.g., by searching for and appraising research on a regular basis). Lack of skills and knowledge was a barrier to using evidence for nine of the 10 participants. Completing critical appraisals and understanding statistics were tasks with which many struggled. However, *Competent Non-Experts* were able to engage in the first three stages of the EBP process at the time of interview and had overcome many difficulties by persisting, practicing, and seeking help. The following quote reflects one participant's recognition of the importance of using her newly acquired skills:

> *The penny started to drop—that with more practice [my skills and knowledge increased] (OT4)*

Five of the 10 participating occupational therapists were actively involved in journal clubs or similar research-focused activities at work, which required them to use their skills and knowledge often:

> *[We] started the new journal club about a year ago... everyone has a group that [they're] in. We meet once a month and pick a topic, and then everyone has a certain task to do in terms of doing the searches, or reading the articles or writing the summary (OT1)*

Competent Non-Experts were more likely than *Novices* or *Apprentices* to be involved in such activities. This involvement was partly due to organizational expectations and a habit of routinely questioning work practices. These participants were motivated to find and use evidence in order to provide the best practice to clients. Although half of the participants hoped to change their practice in some way based on research evidence, none were using published evidence routinely in clinical decision making.

Novices were more likely to maintain the status quo than *Competent Non-Experts*. *Novices* were caught in a cycle of being unable or unwilling to develop their skills because of barriers such as searching difficulties. They felt unable to overcome such deficits and tended to rely on old habits and experience:

> *People rely on their experience more than [they] rely on the research... there's not a great culture of trying to be very clinically objective. It's more about what we've learnt in the past... and putting that into practice than about continually searching for the best methods (OT8)*

Teaching EBP to others helped the *Competent Non-Experts* consolidate and practice their new skills, and develop confidence in their abilities: *it was good doing the in-service... you often learn something better and practice it more than if you're just reading it.* They were expected to educate others in their organization about EBP and about searching and appraisal: *it was very much pushed that we had the responsibility to educate [others].* However, *Novices* did not encounter the same expectations and were less likely to feel they had the skills to educate others.

The role of local opinion leader was one that *Competent Non-Experts* often adopted upon their return to work: *[I was] dobbed in [i.e., nominated] to be the evidence-based champion.* They provided in-services at work for other staff and established journal clubs.

The third way in which participants developed their skills and knowledge was by actively seeking help from others, in person or by phone and email. This help sometimes involved a demonstration of searching techniques from a buddy or mentor or obtaining expert advice about the interpretation of statistics. Librarians were a common source of help and support. Work could be delegated to a librarian in some organizations *to save a bit of time in the process... I develop the clinical question and mail it down to the librarian. She'll do the search for me and send up the result.*

A buddy was someone who worked with participants on their CAT assignment for the research project. A buddy helped maintain motivation, shared the work, and sometimes supplied journal articles:

> *I think the buddy system ...worked really well, with everyone being motivated ... to share out the jobs a little bit, bounce ideas off each other and motivate each other. To also remind each other when deadlines were coming up and that sort of thing. I thinks that's a great system and it helps you to network a little bit too (OT9)*

Three participants worked with a buddy. Those who did not—because of distance or lack of agreement on the CAT topic—appeared to feel more isolated than those with a buddy. However, participants learned to use other experts such as the project outreach support person who conducted support visits, answered email enquiries, and helped with searching over the telephone:

> *Just having M there—knowing that she was on the other end of the [telephone] and email... that was invaluable. I think lots of people probably found that... and the fact that she responded so quickly (OT2)*

In summary, *Competent Non-Experts* in this study developed skills and knowledge by using evidence more often than others, by *teaching EBP to others*, and by *seeking help* in times of difficulty.

Staying Focused

Staying focused was the third strategy used by participants. This strategy involved *making a commitment* to EBP, *being persistent* when barriers were encountered, and *being motivated* about EBP. This strategy involved changing work habits and maintaining these changes over time in spite of the many distractions:

> *...so easy to slip back... because it's just what you've always done, or your supervisor on your 4th year practicum told you so (OT1)*

Staying focused did not mean there was constant activity. The *Competent Non-Experts* who managed to stay focused worked in peaks and troughs; they had periods of continuous activity followed by periods of inactivity. However, despite periods of inactivity and barriers encountered along the way, they did not lose sight of their goals. The first step was *making a commitment.*

Making a commitment meant committing one's self to completing activities such as searching and appraisal because there was an expectation, personally or from the organization, that a summary of evidence would be completed within 8 months. *Making a commitment* also implied that using evidence was valued:

> *I suppose I had… this obligation, having been part of the project… You signed up, and you knew what you were in for. So we needed to finish it. But that was probably a self-imposed obligation, because all along, we were aware we could drop out (OT10)*

The attitude of *Novices* was positive at the end of the 2-day workshop but waned over time. Their commitment was more likely to waiver when barriers emerged, such as lack of time or limited success with searching:

> *just lack of commitment, I suppose, to put in the time when I didn't feel that I could do… a great deal in work time.*

Being persistent involved hard work and continuing with an activity despite failure or obstacles. It was easier for practitioners to persist if they were internally motivated, committed to using evidence, and had organizational support. The following quote provides an example of diminishing enthusiasm and motivation:

> *[I remember] frustration when my first search was unsuccessful …I remember mentioning this to [the project manager]. That was a big turn-off (OT8)*

Being motivated meant having the desire and drive to finish the summary of evidence. Many were motivated by a desire to stay up-to-date. All had been motivated initially to participate in the study and attend the 2-day workshop: *I did the 2-day workshop and came back very motivated and very keen … and did quite a lot of work into my question.* However, as time progressed and deadlines advanced, motivation diminished for most participants. Lack of motivation was characterized by long periods of inactivity and limited time spent searching or appraising evidence, and, therefore, limited time spent developing or practicing skills.

Competent Non-Experts reported being motivated to continue using evidence because of comments made by work colleagues, friends, and managers and by emails sent from the outreach support person. They were also motivated by meeting deadlines for the project, such as completing and then presenting their CAT to others at a 1-day conference. One *Competent Non-Expert* stayed focused because her manager showed great interest in the project and kept asking for email updates on her progress with the CAT. In summary, *Competent Non-Experts* stayed focused on becoming an evidence-based practitioner by *making a commitment*, *being persistent*, and *being motivated*.

Conditions That Helped Practitioners to Change

There were several factors or conditions that helped participants to change and adopt EBP, or conversely, that limited their progress and became barriers (see Table 3-4). These conditions were *readiness for change*, personal and organizational *expectations*, the *presence of deadlines*, and the *availability of support*. If these conditions were present and positive, participants were more likely to progress; if these conditions were absent or negative, progress was limited.

Readiness for Change

Readiness for change facilitated the process of using evidence and refers to participants who were ready to learn and use the skills for EBP. There were different types of readiness; participants could be "time ready," "intellectually ready," "resource ready," and/or "skill ready."

Comments were made by several participants who recognized that they were ready for change:

> *I was probably ready for the change… I was probably mentally ready and I think when you're mentally ready, then you're more likely to take on board new ideas (OT7)*

Competent Non-Experts displayed behaviors that were characteristic of being ready for change. These behaviors included searching and critically appraising evidence, teaching others the skills and knowledge they themselves had acquired, and finding time to use evidence. In contrast, *novices* displayed behaviors that suggested they were not yet ready to change. They had access to the same resources as other participants but did not use these resources to develop their skills and knowledge.

Personal and Organizational Expectations

The term *expectations* appeared frequently in the transcripts. Expectations could be large or small, short or long-term, single or multiple. The *Competent Non-Experts* worked in organizations in which the use of evidence was encouraged and expected. Such organizations had great expectations of individual therapists. *Competent Non-Experts* also had a personal expectation that they would complete the EBP assignment. Following is one such comment from a participant who received encouragement from a senior manager:

> *I didn't feel like I'd just been given a project [the CAT] and that no one was interested in it. I think the manager was very much driving it and was very interested individually in what people's projects were and what we were all up to … I probably think without that … it would have just fallen by the wayside because it's an awful lot of work to do… if you can't see it going back into the system somehow (OT7)*

In contrast, *Novices* typically worked in organizations that did not expect them to use their new knowledge to find, appraise, or teach others about evidence. The focus in such organizations was more on continuing to use experience to guide practice. *Novices* may have started their CAT with a personal expectation of completing the project. However, this intrinsic motivation waned once they returned to work and faced barriers such as lack of time or difficulty with search and appraisal activities.

Presence of Deadlines

The *presence of deadlines* was the third condition that helped participants in the study to become evidence-based practitioners. There were different types of deadlines. They could be intrinsic or extrinsic, negotiable or non-negotiable, urgent or nonurgent. Seven of the 10 participants indicated that having a deadline was one of the main factors that helped them to keep going

> *…it was the … due dates that actually made me complete [the CAT assignment]*

However, only four of the seven participants completed their CAT within the required timeframe. Meeting deadlines sometimes involved delegating part of a task to someone else or working outside of business hours.

Activities involving the use of evidence occurred mainly in bursts rather than consistently. Activity was stimulated by deadlines or by an outreach visit. Despite this mode of working, *Competent Non-Experts* were able to remain focused and complete their CAT. Participants indicated that they were motivated to stay on track because of organizational expectations as well as personal expectations. *Competent Non-Experts* persisted because they wanted to meet deadlines:

The deadline and I think I was sufficiently interested in the topic to find out [the answer to the clinical question] (OT3)

Novices were less likely to consistently meet deadlines. They appeared to lack persistence and did not have the same organizational expectations to complete their CAT as did other participants. Attitudes toward using evidence also played a role. The following comment highlights how the presence of deadlines alone was not a strong enough motivator for novices to engage in EBP:

While we had intentions of doing it [the CAT], when the time passed and you really weren't going to hit the target of getting something in for the workshop or to have it published... we felt "well there's no point now.. it's... past the barrier point" (OT5)

Availability of Support

The *availability of support* was the fourth influencing condition. The presence or absence of support affected participants' ability to become an evidence-based practitioner. There were different types of support available to participants: emotional encouragement, physical resources, and financial assistance. The level of support provided by managers and the organization varied considerably. *Competent Non-Experts* considered their managers and organizations to be supportive of EBP activities. They appeared to receive high levels of support, as reflected by the following quote:

The senior OT ... was just really supportive and ... open to me going to the workshop. She advocated on my behalf for me to get Internet access. Because I didn't automatically have that and it was a cost.... And ... all the way along, like toward the end when I needed to put time aside at work to finish off the summary, she was really open to giving me that time (OT2)

Competent Non-Experts indicated that they were encouraged, even expected, to search for and critically appraise research articles. These occupational therapists were actively involved in journal clubs or other similar activities in their workplace:

Our organization was very motivated and research focused. That certainly helps to drive people along (OT9)

Other participants felt guilty about engaging in these types of activity because they did not receive encouragement and support, as reflected by the following quote:

... If you're trying to read a journal article, you have to have a report that you're writing to slip over the top so that if anyone comes in and sees you, you can pretend you're doing that [writing the report]. Because it's ... frowned upon, to be doing that sort of thing [in work time] (OT1)

Some participants felt their managers were unhelpful in providing concessions for them to complete their CAT in addition to other workload responsibilities:

It was a contract written in blood...it had that feeling. There was a great deal of reluctance initially from our manager who didn't quite understand the importance ... Which surprised me ... "I'll give you the time but only grudgingly" or "I'll be watching." [Which] I think probably made [me] ... a bit reluctant to get in initially and take the time (OT4)

The level of support available to participants seemed to play an important role in helping the *Competent Non-Experts* move further along the continuum to being evidence-based practitioners. Lack of support appeared to limit progress.

Access to physical resources helped participants engage in EBP. Physical resources included access to the Internet, databases, and journals. All participants in the study had access to databases; however, some had limited access because their computer was shared with other staff. Limited access meant that participants were restricted as to when they could conduct a search. Several participants had only gained access to the Internet at work after attending the workshop.

Having access to resources facilitated the process of using evidence. Private practitioners used other people to obtain access to resources such as databases and journal articles. Several practitioners commented that while direct access to resources was not essential, having easy access made the task of becoming an evidence-based practitioner less of a challenge. Those participants who had shared or limited access to resources either delayed commencing the database searching or alternately tried to complete these activities or nonwork time.

In summary, the presence of certain conditions helped participants to engage in EBP. These conditions were *readiness for change,* which involved being ready to change habits and allocate time to search and appraisal activities; *personal and organizational expectations,* which helped participants stay motivated and continue; the *presence of deadlines,* which provided direction and focus for participants; and the *availability of support,* which enabled participants to actually engage in evidence-based activities in their workplace. All participants had at least one of these conditions present. *Competent Non-Experts* typically had at least three if not all of these conditions present.

Conclusion

This chapter has described the journey that occupational therapists took when endeavoring to become an evidence-based practitioner. A typology of practitioners and theory of change have been proposed outlining the characteristics, strategies, and conditions necessary for engagement with EBP. The proposed typology refers to *Novices, Apprentices,* and *Competent Non-Experts* according to their skills, knowledge, behavior, and attitudes. These three types of practitioner exist along a continuum from those who operated more as experience-based practitioners (the *Novices*) to those who were trying to be more evidence based in the way they thought, taught, and practiced (the *Competent Non-Experts*).

Several strategies were used more often and more consistently by the *Competent Non-Experts.* They found time for EBP activities in their busy schedule. They actively worked on developing their skills. They stayed focused over the 18-month period on small projects, answering clinical questions using published research.

Several factors helped these occupational therapists to change and adopt the principles of EBP. Being ready to change was helpful. Holding personal expectations that their skills and knowledge would be used and valued in their organization was a distinct advantage. Working in a department in which searching and reading research was encouraged and expected was helpful, as was a manager who showed support in practical ways. Having deadlines was also beneficial. Lastly, resources such as access to the Internet, electronic databases, and so forth facilitated EBP. Again, managers were important allies in the process of becoming an evidence-based practitioner.

This chapter will conclude with a discussion of key findings and implications for practice, education, and research.

MOVING BEYOND BARRIERS

In previous literature, commonly reported barriers to the adoption of EBP have included lack of time and limited search and appraisal skills (Curtin & Jaramazovic, 2001; McCluskey, 2003; Pollock, Legg, Langhorne, & Sellars, 2000). These barriers are consistent across countries and disciplines (Jette et al., 2003; Metcalfe et al., 2001). There is little need to continue exploring the topic, at least in developed countries. Our task now is to help practitioners address some of these barriers.

In our study, the more optimistic and progressive practitioners spoke very little about barriers. They no longer complained about why they could not look for or read research. Instead, they were actively addressing barriers, particularly lack of time and skills. They described strategies that helped them to find and manage time and prioritize EBP into their work. Educators and managers may wish to share these findings with practitioners. Articles that discuss how to identify and target local barriers may also be useful for discussion at staff meetings (e.g., McCluskey & Cusick, 2002; National Institute of Clinical Studies, 2006). Further research is also needed to confirm whether these attitudinal differences are consistent across health practitioners and in other settings and countries.

IMPROVING CRITICAL APPRAISAL SKILLS

As already noted, difficulty with critical appraisal has been identified as a barrier to EBP (Bennett et al., 2003; McCluskey, 2003). Findings from our study suggest that practitioners need to spend many hours learning and practicing the art of critical appraisal. A 1-day workshop is just the beginning and likely to serve as an introduction only for most practitioners. Journal clubs are a way of improving appraisal skills over a longer period of time. Reading randomized controlled trials and systematic reviews regularly probably helps practitioners to become more efficient at reading methods-and-results sections of published papers. Advanced workshops or master classes on appraisal where challenging studies and Cochrane reviews are discussed in detail may also be beneficial and popular. A similar process is also most likely to be needed for improving understanding of qualitative research methods.

While education in critical appraisal does appear to improve knowledge (Taylor et al., 2000), there are few randomized controlled trials that rigorously evaluate the effectiveness of practitioner education, and almost none involve allied health professionals. One British study that did include allied health professionals delivered a half-day workshop on critical appraisal to a self-selected sample (n = 145) of practitioners, managers, and administrators (Taylor, Reeves, Ewings, & Taylor, 2004). These researchers found that knowledge of appraisal did improve after a half-day workshop (on critical appraisal) but questioned whether a mean difference at follow-up of 2.6 points (95% CI 0.6 to 4.6) was worthwhile, on a Likert scale from –18 to +18, given the cost of the workshop (£250).

As noted earlier in this chapter, knowledge of research methods and critical appraisal did improve in our study involving occupational therapists (McCluskey & Lovarini, 2005). However, analysis of participants' daily diaries revealed that most (60%) were not reading any research articles in an 8-week period and only a small proportion (18%) engaged in critical appraisal. Thus, there are two challenges for educators: helping those who want to learn about critical appraisal to improve their skills and increasing the frequency of reading and appraisal.

THE PROCESS OF CHANGE WAS SLOW

Participants were generally slow to develop the skills and knowledge necessary for EBP. They had 8 months to complete the first three stages of EBP, from writing a structured clinical question to searching databases and completing a critical appraisal. Several participants used most of this time to develop a clinical question and carry out searching activities. Six of the 10 participants completed their CAT after 8 months, but most still had difficulty interpreting statistics. After 18 months, only two participants were actively using research findings to inform policy, local guidelines, and client information sheets. The uptake of EBP and skill development appears to be a slow process. This fact has been acknowledged by other authors (e.g., Forsetlund et al., 2003). As educators, we can alert practitioners to the fact that changes in skill, knowledge, and behavior will be slow, and gains might best be measured in years not weeks or months. Researchers also need to conduct longitudinal studies and plan for extended follow-up periods.

GREATER FOCUS NEEDED ON IMPLEMENTATION

This study highlights a need to focus more on behavior change and help practitioners to implement best evidence using education, case file audits, feedback, and reminders (Grimshaw, Eccles, & Tetroe, 2006; Hysong, Best, & Pugh, 2006; Jamtvedt, Young, Kristoffersen, Thomson O'Brien, & Oxman, 2003). Implementation research is a relatively new form of research in which the focus is on practitioner behavior rather than client outcomes.

One example of implementation research has recently been reported in the occupational therapy literature (Hammond, Jeffreson, Jones, Gallagher, & Jones, 2002; Hammond & Klompenhouwer, 2005). The researcher, Allison Hammond, trained practitioners in rheumatology to deliver an evidence-based joint protection education program. She then investigated whether these practitioners had changed the joint protection education provided to clients. A postal survey was used to evaluate effectiveness. Of the 48 respondents, 45 had changed the education provided to clients. Of the 48, 13 had implemented the evidence-based group program, 25 were still contemplating using the program, and 10 were not. Barriers to change included limited staffing, difficulty accessing appropriate facilities, lack of time to make practice changes, and the cost and time required to deliver the program. The implementers felt that supportive managers and teams helped to overcome these problems.

The perception that supportive managers and teams helped practitioners to implement change is consistent with our study findings. The implementers and champions of EBP in our study—the *Competent Non-Experts*—worked in supportive organizations with encouraging managers. These managers valued time spent on research utilization, helped participants to obtain resources such as Internet access, and generally helped drive change.

TEACHING HELPED TO CONSOLIDATE SKILLS

Teaching EBP to others helped participants to advance their skills and knowledge. Teaching others can facilitate self-learning and is recognized as an effective way of improving performance. Teaching students was recently proposed as a strategy for promoting use of research evidence (Craik & Rappolt, 2003). These researchers found that when experienced occupational therapists taught students in clinical practice or on campus, this teaching role consolidated their skills and knowledge: "Participants reported that students acted as catalysts for their own learning by modeling skills for research retrieval and critical analysis, presenting opportunities for the discussion of the research, and its application to practice" (p. 271).

Yet in the current study, few participants, other than the three *Competent Non-Experts* engaged in teaching others. Perhaps there needs to be an expectation or commitment from health professionals who are learning about EBP that they will teach others what they have learned, as well as seeking help from others when they return to work.

There are many Internet resources and educational Web sites available for those engaged in teaching. These sites include the following:

- Centre for Evidence-Based Medicine (Canada)
  www.cebm.utoronto.ca

- OTseeker (Occupational Therapy Systematic Evaluation of Evidence)
  www.otseeker.com

- The Critical Appraisal Skills Program (CASP)
  www.phru.org.uk/~casp/casp.htm

- The Centre for Evidence-Based Medicine (UK)
  www.cebm.net/index.asp

- The Centre for Evidence-Based Practice (CEBP) (Australia)
  www.cebm.net

Many of these Web sites contain presentations and tutorials that can be downloaded for teaching purposes.

FUTURE RESEARCH

The current study involved a small sample of participants. Confirmation of the categories and typology should be sought with other groups of occupational therapists and health disciplines. For example, does this theory adequately explain how physiotherapists and speech pathologists experience the change process and how practitioners in developing countries learn about and adopt EBP? And what are the similarities and differences in the experiences of new graduates versus those of more experienced practitioners? Longitudinal studies are also required that collect quantitative data (measures of knowledge and skill, frequency of searching and appraisal) as well as qualitative data about the process of change. More implementation research is required so that clients ultimately benefit from the process.

CONCLUSION

In this chapter, we presented findings from a qualitative study involving occupational therapists. Becoming an evidence-based practitioner involved readiness for change, the ability to prioritize time, set deadlines and use research, a willingness to practice new skills and teach others what had been learned, and persistence. Managers who valued research in addition to experience, and who encouraged staff to spend time on EBP facilitated the change process. We look forward to reading more about the experiences of practitioners and managers who are embarking on this journey together.

TAKE-HOME MESSAGES

Practitioners who wish to pursue EBP should aim to do the following:

✔ Record the number and type of clinical questions that will be answered in a 12-month period.

✔ Set deadlines and discuss these with peers and managers.

✔ Teach colleagues how to search for and appraise research.

✔ Practice searching for and appraising research.

✔ Avoid complaining about lack of time.

✔ Persist, practice, and expect skill development to be slow but steady.

✔ Move beyond searching and appraisal activities and consider how evidence can be incorporated into practice.

Managers who wish to develop a culture of EBP should aim to:

✔ Encourage staff who show an interest by asking about progress with projects and inviting them to teach other staff what they know.

✔ Value time spent by staff seeking, reading, and discussing research.

✔ Show support by attending education sessions and journal clubs.

✔ Lobby for important resources such as Internet access, databases, and a reasonable number of fast, readily available computers for staff.

Acknowledgement

This research was funded by a project grant from the Motor Accidents Authority of New South Wales, Australia.

LEARNING AND EXPLORATION ACTIVITIES

Exercise 1: Values Clarification

This exercise is based on the contention that human behavior is shaped by the beliefs and values held by the individual. Thus behaviors taken as therapists are shaped by their own beliefs and values. We are, however, often unaware of these values and, therefore, unable to analyze their influence on our practice. Many fields of endeavor, from business practices to personal relationships, recommend exercises to allow for clarification of one's personal values (Levoy, 1997; Pfeiffer & Jones, 1973; Senge, Roberts, Ross, Smith, & Kleiner, 1994). This exercise, adapted from several works, should be done alone and can help you to uncover your own values and begin to analyze their impact on your work with clients. The process of doing this will inform how you view EBP.

From the following list of values (both work and personal), select the 15 that are most important to you. Feel free to add important values that are missing from the list in the spaces at the end.

Step 1: Make a list of your most strongly held values—choose 15

___advancement	___change and variety	___competition
___power	___fame	___pleasure
___challenges	___excellence in practice	___helping myself
___collaborating with others	___the affections of others	___wisdom
___peace of mind	___professional growth	___decisiveness
___community recognition	___supervising others	___self-respect
___meaningful work	___stability and predictability	___excitement
___new learning	___physical activity	___freedom
___being sure of myself	___family connections and time	___integrity

___achievement	___economic security	___the gratitude of others
___friendship	___efficiency	___personal growth
___leadership	___thought-provoking work	___cooperation
___helping others	___improving society	___responsibility
___loyalty	___honesty	___privacy
___financial gain	___independence	___creativity
___ethical practice	___knowledge acquisition	___cooperation
___security	___working alone	___sophistication

Step 2: Reduce the list

Now that you have identified 15 values, imagine that you can only have 5. Which 10 would you give up? What are you left with? Now try to reduce your list to only 3.

Step 3: Analysis

Take a look at the three values remaining on your list. Consider the four following questions and write a paragraph relating to each to capture your reaction. What do you think these values say about you as a person? What do they tell you about you as a therapist? What picture develops regarding what kind of work you value most? Are your values congruent with those of your supervisor, manager, and/or organization?

Exercise 2: Letter to a Learning Partner

This exercise is best applied by students during their fieldwork experiences or by novice therapists. You will need a partner to work with on this exercise. It will be important to choose someone with whom you feel comfortable and trust so that you can have open dialogue and share your ideas without fear or criticism. This dialogue will span an expanded period of time, so choose your learning partner accordingly.

Over the course of a few weeks, you are going to write several letters to your partner. Ideally, your partner will do the same, thus using you to help him or her reflect on practice. The letters are written about your reactions to *significant experiences* during your clinical encounters. They will be snapshots of your reactions at one point in time. At each interval, you will describe what occurred, how you felt about the experience, and what conclusions you drew at that moment. At the end of the overall time period, you will be guided through your own analysis of the letters as a group.

Before starting, you and your partner must decide whether both of you are participating and how long you are contracting to work together. It may be for 1 week, the course of the clinical practice, or for all practice at preset intervals. You may also set some rules for feedback that will be followed, perhaps regarding the need for a balance for frankness and respectfulness of communication style.

Definition of *significant experience*: A significant experience is one that has emotional impact. You may recognize that it has occurred because it makes you stop and think, makes your heart skip a beat, rocks your sense of rightness or confidence, makes you blush, or makes your stomach lurch. Whatever your reaction, if it makes you take notice. Such experiences are often called "aha" moments.

Step 1: Writing the letters

Right after a significant experience occurs, jot it down. If possible, immediately take 10 minutes to write your letter. If you cannot do it right away, use your jotting to jog your memory at some later time. Do not take any longer than that, as the exercise is intended to capture your immediate reaction. Try to choose different types of experiences to write about over the course of the contracted time.

Format for Each Letter:

Dear_____,

Write a few sentences to describe briefly what happened using action language.
To get started, complete the following sentences:
"I felt....................."
"I have felt this way before when..............."
"From this experience, I think the following is true................."

Complete your letter quickly, put it away, and repeat the exercise at least five or six times over the course of a few weeks or longer, depending on the terms of your contract with your partner. The analysis can occur once you have collected at least five letters.

Step 2: Analysis

This step is done in conjunction with your learning partner. Each partner does this step separately, then compares each other's reaction to the same set of letters. Read over one person's collection of letters. Is there anything that jumps out at you? Are there insights there that surprise you? What do you think these tell you about the person? What values seem to emerge? How was evidence used, if at all? In the experiences described, were any values shaken or reinforced? What does it seem that he or she believes about effective practice? Were there any particular situations in which the person seemed to feel most comfortable? Are there types of clients where he or she seemed to feel most skilled? Do you see any patterns? How do your conclusions hold up with the passage of time?

As the writer, consider these questions: How do you react to the feedback from your partner? Do you agree or disagree with his or her conclusions? Were there things that you felt were true at the time that you now question? What has happened in the interim to change your thinking? Have your perspectives broadened or narrowed? When do you feel most vulnerable? When do you feel most capable? What does this tell you about factors that shape your practice as a therapist?

Sources: Hunt, 1988; Rochon, 1994; Wilkins, Pollock, Rochon & Law, 2001.

Exercise 3: Video Case Analysis

Step 1: One therapist/student therapist will be the subject of the video. That person, chooses a client and seeks his/her consent to participate in a videotaped case analysis. Prior to taping the client, the therapist answers some questions on the videotape, either alone or through an interview conducted by a colleague.

On the tape, briefly describe the client who will be taped, then answer these questions:

What are the client's current goals for therapy?

What are the immediate goals for this session?

What assumptions have you made about the client?

What theoretical approach or practice model are you using?

What hypotheses do you have about the client?

What do you expect to happen in the therapy session and why?

Step 2: Videotape the therapy session with the client.

Step 3: Show the tape to your colleagues and discuss what happened, how it relates to your prior assumptions, how it differed from your expectations and why. Draw some conclusions and summarize your insights. How will this impact your next encounter with this client? What general insights can you take to all of your client encounters?

Exercise 4: Experiential/Evidence-Based Practice

This chapter discusses two broad categories of practitioners: those who have a more experience based approach to their practice, and those who have a more evidence-based approach. Reflect on your own stage of learning or practice: are you more evidence-based or experience based? What do you think are the key characteristics of each?

With a partner, read the scenario below:

> *Ms. Smith is a 75-year-old woman who has just had a right above knee amputation as a result of a motor vehicle accident. Prior to the accident, Ms. Smith used a cane for ambulation due to instability and pain in her feet. She lives alone in an apartment, and has had her driver's license removed due to deteriorating vision. Ms. Smith is currently undergoing rehabilitation at the local hospital, and expects to return home. She is currently using a wheelchair for mobility and a decision has not yet been made about her prosthetic limb. You are a clinician on the rehab team who will make recommendations as to Ms. Smith's future mobility options.*

Decide between you and your partner who will discuss the scenario from each approach. How do you feel an experience based clinician might approach this scenario? How might this differ from an evidence-based clinician? Are there times where both approaches may be valuable?

Exercise 5: SWOT Analysis

In addition to identifying values, it can be helpful to consider the strengths and weaknesses within your organization, as well as opportunities and threats associated with the introduction of EBP. List examples for each of the SWOT categories that relate to your organization. Perhaps you can conduct this exercise as a group (e.g., during a staff meeting). Discuss ways in which opportunities (e.g., employment of a new graduate with knowledge of EBP or a keen librarian) can be used to overcome lack of skills and knowledge within an organization (a potential weakness).

Reference

McCluskey, A., & Cusick, A. (2002). Strategies for introducing EBP and changing clinician behavior: A manager's toolbox. *Australian Occupational Therapy Journal, 49*(2), 63-70.

REFERENCES

Bennett, S., Tooth, L., McKenna, K., Rodger, S., Strong, J., Mickan, S., et al. (2003). Perceptions of EBP: A survey of Australian occupational therapists. *Australian Occupational Therapy Journal, 50*, 13-22.

Craik, J., & Rappolt, S. (2003). Theory of research utilization enhancement: A model for occupational therapy. *Canadian Journal of Occupational Therapy, 70*, 266-275.

Curtin, M., & Jaramazovic, E. (2001). Occupational therapists' views and perceptions of EBP. *British Journal of Occupational Therapy, 64*(5), 214-222.

Fagerhaugh, S. (1986). Analyzing data for basic social processes. In W. Chenitz & J. Swanson (Eds.), *From practice to grounded theory: Qualitative research in nursing* (pp. 133-145). Menlo Park, CA: Addison-Wesley.

Forsetlund, L., Bradley, P., Forsen, L., Nordheim, L., Jamtvedt, G., & Bjorndal, A. (2003). Randomised controlled trial of a theoretically grounded tailored intervention to diffuse evidence-based public health practice. *BMC Medical Education, 3*, 2.

Glaser, B. G. (Ed.). (1996). *Gerund grounded theory: The basic social process dissertation*. Mill Valley, CA: Sociology Press.

Glaser, B. G., & Strauss, A. (1967). *Discovery of grounded theory*. Chicago, IL: Aldine.

Grimshaw, J., Eccles, M. P., & Tetroe, J. (2006). Implementing clinical guidelines: Current evidence and future implications. *Journal of Continuing Education in the Health Professions, 24* (Suppl. 1), S31-S37.

Hammond, A., Jeffreson, P., Jones, N., Gallagher, J., & Jones, T. (2002). Clinical applicability of an educational-behavioural joint protection program for people with rheumatoid arthritis. *British Journal of Occupational Therapy, 65*(9), 405-412.

Hammond, A., & Klompenhouwer, P. (2005). Getting evidence into practice: Implementing a behavioural joint protection education program for people with rheumatoid arthritis. *British Journal of Occupational Therapy, 68*(1), 25-33.

Hunt, D. E. (1988). *Beginning with ourselves: In practice, theory and human affairs.* Cambridge, MA: Brookline Books.

Hysong, S. J., Best, R. G., & Pugh, J. A. (2006). Audit and feedback and clinical practice guideline adherence: Making feedback actionable. *Implementation Science, 1*, 9.

Jamtvedt, G., Young, J.M., Kristoffersen, D.T., Thomson O'Brien, M.A., & Oxman, A.D. (2003). Audit and feedback: Effects on professional practice and health care outcomes. *The Cochrane Database of Systematic Reviews*, Issue 3.

Jette, D. U., Bacon, K., Batty, C., Carlson, M., Ferland, A., Hemingway, R. D., et al. (2003). EBP: Beliefs, attitudes, knowledge, and behaviours of physical therapists. *Physical Therapy, 83*(9), 786-805.

Levoy, G. (1997). *Callings: Finding and following an authentic life.* New York: Three Rivers Press.

McCluskey, A. (2003). Occupational therapists report a low level of knowledge, skill and involvement in EBP. *Australian Occupational Therapy Journal, 50*, 3-12.

McCluskey, A. (2004). *Increasing the use of research evidence by occupational therapists.* Final Research Report; Penrith South, Sydney; University of Western Sydney.

McCluskey, A., & Cusick, A. (2002). Strategies for introducing EBP and changing clinicians' behavior: A manager's toolbox. *Australian Occupational Therapy Journal, 49*(2), 63-70.

McCluskey, A., & Lovarini, M. (2005). Providing education on EBP improved knowledge but did not change behavior: A before and after study. *BMC Medical Education, 5*, 40.

Metcalfe, C., Lewin, R., Wisher, S., Perry, S., Bannigan, K., & Moffett, J. (2001). Barriers to implementing the evidence base in four NHS therapies. *Physiotherapy, 87*(8), 433-441.

National Institute of Clinical Studies. (2006). *Identifying barriers to evidence uptake.* Melbourne, Australia: Author.

Pfeiffer, J. W., & Jones, J. (1973). *A handbook of structured experiences for human relations training.* La Jolla, CA: University Associates.

Pollock, A. S., Legg, L., Langhorne, P., & Sellars, C. (2000). Barriers to achieving evidence-based stroke rehabilitation. *Clinical Rehabilitation, 14*, 611-617.

Rochon, S. (1994). Theory from practice: A reflective curriculum for occupational therapists. Unpublished master's thesis, McMaster University, Hamilton, Ontario, Canada.

Schreiber, R. S. (2001). The "how to" of grounded theory: Avoiding the pitfalls. In R. Schreiber & P. Stern (Eds.), *Using grounded theory in nursing* (pp. 55-83). New York, NY: Springer.

Senge, P.M., Roberts, C., Ross, R., Smith, B., & Kleiner, A. (1994). *The fifth disciplne fieldbook.* New York: Doubleday.

Strauss, A. L., & Corbin, J. (1998). *Basics of qualitative research: Techniques and procedures for developing grounded theory* (2nd ed.). Thousand Oaks, CA: Sage.

Taylor, R., Reeves, B., Ewings, P., Binns, S., Keast, J., & Mears, R. (2000). A systematic review of the effectiveness of critical appraisal skills training for clinicians. *Medical Education, 34*, 120-125.

Taylor, R., Reeves, B., Ewings, P., & Taylor, R. (2004). Critical appraisal skills training for health care professionals: A randomized controlled trial. *BMC Medical Education, 4*(30), 1-10.

Wilkins, S., Pollock, N., Rochon, S., & Law, M. (2001). Implementing client-centred practice: Why is it so difficult to do? *Canadian Journal of Occupational Therapy, 68*(2), 70-79.

SECTION II:
FINDING THE EVIDENCE

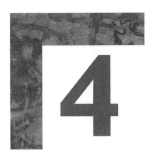

Incorporating Outcomes Measures Into Evidence-Based Practice

Joy MacDermid, PT, PhD and Susan Michlovitz, PT, PhD, CHT

LEARNING OBJECTIVES

After reading this chapter, the student/practitioner will be able to:

- Describe how and why outcome measures are utilized in evidence-based practice (EBP).
- Relate outcome measurement to conceptual models of health.
- Differentiate between health and quality of life (QOL).
- Differentiate different types of outcome measures for clinical practice.
- Use available resources to find appropriate outcome measures.
- Use a critical appraisal process to select appropriate measures or tests for outcome evaluations.
- Use outcomes data to evaluate the impact of EBP on individual patients or rehabilitation programs.
- Identify barriers to implementing outcome measures in practice and recognize potential solutions and opportunities.

The purpose of this chapter is to provide the practitioner with the foundations for selecting and using evidence-based outcome measures as a means of evaluating the impact of evidence-based clinical decisions.

OUTCOME MEASURES ARE NEEDED IN EVIDENCE-BASED PRACTICE

If EBP has value, it must be measurable in terms of better outcomes for patients. Surprisingly, few studies address whether an EBP approach actually improves outcomes for groups of patients when compared to traditional practice. However, results from these limited number of studies suggest that improved patient outcomes are possible with an EBP approach (Bedard, Purden, Sauve-Larose, Certosini, & Schein, 2006). Clinicians using EBP principles are interested in evaluating the impact of their decisions both for individual patients as well as for rehabilitation programs provided to groups of patients. An effective strategy for implementing the tenets of EPB should be based on selecting outcome measures that are valid and reliable, as well as relevant to patient values and goals. The measures should have the following attributes:

- Easy to apply, provide minimal inconvenience or discomfort for the patients
- Sensitive to detecting changes induced by the rehabilitation program
- Useful for guiding clinical practice at the individual level
- Help establish diagnosis, prognosis, and the extent to which health or participation outcomes were achieved
- Useful in goal setting
- Useful at the group level for assessing the impact of programmatic changes on how care is delivered

No single measure can fulfill these multiple and often competing purposes. However, a spectrum of tools is available with varying ability to support these elements of practice. Practice that is evidence-based is by definition reflective, as it incorporates formal evaluation of the impact of your decision making. Further benefits of incorporating formal evaluation as a routine part of clinical practice are that it will demonstrate the value of the service to other health care stakeholders or payers and will institute an ongoing renewal process that supports the scientific foundation of the discipline.

Not only is outcome evaluation critical to EBP, it is also mandated by the challenges of our health care systems. Needs of an aging population with expectations of optimal health provide huge expansionary pressures on health care systems. Rapid improvements in technology and specialty services increase these pressures. The economy cannot support unchecked expansion, and it is inevitable that there will be an ever-increasing need to prove to payers and administrators that health care dollars are being allocated to "worthy" services. Practitioners who have an integrated evidence-based approach that includes outcome evaluation into their clinical practice will be prepared to justify their services.

CONCEPTUAL MODELS OF HEALTH PROVIDE A FRAMEWORK FOR SELECTING OUTCOME MEASURES

The biomedical model defines health as the absence of disease. It assumes that diseases lead to defects, which result in reduced health. Historically, the biomedical model has significantly influenced rehabilitation and its approach to outcome measurement. While there is inherent value in this model, it implies that accurate diagnosis and identification of the biological defects will allow clinicians to select the intervention that best restores integrity to the structure or system and thereby maximize health. In this biomedical framework, it is important to focus measurement on structural or system integrity to evaluate the success of an intervention. The influence of this model on rehabilitation practice is seen in areas that are highly reliant on measures of impairment.

As we evolve into other models, the importance of this model should not be minimized. The biomedical model has led to scientific advancements in recognizing pathology, defining physical impairment, and ameliorating physical abnormalities. It has challenged rehabilitation practitioners to adopt more accurate measures of impairment. However, rehabilitation practice focuses on more than just impairments. Rather, rehabilitation focuses on maximizing functional movement, activity, and communication as a means of restoring meaningful participation. Despite the holistic philosophical orientation, many rehabilitation practitioners continue to rely on the medical model when it comes to evaluating outcomes by focusing on impairment measures to evaluate their treatment programs. The benefits of rehabilitation may be under appreciated when outcome assessments focus only on impairments. Furthermore, the medical model is less well suited to chronic or episodic health care problems, which comprise the majority of rehabilitation practice. The lack of fit is further exacerbated when the biological basis for the disorders is inadequately understood (such as impaired mental health or chronic pain).

HEALTH VERSUS QUALITY-OF-LIFE

Terms like health, QOL, and health-related QOL (HRQOL) are often used interchangeably without considering differences in meaning among these terms. A systematic review (Post, de Witte, & Schrijvers, 1999) on this topic discussed three applications of the quality-of-life concept in the literature: as health, as well-being, or as a superordinate construct that encompasses both. These authors found that the concept of QOL has been used as synonymous with a variety of terms: "health status, physical functioning, perceived health status, subjective health, health perceptions, symptoms, need satisfaction, individual cognition, functional disability, psychiatric disturbance, well-being and often, several of these at the same time." While there are no standard definitions for all of these terms, rehabilitation practitioners usually do not view these terms as interchangeable.

QOL refers to the broad context concerned with a person's overall satisfaction with respect to the aspects of his or her life that he or she considers to be important. HRQOL is concerned with QOL in the context of a given health status affecting that person. This may explain why health status measures such as the SF-36 are sometimes referred to as quality-of-life measures.

Some of the leading health organizations have put forth definitions for QOL and/or HRQOL:

- The Centre for Disease Control defines HRQOL as "a person or group's perceived physical and mental health over time" (Centers for Disease Control and Prevention, n.d.).

- The National Institutes of Health (NIH) define QOL as "the overall enjoyment of life" (National Cancer Institute, n.d.).

- The World Health Organization (WHO) defines it as "an individual's perception of their position in life in the context of the culture and value systems in which they live and in relation to their goals, expectations, standards and concerns" (www.who.int/evidence/assessment-instruments/qol/ql1.htm).

- The QOL research unit at the Center for Health Promotion, University of Toronto has defined QOL as "the degree to which the person enjoys the important possibilities of his or her life," and has a number of domains that fall under "being, becoming and belonging" (Raeburn & Rotman, 1996) (Figure 4-1).

The WHO considers QOL to be subjective and they do not feel that it can be "simply equated with the terms health status, life style, life satisfaction, mental state, or well-being. Rather, it is a multidimensional concept incorporating the individual's perception of these and other aspects of life" (www.who.int/evidence/assessment-instruments/qol/ql1.htm). They have developed a quality-of-life measure (WHOQOL-100 and a shorter version) (Ackerman, Graves, Bennell, & Osborne, 2006; Anderson, Aaronson, Bullinger, & McBee, 1993, 1996; Cieza & Stucki, 2005; Hanestad, Rustoen, Knudsen, Jr., Lerdal, & Wahl, 2004; Huang, Wu, & Frangakis, 2006; Hwang & Wang, 2004; Jang, Hsieh, Wang, & Wu, 2004; Li, Young, Xiao, Zhou, & Zhou, 2004; Lin, 2006;

Figure 4-1. Health as a component of quality of life. (Reprinted with permission from Raeburn, J. M., & Rotman, I. (1996). Quality of life and health promotion. In R. B. I. Renwick, & M. Nagler (Eds.), *Quality of life in health promotion and rehabilitation: Conceptual approaches, issues and applications* (pp. 14-25). London: Sage publications. This work is protected by copyright and it is being used with the permission of Access Copyright. Any alteration of its content or further copying in any form whatsoever is strictly prohibited.)

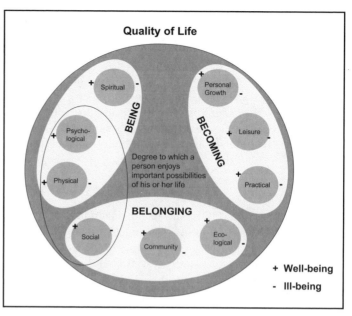

Naumann & Byrne, 2004; Norholm & Bech, 2001; Ohaeri, Olusina, & Al Abassi, 2004; Power, Harper, & Bullinger, 1999; Power, Quinn, & Schmidt, 2005; Skevington, 1999; Skevington, Bradshaw, & Saxena, 1999; Skevington, Lotfy, & O'Connell, 2004; Skevington & O'Connell, 2004; Trompenaars, Masthoff, Van Heck, Hodiamont, & De Vries, 2005; Williams, 2000; Yao & Wu, 2005; that includes the following domains: physical capacity, psychological, social relationships, environment, independence, and spirituality. The WHO has not defined HRQOL as such; however, their definition of health ("a state of complete physical, mental and social well-being and not merely the absence of disease and infirmity") is used by many researchers to define HRQOL and measures of HRQOL tend to focus on physical, mental, and social domains (Jette, 1999).

Figure 4-1 illustrates how health contributes to the larger concept of QOL as described by John Raeburn and Irving Rootman (Raeburn & Rootman, 1996). Whereas "being, becoming, and belonging" are domains of QOL; physical, psychological, and social components are domains of health. These domains of health are also consistent with the domains of health as recently defined by PROMIS (see below). As rehabilitation is a health discipline that is primarily directed at facilitating our broad view of health, then conceptual frameworks of health are important foundations for outcome assessment.

HEALTH MODELS

International Classification of Functioning Model

The WHO introduced a classification system in 2001 for understanding functioning and disability: the International Classification of Functioning (ICF) Model (2003b) (Figure 4-2). This model portrays the relationships among impairments, activities, and participation nested in the environmental context. This model is an important framework because emphasis is placed on the influence of personal and environmental factors on the three dimensions of body functions and structures, activities, and participation. Whereas the biomedical model suggests

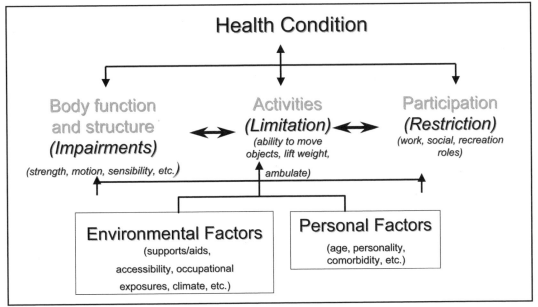

Figure 4-2. Interaction of concepts. (ICF, 2001.)

relationships are linear so that disability results from impairments, the ICF model recognizes that interrelationships are interlinked. Impairments can cause activity limitations (e.g., reduced ability to walk, communicate, or perform self-care). Conversely, activity can also cause impairment (e.g., repetitive work or sports participation can lead to injury). The ICF also frames functioning and disability in more positive terminology rather than older and more negative terms like disability and handicap.

The ICF model was devised as a classification, not as a system for measuring outcomes. However, it is increasingly being used as a conceptual framework to assist practitioners and researchers to establish relevant goals and observable outcome measures (Barbier, Penta, & Thonnard, 2003; Salter et al., 2005; Salter, Jutai, Teasell, Foley, & Bitensky, 2005; Schasfoort, Bussmann, & Stam, 2000; Stucki et al., 2004; Weigl et al., 2003). Some interventions are designed to change impairments and the direct impacts of these interventions are indicated by outcome measures that focus on the body function (impairment) level (e.g., improving range of motion, reducing tone). In addition, the practitioner may also want to know that changing this impairment will directly or indirectly influence performance at the activity or at the participation level (e.g., increasing range of motion may provide the foundational skills for the individual to place an object on a shelf [activity] and return to regular employment [participation]). Table 4-1 provides definitions of and illustrates some examples of desired outcomes at each level. In some circumstances, practitioners are not concerned with changing impairments but may be working on the environmental aspects of the health problem. Measures at the participation level are appropriate primary outcomes in this case.

PROMIS

The National Institutes of Health (NIH) recognized the need for better patient-reported outcome measures as a foundation for better quality clinical research and practice. In 2004, NIH funded a network whose mandate was development of clinical outcomes as an adjunct to the NIH roadmap for clinical research initiatives. The patient-reported outcomes measurement

Table 4-1

ICIDH-2. DEFINITIONS OF THE DIMENSIONS CONSIDERED IN THE CONTEXT OF A HEALTH CONDITION

Dimensions	Definitions	Limitations	Examples of Target Outcomes
Body functions and structure	Body functions are the physiological and psychological functions of the body systems. Body structures are the anatomical parts of the body such as organs, limbs, and their components.	Impairments are problems in body function or structure such as a significant deviation or loss.	• Range of motion • Balance • Strength • Sensibility • Muscle tone • Wound size • Visual tracking • Praxis • Tidal volume • Heart rate • Nerve conduction • Imaging results
Activity	The performance of a task or action by an individual.	Activity limitations are difficulties an individual may have in the performance of activities.	• Walking • Lifting a glass • Dexterity • Functional capacity • Overhead lift • Transferring • Eating • Dressing • Toileting • Throwing a ball • Making a bed
Participation	An individual's involvement in life situations in relation to health conditions; body functions; and structures, activities, and contextual factors.	Participation restrictions are problems an individual may have in the manner or extent of involvement in life situations.	Ability to participate in: • Work • Community • Family life • Advocacy • Lived experiences • Usual social roles

Contextual factors: An integral component of the classification, consisting of environmental factors (the physical, social, and attitudinal environment in which people live and conduct their lives) and personal factors.

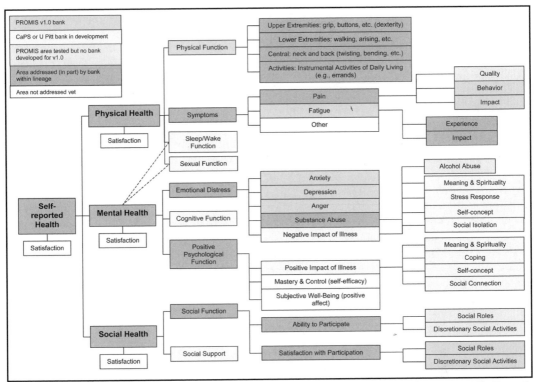

Figure 4-3. Patient Reported Outcomes Measurement Information Systems (PROMIS) Domain Framework. (Reprinted with permission of the PROMIS Health Organization and the PROMIS Cooperative Group © 2007.)

information system (PROMIS), which can be found at www.nihpromis.org, purposed to revolutionize the way patient-reported outcomes, are selected and employed in clinical research and practice. Six primary research sites are currently working on developing patient-reported outcome measures that will assess important aspects of HRQOL across a wide variety of chronic diseases and conditions (Bruce & Fries, 2005; Fries, Bruce, & Cella, 2005). The broad objectives of this initiative are to develop and test a large bank of items that can be used to create a computerized adaptive testing system that will allow for efficient, reliable, and valid assessment across a wide range of disorders. At the inaugural conference in September 2006, preliminary progress in developing item banks within a conceptual framework was shared (conference presentations are available for viewing on the Web site; outcome instruments to be available in 2007). The intent is to have ongoing updating and enhancement of item banks based on experience and data acquired as the system evolves. In keeping with the objective of enhancing both clinical and research evaluation, PROMIS measures are intended for public use.

Figure 4-3 illustrates a conceptual framework underlying PROMIS. Similar to other health models, physical, mental, and social health are viewed as the three primary domains. In addition, every domain of health may have a related satisfaction rating.

Patients typically seek care due to symptoms that limit function. These two concepts are reflected in physical health domain as is it divided into symptoms and function/disability. The category of "Symptoms" has been subdivided into pain and fatigue and others. Physical function is considered as "one's ability to carry out various activities, ranging from self-care (activities of daily living) to more challenging and vigorous activities that require increasing degrees of mobility, strength, or endurance" (PROMIS, n.d.). Some decisions have been made on the optimal way of measuring physical function outcomes within this framework. For example, question stems will focus on capability rather than performance. At least four subdomains are currently identified: mobility (lower extremities), dexterity (upper extremities and hands), axial (neck and back), and integrated activities of daily life (IADL).

Mental health has been divided into three domains: emotional distress, cognitive function, and positive psychological functioning. Cognitive function and positive psychological functioning item banks were not fully developed at the time of writing this book. Databanks were more well-developed for emotional distress aspects, including anxiety, depression, anger/aggression, substance abuse, and negative impacts of illness. Emotional distress defined as unpleasant emotions are cognitions that may interfere with the ability to cope with the disease, its physical symptoms, and its treatment.

The social health domain has been subdivided into role participation and social support. Social health is operationally defined as "perceived well-being regarding social activities and relationships, including the ability to relate to individuals, groups, communities and society as a whole" (PROMIS, n.d.). The term social health is used as a synonym for social function and refers to a higher order domain with measurable subdomains that would include understanding and communication, getting along with people, participation in society, and performance of social roles.

TYPES OF OUTCOME MEASURES

Outcome measures vary according to their structure, purpose, domain, and measurement methods and properties. Outcome scales require that measurements or ratings be performed. Measurements can be observer-based (sometimes called clinician-based outcomes or CBOs) or self-reported (sometimes called patient-reported outcomes or PROs). PROs can actually be self-reported (using questionnaires) or based on interviews that use structured or semi-structured inquiry to obtain patient responses.

Traditionally, in medicine and, subsequently, in rehabilitation, there has been a strong reliance on CBOs ranging from physical impairment measures to composite observer-based scales where clinicians rate performance while observing patients performing a task. The assumption by many clinicians has been that these measures are more reliable than self-report measures. In fact, studies indicate the contrary. Well-constructed, self-reported measures generally demonstrate a higher level of reliability than physical impairment measures assessed at the same time (MacDermid, Ramos, Drosdowech, Faber, & Patterson, 2004; Marx, Bombardier, & Wright, 1999). Some impairment measurements are associated with a high degree of tester or occasion variability. For example, strength and endurance can vary substantially even within a single day in a medically stable person (Boadella, Sluiter, & Frings-Dresen, 2003; Coldwells, Atkinson, & Reilly, 1994).

Agreement between CBOs (particularly at the impairment level) and self-reported measures of pain and disability has been shown to be only moderate across a wide spectrum of patient problems, suggesting that these are distinct perspectives. In some subdisciplines, it is popular to use overall indices of outcome that combine clinician-based and patient reported outcomes into a composite score. For example, the Mayo Elbow Performance Index (MEPI) (Morrey, An, & Chao, 2000) combines patient-based functional items with impairment-based measures of range of motion, strength, and stability to formulate a single score that ranges from 0 to 100. Different score ranges are provided with subjective ratings of either excellent, good, fair, or poor. While combined scales are popular in some areas of practice, caution is advised because the assignment of the qualitative ratings to a specific range of scores has usually been performed in an arbitrary fashion and has not been validated against an external standard. The weighting of different impairments is usually arbitrarily set and may not relate to the role of these specific impairments as contributors to function (Turchin, Beaton, & Richards, 1998). Finally, as self-rated and clinician-based impairment measures tap into different concepts, combining them in a composite score may be uninformative.

Types of Measures Based on Intended Purpose

Outcome scales can serve three different clinical purposes, including the following:

1. Evaluate change over time

2. Discriminate between different groups

3. Predict future status

By far, the most common clinical purpose for using outcome measures is to evaluate change following interventions. In fact, most of the measures accepted into clinical practice were designed for this purpose.

The second most common purpose for using an "outcome" instrument is actually for discrimination into subgroups. Discrimination may be in the form of classification or diagnosis. For example, hand diagrams (Katz & Stirrat, 1990) and diagnostic questionnaires (Kamath & Stothard, 2003) have been developed to assist with making the diagnoses of carpal tunnel syndrome. These tools have been shown to have acceptable levels of sensitivity and specificity in separating individuals with or without carpal tunnel syndrome as defined by an external comparator. Classification may also be used to separate different clinical subgroups to establish their (treatment) needs or capability. For example, it has been shown that a classification system is useful to divide patients with low back pain into different clinical subgroups that require different treatment approaches (Fritz, Delitto, & Erhard, 2003). Others have developed a staging system for functional independence across the activities of daily living (ADLs), sphincter-management, mobility, and executive-function domains (ASME) using the Functional Independence Measure (FIM) in a manner consistent with the ICF model as method for "assessment and goal setting in terms that are meaningful to patients and their care givers" (Stineman, Ross, Fiedler, Granger, & Maislin, 2003).

Finally, outcome instruments are sometimes used to predict a patient's future status. For example, the Movement Assessment of Infants (MAI), a neuromotor assessment tool, has been used to predict which infants will be diagnosed with cerebral palsy at a future follow-up (Harris et al., 1984). The FIM has been used to predict discharge status for stroke patients, correctly predicting outcome in 70% of cases (Mauthe, Haaf, Hayn, & Krall, 1996).

Types of Outcome Measures Based on Underlying Theory

Two distinct theoretical approaches to assessment of outcomes have evolved over the years. Psychometric methods are most prevalent and rely on years of research in psychological measurement. These approaches are concerned with creating instruments in which a specific domain of content is sampled and items are developed to represent this domain. Multivariate statistical methods, like factor analysis, are often used to determine the validity of these domain structures. Classical test theory has provided many of the methods used to evaluate these outcome measures. More modern test theories are emerging, like item response theory, to provide alternative methods to evaluate attributes. However, all psychometric-based methods remain dependent on test items as a means of estimating some underlying conceptual construct. Although the psychometric approach has been instrumental in making outcome evaluation more precise, a conceptual conundrum remains. The fact is that the psychometric approach does not directly address how a person evaluates his or her QOL.

As QOL is a subjective evaluation, other methods have focused on decision theory as a basis for understanding how people value their life or health state. These methods are common in health economics where a unidimensional measure of quality/utility is important to costing out interventions and associated changes in health state. Utility scores range from 0 to 1, usually with 0 representing the worst-case scenario (death or worst possible health state) and 1 representing the best-case scenario (full health or best possible health). A variety of techniques like standard-gamble or time-trade-off (Bakker, Rutten van Molken, van Doorslaer, Bennett, & van der Linden, 1993; Feeny et al., 2004; Sackett & Torrance, 1978; Smith & Dobson, 1993; Torrance, 1987) are used to establish a valuation for given health states. These techniques relate back to decision theory by using methods that ask the person to make an inherently value-laden decision about "the value" he or she places on a given health state by using a series of decisions (choice options) to find a point of uncertainty or equivalence. For example, standard gamble patients might be asked whether they were willing to accept a specific probability of death or total disablement to attain a specific probability of optimal health. A similar approach is used in the time trade-off technique, but utility is calibrated by determining the amount of time people would be willing to trade off (loss of years of life) to achieve a better current QOL. Utility can also be measured using specific utility questionnaires (Torrance, 1987) or overall rating scales. Quality-adjusted life years (Dolan, Shaw, Tsuchiya, & Williams, 2005; Richardson & Manca, 2004; Ventegodt, Merrick, & Andersen, 2003) are measures of life expectancy adjusted for QOL. In economic studies, these types of outcome measures are used to evaluate how interventions affect the duration and quality of remaining life (Kaplan, Alcaraz, Anderson, & Weisman, 1996; Russell, Gold, Siegel, Daniels, & Weinstein, 1996).

TYPES OF OUTCOME MEASURES BASED ON SCOPE

Different types of outcome measures arise based on the domain structures. The most common types of instruments seen in rehabilitation include the following:

- Generic instruments (like QOL, general health, utility or participation)
- Disease or symptom-specific measures that focus on the key aspects of a disease or symptom (like stroke or pain)
- Regional or body part-specific measures that focus on a body area (like the DASH [American Academy of Orthopaedic Surgeons, 2002; Beaton et al., 2001a; Solway, Beaton, McConnell, & Bombardier, 2002]) or the Shoulder Pain and Disability Index ([Heald, Riddle, & Lamb, 1997; MacDermid, Solomon, & Prkachin, 2006; Roach, Budiman-Mak, Songsiridej, & Lertratanakul, 1991; Williams, Holleman, & Simel, 1995])
- Patient-specific measures in which items are selected to be meaningful to the patient (like the Canadian Occupational Performance Measure ([Carswell et al., 2004; Law et al., 1990, 1994, 1998; McColl, Paterson, Davies, Doubt, & Law, 2000) or Patient Specific Functional Scale [Chatman et al., 1997; Westaway, Stratford, & Binkley, 1998])

STRUCTURAL CHARACTERISTICS OF OUTCOME MEASURES

Developers of outcome measures make fundamental decisions on the structure of scales/subscales, individual items, and response options when creating instruments. All of these decisions will impact the psychometric properties, clinical utility, and acceptability of the instrument to patients and clinicians.

The structure of the instrument includes the instructions provided to respondents about how to attribute their symptom or function. Instruments vary in how they attribute responses to either a specific timeframe or to a specific construct. Some instruments inquire about the person's difficulty performing a task without attribution, while another scale might ask the same question but would frame the question by attributing it to an affected area or health problem. We can imagine that these two questions might be answered quite differently depending on the task and the extent to which the person had adapted to his or her health problem. Patients with upper extremity problems will report higher levels of disability when questions are attributed to their upper extremity than when responding to general questions (Marx et al., 2001). For example, we observed that patients reported high levels of emotional impact on a disease-specific, quality-of-life instrument for rotator cuff, but low levels on the SF-36 where emotional health was placed in a global context (MacDermid et al., 2004).

Similarly, patients may respond differently depending on whether questions are framed in terms of capability or performance. Asking a person whether he or she can do something may elicit a different response that asking if he or she did something. For example, a study comparing relationship between capability and performance administered two versions of the Activities Scale for Kids (ASK) to 28 physically disabled children. The capability version asked children what they "could do," whereas the performance version asked what they "did do." Capability was found to exceed performance by approximately 18%, which the authors attributed to environmental context (Young, Williams, Yoshida, Bombardier, & Wright, 1996). This conclusion was supported in a separate study in which children with cerebral palsy where children performed crawling or walking more often at home than in school or community environments (Tieman, Palisano, Gracely, & Rosenbaum, 2004).

Outcome scales may be one-dimensional or have subscales that reflect different aspects of the health domain. For example, the SF-36 has eight different subscales that address different subdomains of health (Ware & Sherbourne, 1992; Ware, 2003; Ware, Gandek, et al., 1998). The physical and mental summary scores are intended to provide overall scores for two global and independent aspects of health. Factor analysis is a statistical process used to group items that behave similarly when a test is administered. This analysis is often used to determine whether items on a self-report measure follow the subscales structure defined by the authors. In general, correlations between physical and mental summary scores on the SF-36 are quite low, suggesting that the questionnaire is able to differentiate these two separate components of health (Ware, Kosinski, et al., 1998).

Instruments will also vary on how individual questions and subscales are scored. Many patient-based outcomes are determined on the basis of questionnaires containing a range of scored items using Likert scaling or visual analog responses. Likert scaling of items provides a range of subjective options in an ordinal scale. Other instruments used a numeric 0 to 10 or visual analog scale response scale. In some cases, Likert and visual analog versions of the scale are available. In some pediatric scales, pictorial representations are used to represent different response options as a means of allowing young nonreaders to communicate their ratings.

Instruments should provide instructions on how missing items are handled and other procedural elements. Regardless of the measurement approach, it is important that instructions contain sufficiently detailed instructions on how to score items, subscales, and total scores to ensure consistency across centers and clinical studies when instruments are applied in different situations.

IDENTIFYING OUTCOME MEASURES FOR USE IN CLINICAL PRACTICE

One of the first steps in using outcome measures to determine whether an intervention is effective is selecting the appropriate measure. Methods for searching for these instruments have been defined in Chapter 3 of this text and will not be reviewed here. However, it is worth noting some special considerations that apply to outcome measures. Many outcome measures may be mentioned in treatment studies or psychometric studies, but it is less common for the actual instruments themselves to be readily accessible. It may be necessary to contact the instrument developer to gain this access. Some textbooks and Web sites are specifically focused on the need to obtain the instruments and a number of these resources are listed in an annotated bibliography below. One of the advantages of these resources is that they allow clinicians to overview a large number of potential scales to gain the breadth of instruments available. For example, the *AO Handbook: Musculoskeletal Outcome Measures and Instruments* provides and reviews more than 150 different outcome scales. Clinicians should be aware that books are often out of date by the time they are in print, thus database searching for scientific articles is necessary to be aware of advances in the field.

The steps to identify an appropriate measure are as follows:

- *Identify the conceptual framework and/or concepts that are important to measure.*

- *Use searching of scientific articles on outcome measures, articles addressing treatment effectiveness in a similar patient population, textbooks, online outcome measure resources to identify a potential list of outcome measures/instruments.*

- *Remove any outcome measures that are not standardized, clearly not suited to your purpose or situation, or that have been shown to be unreliable or invalid for your purpose.*

- *Critically appraise your potential outcome scale(s) using a standardized process or instrument OR basic principles to ascertain reliability, validity, and clinical utility.*

- *Determine whether the instrument can evaluate change, discriminate, or predict in the manner required for your population and purpose.*

- *Obtain the measures of interest, determine the scoring mechanism and any specific instructions on administration (including whether valid translations are available).*

- *Identify copyright, reimbursement issues, and ensure compliance.*

- *Devise and document a strategy as to what procedures will be followed in implementing outcome measures into practice (when will they be applied, who will provide them, how/when will they be scored, where will the data be retained, how will the data be used). Ensure that all parties involved participate in devising the implementation strategy and understand their roles.*

- *Pilot test either one or two instruments for a specified period and re-evaluate the instrument's performance, feasibility, and implementation process.*

- *Finalize your choice and a set timeframe to review outcomes data.*

A number of practical issues must be considered when attempting to incorporate new measures into practice. Expect and prepare for a learning curve. Lack of adequate preparation will inevitably lead to frustration and an inability to use outcome measure scores in clinical decision-making. Facilitators when implementing the use of new outcomes measures into practice may include making the instruments readily available for use when needed, teaching clinicians to value the role of the measure, providing the measures at a standardized time frame, and making sure the forms are filled out entirely by the patients.

Developers of outcome measures have intellectual property rights with respect to their instruments so it is important that these be respected. Many developers do not charge for the use of their instruments. In this case, it is advisable to contact the developer and request permission to use the instrument and inquire if there is any documentation regarding proper administration or interpretation. In some cases, outcome measures and/or their supporting documentation must be purchased. Usually, this is a one-time cost, but in some cases there can be ongoing charges for a license and/or for scoring. These practical issues may determine which measures are feasible in your practice. Some companies have developed platforms for administering, scoring, and providing interpretation of outcome measures in a computer-based format. Ongoing license fees for software and for reports are common in this case.

EVALUATING OUTCOME MEASURES

Critical appraisal of outcome measures is more complicated than critical appraisal of individual effectiveness studies. The value of any given outcome measure is reflected across a spectrum of studies that must address initial development of the instrument and subsequent reliability and validity testing. Individual studies on psychometrics of measures will vary in quality and scope. Furthermore, it is important that reliability and validity be established in the clinical population for which the measure will be used. For example, an instrument designed to assess shoulder disability may be useful in most subgroups but may be inappropriate to assess the high-level athlete or musician. We have appended a scale to assist with evaluating individual psychometric articles (Appendices G and H) and one to summarize a measure (Appendix E).

There are many forms of both reliability and validity, and the importance of each psychometric property varies with the purpose of using the outcome instrument. For example, when using instruments to evaluate change over time, responsiveness is particularly important. When using an instrument to determine which group a patient belongs to (determine a diagnosis or status like "able to return to work"), then discriminative validity is of importance. The ability to detect change and the ability to discriminate are two separate psychometric properties and may in fact compete with each other from a statistical point of view. Perhaps for this reason, there is no system of levels of evidence assigned to outcome measures. Recently, there has been work done to make recommendations for evaluation/acceptable criteria for outcome measures but this work is pending (Mokkink et al., 2006). We will not review the basic concepts of reliability and validity as they apply to outcome measures. These can be reviewed in basic texts of introductory articles on clinical measurement. However, at the end of this chapter, there is a review of some basic terminology as a quick reference.

A number of authors have provided a framework for evaluating outcome measures and in some cases, a compendium of evaluated measures. In the text, *Physical Rehabilitation Outcome Measures*, a guide to critical appraisal is provided and over 70 measures from a variety of areas within rehabilitation are summarized on a standard format that includes information on the developers, purpose, a description of the measure, conceptual basis or construct measured, groups tests, translations available, typical reliability estimates, typical validity estimates, responsiveness, and interpretability. Users of musculoskeletal (MSK) measures can find a rating scale used to report concise and clear 10-item summaries of over 150 MSK measures. These were rated in three fields: content, methodology (reliability/validity), and clinical utility (user and clinicians "friendliness"). We include as Appendix E the framework on evaluating outcome measures developed by Law, which is more open-ended and covers many of the concepts we have discussed in this chapter. This tool and guide will be useful to clinicians when choosing an appropriate outcome measure(s). The time invested in critical appraisal will pay back when it is time to use outcome measures in diagnosis, goal-setting, or other clinical decision making as many of the concepts and data retrieved from primary studies can be applied to the process of making stronger and more precise better quantitative clinical decisions.

The following case example illustrates how outcome measures were selected using these principles for one specific problem.

> *A 46-year-old male, who works in auto manufacturing, has right lateral elbow pain when he moves his arm. This pain is usually "achy" after activity or at the end of the day, but occasionally a "sharper pain" occurs with certain activities. These include using tools at work, wringing out a wet towel, and carrying a heavy pot. After his full examination, you conclude he has tennis elbow and want to select outcome measures to monitor the response to your interventions.*

In selecting an outcome evaluation approach that we might use with this patient and future similar cases, we started with the intent to survey the literature to identify a long list of potential outcome evaluation tools. Our first step was to search the literature to identify outcome measures that were used in clinical studies on rehabilitation of tennis elbow. A full table of interventions and outcome measures used was available in a systematic review providing this broad view (Trudel et al., 2004). From this review, we were able to determine that there was no consensus on appropriate standardized outcome measures for this problem. Furthermore, we noted that a number of nonstandardized measures were used. Despite this setback, it was evident that some core "constructs" were being evaluated in clinical studies, including pain, muscle strength, and function. Knowing that education and exercise were important components of treatment because of the supporting evidence, we decided we wanted outcome measures that would reflect the main impairments this patient was experiencing and that would be addressed by our interventions (pain and loss of strength). We also knew that function and participation, particularly in work, were important to this person. We decided to differentiate short-tem and long-term outcome constructs that were clinically relevant. In the shorter term, outcome evaluations would emphasize impairments so that we can determine if the interventions were leading to changes in symptoms and structural changes in the tendon itself. As clinicians we feel that we can impact on the pathological process happening at the tendon level using controlled exercise and activity but recognize that at the same time it is important to quickly address the primary concern of the patient by achieving pain relief. In the longer term, we would be concerned that our patient resume valued participation (safe and productive work) and that would prevent future reoccurrences.

We find studies that address reliability and validity of outcome measures within these constructs and limit ourselves to those that have supporting evidence. This creates a short-list for an outcomes strategy.

We decide to measure short-term outcomes at baseline and at 2-, 4-, and 6-weeks following our initial intervention.

1. *Pain relief* could be measured using either the Patient-Rated Tennis Elbow Evaluation (PRTEE) (MacDermid, 2005; Newcomer, Martinez-Silvestrini, Schaefer, Gay, & Arendt, 2005; Overend, Wuori-Fearn, Kramer, & MacDermid, 1999), the Pain-Free Function Scale (PFFS) (Stratford, Levy, Gauldie, Levy, & Miseferi, 1987), a Visual Analogue Scale (VAS), or Numeric Pain Rating scale.

2. *Patient function* could be measured using self-report scales that include a functional subscale. These include the PRTEE (MacDermid, 2005; Newcomer et al., 2005; Overend et al., 1999), or Disabilities of the Arm, Shoulder, Hand (DASH) (Beaton et al., 2001a; Solway et al., 2002).

3. *Muscle function* can be measured using quantitative measures of isometric strength.

    a. Functional grip—Pain-free grip strength (Stratford, Levy, & Gowland, 1993) is the most responsive and easily performed as most clinics would have quantitative grip devices.

    b. Tendon integrity—Wrist extensor strength would be the most direct "functional" measurement of tendon integrity and could easily be measured using a hand-held dynamometer (depending on equipment availability).

    c. Endurance for activity (a standardized test has yet to be described that quantifies wrist muscle endurance, although a variety of functional tests would tap into this domain)—Given the lack of specificity of these tests to our problem and potential problems with validity, we do not implement this measure at this time.

We decide to measure longer-term outcomes at baseline, discharge, and 6-month follow-up (the latter to be performed by e-mail and telephone survey). The following outcomes are measured:

1. Reoccurrence of symptoms

    a. Pain/Function (Patient-Rated Forearm Scale [MacDermid, 2005; Newcomer et al., 2005; Overend et al., 1999]) or Pain-Free Function [Stratford et al., 1987])

    b. Requiring additional treatment

2. Work outcomes (lost time, the work subscale of the DASH [Beaton et al., 2001b; Solway et al., 2002]) or a scale similar to The Work Limitation Questionnaire (WLQ) [Lerner et al., 2001; Lerner, Reed, Massarotti, Wester, & Burke, 2002]) which describes the difficulty at work).

3. Resumption of valued regular recreational activity—We would select a patient-specific measure to monitor this (like the Canadian Occupational Performance Measure [Carswell et al., 2004; Law et al., 1990, 1994, 1998; McColl et al., 2000) or Patient Specific Functional Scale [Chatman et al., 1997; Westaway et al., 1998]).

How to Use Outcome Measures to Help Make Clinical Decisions on Individual Patients

Once an outcome measure and associated administration timetable has been established, this template can be used across successive patients as standard practice. There is inherent value in asking patients standardized questions regarding their perceived status as a component of clinical evaluation. Patients appreciate when their perspective is central to the treatment process. There is also inherent value in looking at the individual items scored by specific patients as a means of understanding where their functional difficulties lie. However, the maximum benefit of using standardized outcome measures is achieved as clinicians become comfortable with incorporating actual scores into their clinical decision making. We now provide an example of how that can be approached.

> *A male patient, 55 years of age, attends your clinic for the first time with a diagnosis of shoulder pain from a referring general practitioner. The patient has a diagnostic ultrasound report indicating a partial thickness tear of the supraspinatus tendon. Recently, your clinic has added the DASH self-report outcome measure to its clinic assessment protocol. The patient's score is 44 at this visit.*

This simple scenario provides an opportunity to examine some of the typical questions one might ask when using outcome measures to evaluate the impact of an evidence-based decision. It is important that we understand how outcome measures fit into our conceptual framework of health and QOL but ultimately, quantitative decisions on the meaning of scores are required. Data from reliability and validity studies can help in making those quantitative judgments that contribute to goal setting and re-evaluation. The following example can be used as a template. However, some review of basic statistical knowledge (variability, normal curve, etc.) and principles of psychometrics of measurement (see definitions at the end or texts on outcome measures listed below) make it easier to feel comfortable with adapting the concepts to your practice needs. You may wish to go back and forth between reviewing and applying these concepts until you become comfortable with both. The following fundamental questions are posed:

- What does the score on this outcome measure tell me about the patient's status?

- What is the error associated with the measured value?

- How much will the score need to change on subsequent assessments so I can be confident that a real change has occurred?

- How much will the score need to change on a subsequent assessment so I can be confident that an important amount of change has occurred?

- What is my long-term treatment goal and how does it relate to a score on its outcome measure?

What Does This Measure Tell Me About the Patient's Status?

The DASH (American Academy of Orthopaedic Surgeons, 2002; Beaton et al., 2001a; Solway et al., 2002; The Upper Extremity Collaborative Group, 1999; Upper Extremity Collaborative Group, 1996) was designed to reflect the disability a person experiences as a result of problems with his or her upper extremity. Reliability and validity data are excellent, and substantial comparative data are available for use, including a user's manual. This provides confidence that the DASH is a valid measure of upper extremity disability. When looking at the items (the DASH can be obtained from the Web site www.dash.iwh.on.ca), it can be seen that some items address symptoms, others specific activities, and others participation in normal life roles. The DASH scored as a unidimensional scale, and thus, does not clearly distinguish components of the ICF model of disability but incorporates items across its dimensions. Similarly, the DASH includes aspects of both psychosocial and physical health. We might consider the DASH to be a valid indicator of function in persons with physical disorders of the upper extremity.

Clinicians do not have an innate feel for the meaning of the scores obtained from measures such as the DASH. This could be a barrier to implementing these measures in clinical practice. Understanding the scores that we would expect from a typical patient with an acute rotator cuff problem could assist us to understand the severity of this particular patient's problem. When first using outcome measures, it is advisable to collate published comparative data obtained from the same population at different points in clinical recovery to have data for making comparisons. With relatively little clinical experience using outcome measures, most people quickly develop a "feel" for whether scores reported by a given patient are within an expected range, considering the pathology and point in clinical recovery.

Normative data for the DASH are published on the American Academy of Orthopaedic Surgeons' Web site (American Academy of Orthopaedic Surgeons, 2002) and in the user's manual. The average 55-year-old male or female in the general population reports a DASH score of 12. Atroshi, Gummesson, Andersson, Dahlgreen, and Johansson (2000) reported a mean DASH score of 43 for patients awaiting shoulder surgery, compared to a mean score of 35 for nonsurgical patients. Skutek, Fremerey, Zeichen, and Bosch (2000) reported a mean preoperative DASH score of 49 for persons with rotator cuff tears awaiting surgery. The example DASH score of 44 is consistent with that of other persons reporting substantial disability due to rotator cuff pathology.

What Is the Error Associated With the Measured DASH Value?

To be confident that a measured DASH value is useful, we must have some idea of the consistency of the score in a meaningful way. That is the amount of error associated with a measured value must be known. The standard error of mean (SEM) can be used to describe the error associated with a reported value expressed in the original units of the measure. The SEM is related to the variability of the underlying population and the reliability of the scores on that particular outcome measure in a similar group. Although there are several methods for calculating the SEM, the most popular method is as follows:

$$SEM = (\text{sample standard deviation}) \sqrt{1 - \text{reliability coefficient}}$$

While the DASH has been shown to have high reliability coefficients across a broad number of conditions, the standard deviation can be expected to vary between different conditions and even within conditions over time as the level of disability changes. Thus SEM is an estimate. When faced with a lack of data indicating the SEM appropriate to our patient's condition and level of disability, we extrapolate from data that most closely approximates our patient. When one is interested in estimating the error associated with a score at a single point in time, internal consistency coefficients are used to indicate stability.

Once you determine the SEM, you must decide on the level of precision or your estimate. One SEM is associated with a 68% confidence interval (for a description of the sampling distribution and z-values, see any standard statistical text). To obtain higher confidence levels, the SEM can be multiplied by z-values associated with different confidence levels. For example, 1.65 is the z-value associated with the 90% confidence level and 1.96 is the z-value associated with the 95% confidence level. By multiplying the SEM for the measures taken by this level of confidence (z-value), you can establish a range within which a patient's true score is likely to lie—at the specified confidence level.

A SEM (for one point in time) of 4.4 points has been reported for the DASH. Multiplying the SEM of 4.4 points by the z-value of 1.65 associated with a 90% confidence level yields a value of 7.3 points. The interpretation is that at the time of assessment, there is a 90% chance that a patient's true score is within 7.3 points of the measured score.

How Much Will the Score Need to Change on Subsequent Assessments So I Can Be Confident That a Real Change Has Occurred?

One reason for reassessing patients is to determine whether they have changed as a result of implementing an intervention. The measured changed must exceed the error associated with the measurement process to be reasonably certain that a true change has occurred. Often, the term *minimal detectable change (MDC)* is used to specify this value. The MDC can be useful when setting short-term goals because it can establish a reasonable target for where there should be a real change in status. It can also assist with establishing reassessment intervals as the therapist should reassess at an interval where an expected change should exceed the MDC. However, some clinics standardize the time of reassessments, which may be a reflection of requirements under licensure laws or with third-party payers.

To obtain the minimal level of detectable change at a specified confidence (MDC_{CL}), $SEM_{test-retest}$ is multiplied by the z-value associated with the confidence level of interest and by the square-root of 2. For example, MDC at a 90% confidence level, designated MDC_{90} is obtained as follows:

$$MDC_{90} = SEM_{test-retest} \text{ x z } - \text{value x } \sqrt{2}$$

Estimates of MDC_{90} for the DASH vary, with 11 being a typical value. The interpretation of MDC_{90} is that 90% of stable patients are likely to display a difference on retest less than the value of MDC_{90}. Thus, for the described patient vignette, a change of 11 or more DASH points is required to be reasonably certain that a true change has occurred.

How Many Points Does a DASH Score Need to Change Before We Could Confidently Say That an Important Change in Upper Extremity Disability Has Occurred for This Patient?

Clinicians, payers, and other stakeholders are not usually concerned with the least detectable difference but rather an important difference—one that makes a difference in the life of the patient. The term *clinically important difference (CID)* or *minimal clinically important difference (MCID)* (Beaton et al., 2001b; Beaton, Boers, & Wells, 2002; Guyatt, Walter, & Norman, 1987; Jaeschke, Singer, & Guyatt, 1989) is often used to describe this quantity. Estimates of the clinically important difference require that studies evaluate how much change on a measure is of importance to the patient. This has been established for some measures but may not be available for all outcome measures, or across different stages of disability. Despite the many limitations in setting an arbitrary value for this, a reasonable CID for the DASH is estimated as a change of approximately 15 points and this can serve as a general guidepost when making long-term treatment goals.

What DASH Score Is Required to Meet Our Long-Term Treatment Goals for This Patient?

In an EBP approach to practice, long-term goals are shaped by the following:
- The patient's preferences
- Clinical data on the expected effect sizes and its mediators
- The clinician's experience

These factors determine how this evidence can be applied or extrapolated to their patient. When using standardized outcome measures to set and evaluate progress toward long-terms goals, it is important to have data on patients who have had varying levels of disability to help us to set realistic goals. In this case, we are interested in return to work and obtain data on DASH scores that are consistent with return to work. Data obtained by Beaton et al. (2001a) on scores for working and working patients help us make a reasonable prognosis in this regard. They reported a mean DASH score of 50.7 for persons unable to work because of their upper extremity problem, compared to a mean score of 26.8 for persons able to work with an upper extremity problem. In setting a long-term predicted DASH change (e.g., patient prognosis), we would want to meet the lower score.

How to Use Outcome Measures to Help Make Clinical Decisions on Rehabilitation Programs

Many clinicians can readily see the benefit of using outcome measures on individual patients but are unsure as to how to use them to evaluate their clinic outcomes. Outcomes research, program evaluation, and benchmarking share some commonality in that large pools of observational data on outcomes are used to make decisions about services or programs. Some areas like inpatient rehabilitation have moved toward use of standard measures like the FIM that are collected in many centers to facilitate these comparisons. Increasingly, professional associations are providing mechanisms to support databases for outpatient services. For example, both the American Physical Therapy Association (APTA Connect®) and the American Society of Hand Therapists have partnered with Cedaron Medical to create their own outcomes databases. There is increasing pressure from payers to demonstrate outcomes, making it essential that clinicians be prepared to show that meaningful outcomes were achieved for patients and those outcomes compare favorably to those reported when alternative health care providers or interventions are selected. For those without access to established databases or software, clinic databases can be established using routine office software. In addition, the "Red-book" of Physical Rehabilitation Outcome Measures provides a chapter that assists clinicians with a process for using outcome measures in program evaluation.

With the move toward outcomes databases, it will be important to keep in mind the limitations of observational data. We remember the key benefit of randomization (with large numbers of patients) is that it controls for known and unknown factors that may affect outcome by evenly distributing these across comparison groups. Observational data, no matter how meticulously gathered, does not have this protection. Differences between groups may exist because of differences in the factor of interest—usually treatment. However, alternative sources of difference might be driving the observed differences. The reasons or path taken for individuals to end up in a certain subgroup may be the real factor(s) that underlies the outcomes achieved. These factors are usually called biases because they contaminate the ability to ascribe differences between groups to the (treatment) factor. Differences between groups drawn from an outcome database may be due to variation in the distribution of these "risk factors." Common factors that might vary between subgroups include age (and associated differences in comorbidity and physical demands), sex/gender, severity of the disorder, variations in comorbidity/physical health, occupational demands, access to timely services, socioeconomic, or geographical/environmental factors. When comparisons are made across different health care systems, this can create another source of potential covariation that limits the ability to define a causal relationship between outcomes achieved and interventions provided.

IDENTIFYING AND ADDRESSING BARRIERS USING OUTCOMES INSTRUMENTS OUTCOME EVALUATION

The importance of measuring health outcomes has been recognized by the rehabilitation professions. Concerted effort has been made to transfer available knowledge into practice as a means to provide rigorous evaluation of the impact of rehabilitation interventions. These efforts have included national initiatives by the professional associations of both occupational and physical therapists, traditional workshops; published editorials, scientific articles and textbooks; professional association endorsement; and development of outcomes databases. While agreement with the need for outcome measures is consistently high in surveyed therapists, utilization remains low in many areas of practice (Michlovitz, LaStayo, Alzner, & Watson, 2001).

Others have documented barriers that exist to implementing outcome measures in practice (Abrams et al., 2006; Dunckley, Aspinal, Addington-Hall, Hughes, & Higginson, 2005; Dunckley, Hughes, Addington-Hall, & Higginson, 2003; Horner & Larmer, 2006). The most consistent barriers identified include lack of time, administrative support, and specific knowledge on how to find and apply measures. Time since graduation is often associated with less use of outcome measure or greater discomfort with how to do so, which is not surprising given the recent emergence of EBP and outcome measurement.

TIPS FROM THE AUTHORS

In our experience in teaching clinicians how to incorporate outcome measures into practice, we have found that many people are highly interested in outcome measures while at our workshops but are unable to integrate the information into their practice. The most common problem is that clinicians do not follow the steps we have highlighted. Many wait until outcome measures are demanded by insurers and then incorporate them without a clear plan on how they will be collected or used. A home-grown process is essential to success. Some clinics may have elaborate databases and high-tech equipment, whereas this technology solution may not work in a sole-charge clinic. It is wise to develop a plan with reasonable and attainable interim targets to ensure that the process is not abandoned. Working with therapists who have experience with outcome measures is preferable but not essential. Like all new clinical skills, some protected time to adapt the new processes to your clinic is the primary element of success.

EMERGING ISSUES IN OUTCOMES MEASURES

- Outcome measures may be linked to pay for performance.
- New computer-adaptive testing (PROMIS) outcome measures will be available.
- Increased availability of rehabilitation outcomes databases will bring opportunity and challenges.

CONCLUSION

- Outcome measures can be used to assess the impact of EBP as a means of personal or program quality assurance or to demonstrate effectiveness for payers.
- Contemporary health models are moving away from a biomedical view to acknowledge the contribution of physical, social, and psychological well-being and emphasizing the importance of the interaction between the individual and the environment.
- QOL is a broad concept that relates to overall satisfaction with health and/or life; health has a narrower focus that can be measured with generic health instruments.
- Outcome measures commonly used in rehabilitation are classified based on rater (clinician versus self-report), underlying theory (psychometric versus decision), and scope (generic, disease/symptom, regional/body part, or patient specific).
- Texts, Web sites, and journal articles provide access to information about outcome measures, but contacting developers may be needed to get forms and permissions.
- Outcome measures can be used to discriminate (classify or diagnose), predict (future outcomes), or more commonly to evaluate the impact of interventions over time. There are specific psychometric properties required for these functions that should be considered when selecting or interpreting outcome measures.
- Published data on outcome measures can be used to determine client status, short-term treatment goals that exceed measurement error, and long-term goals that constitute a clinically important difference or are consistent with important participation outcomes.
- Lack of time during clinical practice, access to computers/organizational processes that support data collection, comfort with basic psychometric principles, or difficulty in changing clinical behavior can act as barriers to implementing outcome measures in practice.

TERMS USED IN OUTCOME MEASURES RESEARCH

Reliability

Reliability = consistency or agreement between repeated measurements taken when the underlying phenomenon has not changed.

- *Cautions*: There are many different ways to assess reliability. Reliability by itself is not enough to ensure validity or responsiveness, but poor reliability will compromise both validity and responsiveness.

- *Types of Reliability*

    1. Internal consistency—Homogeneity of items or scores within an instrument (usually assessed using Cronbach's alpha).

    2. Inter-rater—Agreement between different raters.

    3. Intra-rater—Agreement between repeated measurements made by the same rater.

    4. Test-retest—The agreement on scores obtained between different occasions.

Kappa (k)—Intraclass Correlation Coefficient

- *Tells you*: The relative reliability (i.e., the ability to distinguish between nominal measurements made on patients [group; yes/no]).

- *Represents*: A ratio of percent agreement corrected for agreement that would occur by chance given the proportion of yes/no responses in the sample.

- *Interpretation*: Vary from 0 to 1, no units associated.

- *Cautions*: Is affected by rates of yes/no and thus tends to vary as chance agreement changes; may be unstable where chance agreement is high. That is, kappa can seem poor even when percent agreement is high if change agreement is also high (Cohen, 1968, 1990; Landis & Koch, 1977; Maclure & Willet, 1987; Shreiner, 1980).

ICC—Intraclass Correlation Coefficient

- *Tells you*: The relative reliability (i.e., the ability to distinguish between patients).

- *Represents*: A ratio of person variance divided by total variance (between persons + within persons); if variability on repeated measurements is small compared to the variability between people, reliability will be good.

- *Interpretation*: Vary from 0 to 1, no units associated.

- *Cautions*: Can seem good in the face of large errors if group is highly variable; or poor where subject variation is small, even though absolute errors are small (Bartko, 1976; Muller & Buttner, 1995; Shrout & Fleiss, 1979).

Standard Error of Mean

- *Tells you*: Absolute reliability (i.e., consistency of the measure in original units of the measure).

- *Represents*: Is a measure of within-patient variability $\times$ internal consistency.

- *Interpretation*: Provides error margins with a defined amount of confidence; less error being preferable.

- *Cautions*: SEM may not be the same across different ranges of scores (at different time points in rehabilitation).

Validity—Trueness of a Measure

- *Tells you*: Whether an instrument performs as expected within a given context to provide a true estimate of the underlying phenomenon in that circumstance.

- *Cautions*: Validity is specific to the purpose, context, and clinical population. No single study will establish it. It is an ongoing process. You hope to find that an instrument has been validated in a group of people similar to those you wish to apply it to and has been used to make decisions similar to those you wish to make.

- *Types of Validity*

  1. Face—The extent to which an instrument appears to be valid (usually determined by expert review).

  2. Content—The extent to which an instrument addresses and samples relevant aspects within the concept being assessed.

  3. Criterion—The extent to which an instrument agrees with an external criterion measurement of that concept. Where a definitive external criterion is available, it can be called a gold standard. If a gold standard does not exist, criterion validity is often taken as the extent to which a particular measure relates to other similar measures. Convergent validity assesses the extent to which an instrument agrees with similar conceptual scores, and divergent validity assesses the test for a lack of correlation with instruments that address concepts that are believed to be distinct.

  4. Concurrent—The external criterion is measured at same point in time.

  5. Predictive—The external criterion is measured in the future.

  6. Construct—The extent to which instrument scores conform to theoretically derived hypotheses. This is usually performed by testing known group differences (using statistical tests to detect differences between scores obtained for subgroups that are theorized to be different). Some consider convergent and divergent validity a form of construct validity.

Pearson r—Interclass Correlation Coefficient

- *Tells you*: Measures the strength of the linear relationship between two variables.

- *Represents*: The sum of the products of the standard scores of the two measures divided by the degrees of freedom.

- *Interpretation*: Varies from -1 to 1, no units associated; sign indicated the directionality of the relationship (a negative correlation reflects that scores change in the opposite directions to each other; a positive correlation indicates that scores change in the same direction); for validity, the strength of the association should be based on a priori hypothesis of expected relationships.

- *Cautions*: It is important to be careful about the spectrum on which associations are measured; association may not hold true when generalized outside of this range; association does not mean agreement; therefore, Pearson correlations are not generally considered acceptable as a reliability indicator. Do not always assume higher is better in validation; the key is that the correlation should support the concepts and hypothesis upon which the measure is framed/evaluated.

Detection of Clinical Change

- *Responsiveness*—A special kind of validity that reflects the ability of an instrument to detect (real) change over time (Beaton, 2000; Beaton, Bombardier, Katz, & Wright, 2001; Schmitt & Di Fabio, 2004).
- *Cautions*: There are different ways of measuring change or important change; responsiveness depends on the properties of the instrument, as well as the underlying properties of change being measured in the clinical construct.

MDC—Minimal Detectable Change

- *Tells you*: Whether a true change in status has occurred.
- *Represents*: An estimate of the amount of measurement error multiplied by a confidence factor that represents the extent of confidence one wishes to employ in determining whether a measurement has actually changed (e.g., $MDC_{90} = SEM_{test\text{-}retest} \times z\text{ - value} \times \sqrt{2}$).
- *Interpretation*: If the change on the outcomes measure exceeds the minimal detectable change, then you can be certain, within that specific level of confidence, that is unlikely that this change in score would have occurred in the absence of a true clinical change.
- *Cautions*: Varies according to variability of patient population (and sample size upon which estimates were made); changes by condition and point in recovery.

MICD—Minimally Important Clinical Difference

- *Tells you*: Change in a score indicating a change that is important to the patient.
- *Represents*: An estimate of the amount of change required to attain a clinically important change in status multiplied by a confidence factor that represents the extent of confidence one wishes to employ in determining whether a measurement has actually changed importantly.
- *Interpretation*: Is used as a comparator or benchmark to which changes in outcomes are compared to determine whether a clinically relevant outcome has been achieved.
- *Cautions*: There is no gold standard way to determine what important change is; estimates of important change will vary by methods and context in which the assessments were made; should be considered as general estimates.

Effect Size

- *Tells you*: A standardized rate of change.
- *Represents*: Mean change divided by SD of baseline score (as well as other methods).
- *Interpretation*: When comparing competing measures, the one with a larger effect size will have been more able to detect clinical change.
- *Cautions*: Comparability across studies should be performed with caution given that sample size, the underlying clinical construct, and the time points in which measurements are taken will affect observed effect sizes; methods of separating stable from changed patients can be controversial.

Standardized Response Mean

- *Tells you*: A standardized rate of change.
- *Represents*: Mean change divided by SD of change score.

- *Interpretation*: When comparing competing measures, the one with a larger SRM will have been more able to detect clinical change.

- *Cautions*: Comparability across studies should be performed with caution given that sample size, the underlying clinical construct, and the time points in which measurements are taken will affect observed SRM; methods of separating stable from changed patients can be controversial.

ROC—Receiver Operator Curve

- *Tells you*: The ability of a measure to distinguish a clinically important change where it does exist versus detecting that it does not occur (where it does not exist).

- *Represents*: Explores the ability to distinguish between two health states using methodology usually applied to diagnostic test validity (i.e., the ability of the instrument to detect change, sensitivity [y axis], is plotted against 1-specificity [x-axis])

  a. Sensitivity is the number of patients correctly identified as having undergone a clinically important change based on their outcome measures score divided by the total number of patients who truly underwent a clinically important change (as per diagnostic terminology this would represent true positives).

  b. Specificity is the number patients correctly identified as not having achieved a clinically important change (based on their outcome measures score) divided by the total number of patients who truly did not undergo a clinically important change (as per diagnostic terminology this would represent true negatives)

- *Interpretation*: Area under the curve can be interpreted as the probability of correctly identifying a patient who has undergone a clinically important change versus those who have not undergone an important change.

- *Cautions*: Can be more difficult to interpret; remains an uncommon approach; methods of separating stable from changed patients can be controversial.

LEARNING AND EXPLORATION ACTIVITIES

1. Following the models of Case Example 1, select an outcomes approach for an example from your own caseload and discuss how it fits within a conceptual framework described in this chapter.

2. Using the (Law) evaluation instrument provided in this book, evaluate the measure you selected.

3. Using the (MacDermid) psychometric evaluation form, evaluate one study on your measure—list any terms, or methods you do not understand and consult clinical measurement texts or experts to refine your understanding.

4 Search the web and the outcome measure textbook to see if they have evaluated your scale and compare you results.

5. Compile a list of comparative scores that you might use to help make clinical decisions with your chosen scale.

6. Using Example 2 as an exemplar, work through the clinical decision-making questions using your outcome measure and patient scenario.

7. Identify one barrier in your clinical practice that might be a challenge to implementing this measure routinely in your practice and develop a plan to resolve it.

Tools Included in This Book

1. Outcome Measure Rating Form (Law) can be used to summarize the information on an outcome measure as a means of deciding on its value and application.

2. Critical appraisal of study quality for psychometric articles evaluation form (MacDermid) allows the user to evaluate individual articles on outcome measures.

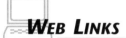

WEB LINKS

- *The official site of the Patient-Reported Outcomes Measurement Information System (PROMIS)*
  www.nihpromis.org/default.asp.
- www.who.int/classifications/icf/site/icftemplates.cfm
  This Web site provides information about the International Classification of Functioning.
- www.canchild.ca/Default.aspx?tabid=188&pid=0
  A site that provides information on outcome measures and products developed by CanChild researchers.
- www.tbims.org/combi
  A site that provides information on outcome measures for brain injuries.
- www.caretrak-outcomes.com
  A site that provides tools for evaluating spinal injuries and diseases (30-day free trial, paid subscription required).
- www.sf-36.org
  A community site that provides news, descriptive information, and demos on the SF tools and products.
- *The official Web site of the Disabilities of the Arm, Shoulder, Hand outcome measure*
  www.dash.iwh.on.ca
- www.csp.org.uk/director/effectivepractice/outcomemeasures.cfm
  A site with an online outcome measures database developed by the Chartered Society of Physiotherapy
- www.proqolid.org
  An online database developed by the Mapi Research Institute that provides descriptive information on QOL outcome instruments.
- *The official Web site of the EuroQol instrument*
  http://gs1.q4matics.com/EuroqolPublishWeb
- www.rand.org/health/surveys_tools.html
  A site that provides information on surveys and tools developed by RAND Health.
- http://phi.uhce.ox.ac.uk
  A site by the National Centre for Health Outcomes Development with a searchable database that provides information and guidance on the selection of patient-reported health measurements.

- www.cebp.nl/?NODE=77
  A site by the National Centre for Health Outcomes Development with a searchable database that provides information and guidance on the selection of patient-reported health measurements.

- http://davidmlane.com/hyperstat/index.html
  Free online stats textbook.

- http://statpages.org
  Free online stats calculations.

- http://nilesonline.com/stats
  Easy reading stats textbook.

Books That Focus on Outcome Assessment/Measures

Bolton, B. (Ed.). (2001). *Handbook of measurement and evaluation in rehabilitation* (3rd ed.). Gaithersburg, MD: Aspen Publication.

Dittmar, S., & Gresham, G. (Eds.). (2005). *Functional assessment and outcome measures for rehabilitation*. Austin: TX: PRO-ED Incorporated.

Enderby, P., John, A., & Petheram, B. (2006). *Therapy outcome measures for rehabilitation professions: speech and language therapy, physiotherapy, occupational therapy* (2nd ed.). Philadelphia: Wiley.

Fayers, P., & Hays, R. (2005). *Assessing quality of life in clinical trials* (2nd ed.). Oxford, UK: Oxford University Press.

Finch, E., Brooks, D., Stratford, P., & Mayo, N. (2002). *Physical rehabilitation outcomes measures: A guide to enhanced clinical decision-making*. Philadelphia: Lippincott Williams & Wilkins.

Hawkins, R. P., Mathews, J. R., & Hamdan, L. (1998). *Measuring behavioral health outcomes: A practical guide*. New York, NY: Kluwer Academic/Plenum Publishers.

Hutchinson, A., McColl, E., Christie, M., & Riccalton, C. (Eds.). (1996). *Health outcome measures in primary and out-patient care*. Amsterdam: Harwood Academic Publishers.

IsHak, W. W., Burt, T., & Sederer, L. (2002). *Outcome measurement in psychiatry: A critical review*. Washington, DC: American Psychiatric Publishing.

Johnson, C. E., & Danhauer, J. L. (2002). *Handbook of outcome measures in audiology*. Clifton Park, NY: Thomson Delmar Learning.

Laurent, D., Lynch, J., Ritter, P., Gonzalez, V., Stewart, A., & Lorig, K. (1996). *Outcome measures for health education and other health care interventions*. Thousand Oaks, CA: Sage Publications.

Law, M., Baum, C., & Dunn, W. (2005). *Measuring occupational performance: Supporting best practice in occupational therapy* (2nd ed.). Thorofare, NJ: SLACK Incorporated.

Law, M., King, G., Russell, D., Stewart, D., Hurley, P., & Bosch, E. (2000). *All about outcomes: An educational program to help you understand, evaluate, and choose adult outcome measures*. Thorofare, NJ: SLACK Incorporated.

Lenderking W. R., & Revicki, D. A. (2005) *Advancing health outcomes research methods and clinical applications. A publication of the International Society for Quality of Life Research*. McLean, VA: Degnon Associates, Inc.

McDowell, I. (2006). *Measuring health: A guide to rating scales and questionnaires* (3rd ed.). New York, NY: Oxford University Press.

References

Abrams, D., Davidson, M., Harrick, J., Harcourt, P., Zylinski, M., & Clancy, J. (2006). Monitoring the change: Current trends in outcome measure usage in physiotherapy. *Manual Therapy, 11*, 46-53.

Ackerman, I. N., Graves, S. E., Bennell, K. L., & Osborne, R. H. (2006). Evaluating quality of life in hip and knee replacement: Psychometric properties of the World Health Organization Quality of Life short version instrument. *Arthritis and Rheumatism, 55*, 583-590.

American Academy of Orthopaedic Surgeons. (2002). DASH normative scoring documentation and scores. Retrieved August 29, 2007, from http://www3.aaos.org/research/normstdy

Anderson, R. T., Aaronson, N. K., Bullinger, M., & McBee, W. L. (1996). A review of the progress toward developing health-related quality-of-life instruments for international clinical studies and outcomes research. *Pharmacoeconomics, 10*, 336-355.

Anderson, R. T., Aaronson, N. K., & Wilkin, D. (1993). Critical review of the international assessments of health-related quality of life. *Quality of Life Research, 2*(6), 369-395.

Atroshi, I., Gummesson, C., Andersson, B., Dahlgren, E., & Johansson, A. (2000). The disabilities of the arm, shoulder and hand (DASH) outcome questionnaire: reliability and validity of the Swedish version evaluated in 176 patients. *Acta Orthopaedica Scandinavica, 71*, 613-618.

Bakker, C. H., Rutten van Molken, M., van Doorslaer, E., Bennett, K., & van der Linden, S. (1993). Health related utility measurement in rheumatology: An introduction. *Patient Education and Counseling, 20*, 145-152.

Barbier, O., Penta, M., & Thonnard, J. L. (2003). Outcome evaluation of the hand and wrist according to the International Classification of Functioning, Disability, and Health. *Hand Clinics, 19*, vii, 371-378.

Bartko, J. J. (1976). On various intraclass correlation coefficients. *Psychological Bulletin, 83*, 762-765.

Beaton, D. E. (2000). Understanding the relevance of measured change through studies of responsiveness. *Spine, 25*, 3192-3199.

Beaton, D. E., Boers, M., & Wells, G. A. (2002). Many faces of the minimal clinically important difference (MCID): A literature review and directions for future research. *Current Opinion in Rheumatology, 14*, 109-114.

Beaton, D. E., Bombardier, C., Katz, J. N., & Wright, J. G. (2001). A taxonomy for responsiveness. *Journal of Clinical Epidemiology, 54*, 1204-1217.

Beaton, D. E., Katz, J. N., Fossel, A. H., Wright, J. G., Tarasuk, V., & Bombardier, C. (2001a). Measuring the whole or the parts? Validity, reliability, and responsiveness of the Disabilities of the Arm, Shoulder and Hand outcome measure in different regions of the upper extremity. *Journal of Hand Therapy, 14*, 128-146.

Beaton, D. E., Bombardier, C., Katz, J. N., Wright, J. G., Wells, G., Boers, M. et al. (2001b). Looking for important change/differences in studies of responsiveness. OMERACT MCID Working Group. Outcome Measures in Rheumatology. Minimal Clinically Important Difference. *Journal of Rheumatology, 28*, 400-405.

Bedard, D., Purden, M. A., Sauve-Larose, N., Certosini, C., & Schein, C. (2006). The pain experience of post-surgical patients following the implementation of an evidence-based approach. *Pain Management Nursing, 7*, 80-92.

Boadella, J. M., Sluiter, J. K., & Frings-Dresen, M. H. (2003). Reliability of upper extremity tests measured by the Ergos work simulator: A pilot study. *Journal of Occupational Rehabilitation, 13*, 219-232.

Bruce, B., & Fries, J. F. (2005). The Arthritis, Rheumatism and Aging Medical Information System (ARAMIS): Still young at 30 years. *Clinical and Experimental Rheumatology, 23*, S163-S167.

Carswell, A., McColl, M. A., Baptiste, S., Law, M., Polatajko, H., & Pollock, N. (2004). The Canadian Occupational Performance Measure: A research and clinical literature review. *Canadian Journal of Occupational Therapy, 71*, 210-222.

Centers for Disease Control and Prevention. (n.d.). *Health-related quality of life*. Retrieved August 29, 2007, from www.cdc.gov/hrqol

Chatman, A. B., Hyams, S. P., Neel, J. M., Binkley, J. M., Stratford, P. W., Schomberg, A., et al. (1997). The Patient-Specific Functional Scale: Measurement properties in patients with knee dysfunction. *Physical Therapy, 77*, 820-829.

Cieza, A., & Stucki, G. (2005). Content comparison of health-related quality of life (HRQOL) instruments based on the international classification of functioning, disability and health (ICF). *Quality of Life Research, 14*, 1225-1237.

Cohen, J. (1968). Weighted kappa: Nominal scale agreement with provision for scaled disagreement or partial credit. *Psychological Bulletin, 70,* 213-220.

Cohen, J. (1990). A coefficient of agreement for nominal scales. *Educational and Psychological Measures, 20,* 37-46.

Coldwells, A., Atkinson, G., & Reilly, T. (1994). Sources of variation in back and leg dynamometry. *Ergonomics, 37,* 79-86.

Dolan, P., Shaw, R., Tsuchiya, A., & Williams, A. (2005). QALY maximisation and people's preferences: A methodological review of the literature. *Health Economics, 14,* 197-208.

Dunckley, M., Aspinal, F., Addington-Hall, J. M., Hughes, R., & Higginson, I. J. (2005). A research study to identify facilitators and barriers to outcome measure implementation. *International Journal of Palliative Nursing, 11,* 218-5.

Dunckley, M., Hughes, R., Addington-Hall, J., & Higginson, I. J. (2003). Language translation of outcome measurement tools: Views of health professionals. *International Journal of Palliative Nursing, 9,* 49-55.

Feeny, D., Blanchard, C. M., Mahon, J. L., Bourne, R., Rorabeck, C., Stitt, L., et al. (2004). The stability of utility scores: Test-retest reliability and the interpretation of utility scores in elective total hip arthroplasty. *Quality of Life Research, 13,* 15-22.

Fries, J. F., Bruce, B., & Cella, D. (2005). The promise of PROMIS: Using item response theory to improve assessment of patient-reported outcomes. *Clinical and Experimental Rheumatology, 23,* S53-S57.

Fritz, J. M., Delitto, A., & Erhard, R. E. (2003). Comparison of classification-based physical therapy with therapy based on clinical practice guidelines for patients with acute low back pain: A randomized clinical trial. *Spine, 28,* 1363-1371.

Guyatt, G., Walter, S., & Norman, G. (1987). Measuring change over time: Assessing the usefulness of evaluative instruments. *Journal of Chronic Diseases, 40,* 171-178.

Hanestad, B. R., Rustoen, T., Knudsen, O., Jr., Lerdal, A., & Wahl, A. K. (2004). Psychometric properties of the WHOQOL-BREF questionnaire for the Norwegian general population. *Journal of Nursing Measurement, 12,* 147-159.

Harris, S. R., Swanson, M. W., Andrews, M. S., Sells, C. J., Robinson, N. M., Bennett, F. C., et al. (1984). Predictive validity of the "Movement Assessment of Infants." *Journal of Developmental and Behavioral Pediatrics, 5,* 336-342.

Heald, S. L., Riddle, D. L., & Lamb, R. L. (1997). The shoulder pain and disability index: The construct validity and responsiveness of a region-specific disability measure. *Physical Therapy, 77,* 1079-1089.

Horner, D., & Larmer, P. J. (2006). Health outcome measures. *New Zealand Journal of Physiotherapy, 34,* 17-24.

Huang, I. C., Wu, A. W., & Frangakis, C. (2006). Do the SF-36 and WHOQOL-BREF measure the same constructs? Evidence from the Taiwan population. *Quality of Life Research, 15,* 15-24.

Hwang, J. S., & Wang, J. D. (2004). Integrating health profile with survival for quality of life assessment. *Quality of Life Research, 13,* 1-10.

Initial steps to developing the World Health Organization's Quality of Life Instrument (WHOQOL) module for international assessment in HIV/AIDS. (2003). *AIDS Care, 15,* 347-357.

International Classification of Functioning, Disability and Health. (2003). Retrieved August 29, 2007, from http://www3.who.int/icf/icftemplate.cfm?myurl=homepage.html&mytitle=Home%20Page

Jaeschke, R., Singer, J., & Guyatt, G. H. (1989). Measurement of health status: Ascertaining the minimal clinically important difference. *Controlled Clinical Trials, 10,* 407-415.

Jang, Y., Hsieh, C. L., Wang, Y. H., & Wu, Y. H. (2004). A validity study of the WHOQOL-BREF assessment in persons with traumatic spinal cord injury. *Archives of Physical Medicine and Rehabilitation, 85,* 1890-1895.

Jette, A. M. (1999). Disentangling the process of disablement. *Social Science and Medicine, 48,* 471-472.

Kamath, V., & Stothard, J. (2003). A clinical questionnaire for the diagnosis of carpal tunnel syndrome. *Journal of Hand Surgery* (Edinburgh, Lothian), *28,* 455-459.

Kaplan, R. M., Alcaraz, J. E., Anderson, J. P., & Weisman, M. (1996). Quality-adjusted life years lost to arthritis: Effects of gender, race, and social class. *Arthritis Care and Research, 9,* 473-482.

Katz, J. N., & Stirrat, C. R. (1990). A self-administered hand diagram for the diagnosis of carpal tunnel syndrome. *Journal of Hand Surgery, 15,* 360-363.

Landis, J. R., & Koch, G. G. (1977). The measurement of observer agreement for categorical data. *Biometrics, 33,* 159-174.

Law, M., Baptiste, S., Carswell, A., McColl, M., Polatajko, H., & Pollock, N. (1998). *Canadian Occupational Performance Measure* (3rd ed.). Ottawa, ON: CAOT Publications.

Law, M., Baptiste, S., McColl, M., Opzoomer, A., Polatajko, H., & Pollock, N. (1990). The Canadian occupational performance measure: An outcome measure for occupational therapy. *Canadian Journal of Occupational Therapy, 57,* 82-87.

Law, M., Polatajko, H., Pollock, N., McColl, M. A., Carswell, A., & Baptiste, S. (1994). Pilot testing of the Canadian Occupational Performance Measure: Clinical and measurement issues. *Canadian Journal of Occupational Therapy, 61,* 191-197.

Lerner, D., Amick, B. C., Rogers, W. H., Malspeis, S., Bungay, K., & Cynn, D. (2001). The Work Limitations Questionnaire. *Medical Care, 39,* 72-85.

Lerner, D., Reed, J. I., Massarotti, E., Wester, L. M., & Burke, T. A. (2002). The Work Limitations Questionnaire's validity and reliability among patients with osteoarthritis. *Journal of Clinical Epidemiology, 55,* 197-208.

Li, L., Young, D., Xiao, S., Zhou, X., & Zhou, L. (2004). Psychometric properties of the WHO Quality of Life questionnaire (WHOQOL-100) in patients with chronic diseases and their caregivers in China. *Bulletin of the World Health Organization, 82,* 493-502.

Lin, T. H. (2006). Missing data imputation in Quality-of-Life Assessment: Imputation for WHOQOL-BREF. *Pharmacoeconomics, 24,* 917-925.

MacDermid, J. (2005). Update: The patient-rated forearm evaluation questionnaire is now the patient-rated tennis elbow evaluation. *Journal of Hand Therapy, 18,* 407-410.

MacDermid, J. C., Ramos, J., Drosdowech, D., Faber, K., & Patterson, S. (2004). The impact of rotator cuff pathology on isometric and isokinetic strength, function, and quality of life. *Journal of Shoulder and Elbow Surgery, 13,* 593-598.

MacDermid, J. C., Solomon, P., & Prkachin, K. (2006). The Shoulder Pain and Disability Index demonstrates factor, construct and longitudinal validity. *BMC Musculoskeletal Disorders, 7,* 12.

Maclure, M., & Willet, W. C. (1987). Misinterpretation and misuse of the kappa statistic. *Journal of Epidemiology, 126,* 161-168.

Marx, R. G., Bombardier, C., & Wright, J. G. (1999). What do we know about the reliability and validity of physical examination tests used to examine the upper extremity. *Journal of Hand Surgery, 24A,* 185-193.

Marx, R. G., Hogg-Johnson, S., Hudak, P., Beaton, D., Shields, S., Bombardier, C., et al. (2001). A comparison of patients' responses about their disability with and without attribution to their affected area. *Journal of Clinical Epidemiology, 54,* 580-586.

Mauthe, R. W., Haaf, D. C., Hayn, P., & Krall, J. M. (1996). Predicting discharge destination of stroke patients using a mathematical model based on six items from the Functional Independence Measure. *Archives of Physical Medicine and Rehabilitation, 77,* 10-13.

McColl, M. A., Paterson, M., Davies, D., Doubt, L., & Law, M. (2000). Validity and community utility of the Canadian Occupational Performance Measure. *Canadian Journal of Occupational Therapy, 67,* 22-30.

Michlovitz, S. L., LaStayo, P. C., Alzner, S., & Watson, E. (2001). Distal radius fractures: Therapy practice patterns. *Journal of Hand Therapy, 14,* 249-257.

Mokkink, L. B., Terwee, C. B., Knol, D. L., Stratford, P. W., Alonso, J., Patrick, D. L., et al. (2006). Protocol of the COSMIN study: Consensus-based standards for the selection of health measurement instruments. *BMC Medical Research Methodology, 6,* 2.

Morrey, B. F., An, K. N., & Chao, E. Y. S. (2000). Functional evaluation of the elbow. In B. F. Morrey (Ed.), *The elbow and its disorders* (2nd ed., pp. 86-97). Philadelphia, PA: W. B. Saunders.

Muller, R., & Buttner, P. (1995). A critical discussion of intraclass correlation coefficients. *Statistics in Medicine, 13*, 2465-2476.

National Cancer Institute. (n.d.). Dictionary of cancer terms. Retrieved October 22, 2007, from http://www.cancer.gov/templates/db_alpha.aspx?CdrID=45417

Naumann, V. J., & Byrne, G. J. (2004). WHOQOL-BREF as a measure of quality of life in older patients with depression. *International Psychogeriatrics, 16*, 159-173.

Newcomer, K. L., Martinez-Silvestrini, J. A., Schaefer, M. P., Gay, R. E., & Arendt, K. W. (2005). Sensitivity of the Patient-Rated Forearm Evaluation Questionnaire in lateral epicondylitis. *Journal of Hand Therapy, 18*, 400-406.

Norholm, V., & Bech, P. (2001). The WHO Quality of Life (WHOQOL) Questionnaire: Danish validation study. *Nordic Journal of Psychiatry, 55*, 229-235.

Ohaeri, J. U., Olusina, A. K., & Al Abassi, A. H. (2004). Factor analytical study of the short version of the World Health Organization Quality of Life Instrument. *Psychopathology, 37*, 242-248.

Overend, T. J., Wuori-Fearn, J. L., Kramer, J. F., & MacDermid, J. C. (1999). Reliability of a patient-rated forearm evaluation questionnaire for patients with lateral epicondylitis. *Journal of Hand Therapy, 12*, 31-37.

Post, M. W., de Witte, L. P., & Schrijvers, A. J. (1999). Quality of life and the ICIDH: Toward an integrated conceptual model for rehabilitation outcomes research. *Clinical Rehabilitation, 13*, 5-15.

Power, M., Harper, A., & Bullinger, M. (1999). The World Health Organization WHOQOL-100: Tests of the universality of Quality of Life in 15 different cultural groups worldwide. *Health Psychology, 18*, 495-505.

Power, M., Quinn, K., & Schmidt, S. (2005). Development of the WHOQOL-old module. *Quality of Life Research, 14*, 2197-2214.

PROMIS. (n.d.). Retrieved October 22, 2007, from http://www.nihpromis.org

Raeburn, J. M., & Rootman, I. (1996). Quality-of-life and health promotion. In R. Renwick, I. Brown, & M. Nagler (Eds.), *Quality-of-life and health promotion and rehabilitation: Conceptual approaches, issues and applications* (pp. 14-25). London: Sage Publications.

Richardson, G., & Manca, A. (2004). Calculation of quality adjusted life years in the published literature: a review of methodology and transparency. *Health Economics, 13*, 1203-1210.

Roach, K. E., Budiman-Mak, E., Songsiridej, N., & Lertratanakul, Y. (1991). Development of a shoulder pain and disability index. *Arthritis Care Research, 4*, 143-149.

Russell, L. B., Gold, M. R., Siegel, J. E., Daniels, N., & Weinstein, M. C. (1996). The role of cost-effectiveness analysis in health and medicine. Panel on Cost-Effectiveness in Health and Medicine. *Journal of the American Medical Association, 276*, 1172-1177.

Sackett, D. L., & Torrance, G. W. (1978). The utility of different health states as perceived by the general public. *Journal of Chronic Disability, 31*, 697-704.

Salter, K., Jutai, J. W., Teasell, R., Foley, N. C., & Bitensky, J. (2005). Issues for selection of outcome measures in stroke rehabilitation: ICF body functions. *Disability and Rehabilitation, 27*, 191-207.

Salter, K., Jutai, J. W., Teasell, R., Foley, N. C., Bitensky, J., & Bayley, M. (2005). Issues for selection of outcome measures in stroke rehabilitation: ICF participation. *Disability and Rehabilitation, 27*, 507-528.

Schasfoort, F. C., Bussmann, J. B., & Stam, H. J. (2000). Outcome measures for complex regional pain syndrome type I: An overview in the context of the international classification of impairments, disabilities and handicaps. *Disability and Rehabilitation, 22*, 387-398.

Schmitt, J. S., & Di Fabio, R. P. (2004). Reliable change and minimum important difference (MID) proportions facilitated group responsiveness comparisons using individual threshold criteria. *Journal of Clinical Epidemiology, 57*, 1008-1018.

Shreiner, S. C. (1980). Agreement or association: Choosing a measure of reliability for nominal data in the 2 x 2 case—A comparison of phi, kappa, and G. *International Journal of Addiction, 15*, 915-920.

Shrout, P. E., & Fleiss, J. L. (1979). Intraclass correlations: Uses in assessing rater reliability. *Psychological Bulletin, 86*, 420-428.

Skevington, S. M. (1999). Measuring quality of life in Britain: introducing the WHOQOL-100. *Journal of Psychosomatic Research, 47*, 449-459.

Skevington, S. M., Bradshaw, J., & Saxena, S. (1999). Selecting national items for the WHOQOL: Conceptual and psychometric considerations. *Social Science and Medicine, 48*, 473-487.

Skevington, S. M., Lotfy, M., & O'Connell, K. A. (2004). The World Health Organization's WHOQOL-BREF Quality of Life Assessment: Psychometric properties and results of the international field trial: A report from the WHOQOL group. *Quality of Life Research, 13*, 299-310.

Skevington, S. M., & O'Connell, K. A. (2004). Can we identify the poorest quality of life? Assessing the importance of quality of life using the WHOQOL-100. *Quality of Life Research, 13*, 23-34.

Skutek, M., Fremerey, R. W., Zeichen, J., & Bosch, U. (2000). Outcome analysis following open rotator cuff repair: Early effectiveness validated using four different shoulder assessment scales. *Archives of Orthopaedic and Trauma Surgery, 120*, 432-436.

Smith, R., & Dobson, M. (1993). Measuring utility values for QALYs: Two methodological issues. *Health Economics, 2*, 349-355.

Solway, S., Beaton, D. E., McConnell, S., & Bombardier, C. (2002). *The DASH outcome measure user's manual* (2nd ed.). Toronto, ON: Institute for Work and Health.

Stineman, M. G., Ross, R. N., Fiedler, R., Granger, C. V., & Maislin, G. (2003). Functional independence staging: Conceptual foundation, face validity, and empirical derivation. *Archives of Physical Medicine and Rehabilitation, 84*, 29-37.

Stratford, P., Levy, D. R., Gauldie, S., Levy, K., & Miseferi, D. (1987). Extensor carpi radialis tendonitis: A validation of selected outcome measures. *Physiotherapy Canada, 39*, 250-255.

Stratford, P. W., Levy, D. R., & Gowland, C. (1993). Evaluative properties of measures used to assess patients with lateral epicondylitis at the elbow. *Physiotherapy Canada, 45*(3):160-164.

Stucki, G., Cieza, A., Geyh, S., Battistella, L., Lloyd, J., Symmons, D., et al. (2004). ICF core sets for rheumatoid arthritis. *Journal of Rehabilitation Medicine*, 87-93.

Study protocol for the World Health Organization project to develop a quality of life assessment instrument (WHOQOL) (1993). *Quality of Life Research, 2*, 153-159.

The Upper Extremity Collaborative Group. (1999). Development of an upper extremity outcome measure: The "DASH" (Disabilities of the arm, shoulder and hand). *American Journal of Industrial Medicine, 29*, S112.

Tieman, B. L., Palisano, R. J., Gracely, E. J., & Rosenbaum, P. L. (2004). Gross motor capability and performance of mobility in children with cerebral palsy: a comparison across home, school, and outdoors/community settings. *Physical Therapy, 84*, 419-429.

Torrance, G. W. (1987). Utility approach to measuring health-related quality of life. *Journal of Chronic Diseases, 40*, 593-603.

Trompenaars, F. J., Masthoff, E. D., Van Heck, G. L., Hodiamont, P. P., & De Vries, J. (2005). Content validity, construct validity, and reliability of the WHOQOL-Bref in a population of Dutch adult psychiatric outpatients. *Quality of Life Research, 14*, 151-160.

Trudel, D., Duley, J., Zastrow, I., Kerr, E. W., Davidson, R., & MacDermid, J. C. (2004). Rehabilitation for patients with lateral epicondylitis: A systematic review. *Journal of Hand Therapy, 17*, 243-266.

Turchin, D. C., Beaton, D. E., & Richards, R. R. (1998). Validity of observer-based aggregate scoring systems as descriptors of elbow pain, function, and disability. *Journal of Bone and Joint Surgery, 80*, 154-162.

The Upper Extremity Collaborative Group. (1996). Measuring disability and symptoms of the upper limb: A validation study of the DASH questionnaire. *Arthritis & Rheumatism, 39*(9), S112.

Ventegodt, S., Merrick, J., & Andersen, N. J. (2003). Measurement of quality of life VI: Quality-adjusted life years (QALY) is an unfortunate use of the quality-of-life concept. *Scientific World Journal, 3*, 1015-1019.

Ware, J. E., Jr. (2003). Conceptualization and measurement of health-related quality of life: Comments on an evolving field. *Archives of Physical Medicine and Rehabilitation, 84,* S43-S51.

Ware, J. E., Jr., Gandek, B., Kosinski, M., Aaronson, N. K., Apolone, G., Brazier, J., et al. (1998). The equivalence of SF-36 summary health scores estimated using standard and country-specific algorithms in 10 countries: Results from the IQOLA Project. International Quality of Life Assessment. *Journal of Clinical Epidemiology, 51,* 1167-1170.

Ware, J. E., Jr., Kosinski, M., Gandek, B., Aaronson, N. K., Apolone, G., Bech, P., et al. (1998). The factor structure of the SF-36 Health Survey in 10 countries: Results from the IQOLA Project. International Quality of Life Assessment. *Journal of Clinical Epidemiology, 51,* 1159-1165.

Ware, J. E., Jr., & Sherbourne, C. D. (1992). The MOS 36-item short-form health survey (SF-36). I. Conceptual framework and item selection. *Medical Care, 30,* 473-483.

Weigl, M., Cieza, A., Harder, M., Geyh, S., Amann, E., Kostanjsek, N., et al. (2003). Linking osteoarthritis-specific health-status measures to the International Classification of Functioning, Disability, and Health (ICF). *Osteoarthritis and Cartilage, 11,* 519-523.

Westaway, M. D., Stratford, P. W., & Binkley, J. M. (1998). The patient-specific functional scale: Validation of its use in persons with neck dysfunction. *Journal of Orthopaedic and Sports Physical Therapy, 27,* 331-338.

WHOQOL Group. (1996). What quality of life? World Health Organization Quality of Life Assessment. *World Health Forum, 17,* 354-356.

WHOQOL Group. (1998a). Development of the World Health Organization WHOQOL-BREF Quality of Life Assessment. *Psychological Medicine, 28,* 551-558.

WHOQOL Group. (1998B). The World Health Organization Quality of Life Assessment (WHOQOL): Development and general psychometric properties. *Social Science and Medicine, 46,* 1569-1585.

World Health Organization. (n.d.). WHOQOL: measuring quality of life. Retrieved October 22, 2007, from http://www.who.int/entity/mental_health/media/68.pdf

Williams, J. I. (2000). Ready, set, stop: Reflections on assessing quality of life and the WHOQOL-100 (U.S. version). World Health Organization Quality of Life. *Journal of Clinical Epidemiology, 53,* 13-17.

Williams, J. W., Jr., Holleman, D. R., Jr., & Simel, D. L. (1995). Measuring shoulder function with the Shoulder Pain and Disability Index. *Journal of Rheumatology, 22,* 727-732.

World Health Organization. (1995). The World Health Organization Quality of Life Assessment (WHOQOL): Position paper from the World Health Organization. *Social Science and Medicine, 41,* 1403-1409.

Yao, G., & Wu, C. H. (2005). Factorial invariance of the WHOQOL-BREF among disease groups. *Quality of Life Research, 14,* 1881-1888.

Young, N. L., Williams, J. I., Yoshida, K. K., Bombardier, C., & Wright, J. G. (1996). The context of measuring disability: does it matter whether capability or performance is measured? *Journal of Clinical Epidemiology, 49,* 1097-1101.

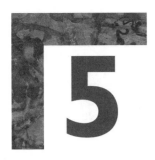

Asking Clinical Questions and Searching for the Evidence

Jennie Q. Lou, MD, MSc, OTR and Paola Durando, BA, MLS

Learning Objectives

After reading this chapter, the student/practitioner will be able to:

- Explain the origin of clinical research questions and identify the constituent elements of successful questions.
- Develop skills in generating answerable clinical questions when searching for evidence.
- Identify and understand the distinctions between various sources of evidence.
- Critically evaluate the value of Internet-based sources.
- Outline the key components and effective methods for a literature search.
- Describe different electronic databases and their various search mechanisms.

In our daily clinical practice, questions about the best care for our clients arise frequently. As the current best evidence on a given topic changes at an unpredictable rate, even the most experienced practitioners cannot assume that they know the answer without looking into the most current literature. It has become increasingly obvious that the pace of development of new evidence from research is too quick for standard textbooks to be dependable. When questions do arise, it is unlikely that they will be answered by these textbooks accurately and quickly. Fortunately, the advent of better research, better information resources, and better information technology makes it possible for us to respond to these challenges by learning some basic literature search skills and acquiring access to key evidence resources in the hospital, clinic, or at home. Figure 5-1 illustrates the steps in acquiring the evidence. This chapter will describe some of the skills and resources for answering questions of relevance to the care of clients in occupational and physical therapy practice.

Figure 5-1. Steps of acquiring the evidence.

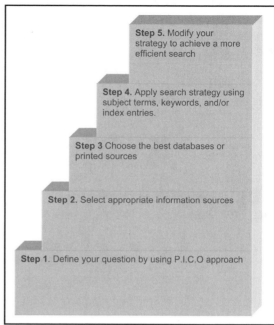

Step 5. Modify your strategy to achieve a more efficient search

Step 4. Apply search strategy using subject terms, keywords, and/or index entries.

Step 3 Choose the best databases or printed sources

Step 2. Select appropriate information sources

Step 1. Define your question by using P.I.C.O approach

Define Your Question by Using P.I.C.O. Approach

The first step for any evidence search is to formulate a "well-built question." This entails identifying a question that is important to the client's well being, is interesting to you, and that you are likely to encounter on a regular basis in your practice. For practical purposes, it is sometimes more efficient if you seek consultants for questions that you seldom address in your practice. The process of formulating an answerable question is a very critical step because the more clearly you can state your question the more likely your will be able to obtain answers that are directly relevant to your clinical situation.

Where Does the Question Come From?

The most common origin of questions is *professional practice*. For example, you may have a client who has a specific visual perceptual problem and you do not know how to treat him or her, and none of your colleagues are able to help. You could develop a clinical question based on the clinical situation, such as what is the most appropriate intervention for your client. Another common source for questions is *professional trends*. For example, in occupational therapy there is a push to understand "the form, function, and meaning of occupation" (Zemke & Clark, 1996). From this knowledge, you could form a question to develop a better understanding of a particular occupation. You may also develop a question from the *existing published research.* For example, reading an article in an occupational or physical therapy journal might raise more questions for you. You could use one of these questions to further explore the literature. Alternatively, you might read a body of literature, realize that there are gaps in your knowledge, and develop a question to explore one of these gaps in more details. *Existing theory is another area where questions can be developed*. For example, you might use a particular model and frame of reference in practice, and want to critically compare it to what happens in the real world. You could develop a question based on your own curiosity. For the purpose of this book, the following discussion will focus on questions that are generated from clinical practice.

How to Formulate an Answerable Question

One of the benefits of forming a careful and thoughtful question is to make the search for evidence easier. The well-built question makes it relatively straightforward to elicit and combine the appropriate terms needed in the query language. To be answerable, the question must be specified clearly so that it includes (a) a specific client group or population; (b) the assessment, treatment, or other clinical issues that you are addressing; (c) the comparison; and (d) the outcome in which you are interested. Basically, when you develop the question, you are preparing a checklist or writing a search strategy for your literature search. Essentially, you must convert a gap in your knowledge into a precise question so that you can then seek the best answer for it.

In practice, well-built clinical questions usually contain four elements—*client/population (P), intervention or exposure (I), comparison (C), and outcome (O).* This is a way of breaking down a clinical problem into a question that can be answered. P.I.C.O. is a mnemonic used to describe these four elements; we sometimes refer to this as the anatomy of a question. If you use this "anatomy," it will help you become more clear about the question you are trying to answer and facilitate in identifying elements that are of particular importance. Clinical Scenario #1 is used as an example to take you through the question-developing process.

> ## Clinical Scenario #1
> Recently, several elderly clients have suffered falls, leading to hospital admissions and surgery. The clients, although frail, had all been self-caring before their falls. Getting them back to their own homes was a slow process and two have ended up in long-term institutional care. You wonder if there is a benefit in initiating a program to prevent elderly clients from falls at homes.

Patient/Population/Problem

Who or what is your question about? In EBP, this involves defining the client/patient as a member of a population in terms of the most important characteristics of the patient/population/problem such as disease, age, sex, ethnic group, etc. But it could also deal with any aspect of health care delivery (e.g., how do we manage our appointments system?). Remember that the articles you search for should be explicit in describing the criteria used to select their subjects. In real life, however, you would be very lucky to find a study that selected exactly the sort of situation you are dealing with. Therefore, you always need to keep this question in mind, "Are the subjects in this study so different from my situation that I cannot generalize its findings?"

P	I	C	O
Elderly clients who live independently at home			

Intervention

Intervention is what you wish to do. This covers anything you plan to do. It also involves what you may be doing at present and wish to assess. This would be therapy (e.g., choice of specific intervention), assessments (e.g., which specific assessment tool is more appropriate to use for your client with visual perceptual deficits?), preventative measures (e.g., counseling on lifestyle or risk factors), and/or management (e.g., when to refer your client to a cardiac rehabilitation program). You may wish to look for a comparison of two or more interventions, particularly to see if some innovative intervention is "better" than your current practice or beats the accepted "gold standard."

P	I	C	O
Elderly clients who live independently at home	Fall prevention program		

Comparison

Is there an alternative intervention to compare, or a no-treatment control group? Please note that your <u>clinical question does not have to always have a specific comparison</u>.

P	I	C	O
Elderly clients who live independently at home	Fall prevention program	Education on safety at home upon discharge from acute care	

Outcomes

Outcomes are what you wish to achieve. This may also include possible adverse effects you wish to avoid or minimize. Prevention of disability, recovery of function, and saving of time, money, and effort are some examples of outcomes. Remember that outcomes should define something that is important to the client, such as recovery of function (e.g., combing hair), rather than merely of interest to the health care providers, such as controlling upper extremity spasticity.

P	I	C	O
Elderly clients who live independently at home	Fall prevention program	Education on safety at home upon discharge from acute care	Decreased incidence of falls at home

Once you have listed the three (or four) elements of the question, the question should be fairly straightforward.

P	I	C	O
Elderly clients who live independently at home	Fall prevention program	Education on safety at home upon discharge from acute care	Decreased incidence of falls at home

Question 1: Is a fall prevention program more effective than education upon discharge from an acute care in decreasing the incidence of falls in elderly clients who live independently at home?

OR, if you do not use a comparison,

Question 2: Does a fall prevention program decrease the incidence of falls in elderly clients who live independently at home?

When preparing your question, remember that your question should be *relevant, direct and clear,* and *focused.* A common mistake that clinicians often make is to seek answers to questions about a whole process of care rather than a focused clinical issue. Searching for answer to a generic question is often very difficult. Rather than asking, "What is the impact of a rehabilitation program on the quality of life for my clients?," the clinician may ask, "Can the incidence of falls be decreased by a fall prevention program?" Another example would be instead of asking, "Is occupational therapy effective in treating children with autism?," the clinician may ask, "Does sensory integration improve social behavior in children with autism?" Questions do not have to relate specifically to intervention but can also address issues of prevention, prognosis, or diagnosis. For example, does a chronic disease self-management program prevent falls for older adults?

SELECT APPROPRIATE INFORMATION SOURCES

Now that you have developed the answerable question, you will need to identify different sources for your search. During your search, you must be able to organize and evaluate the information that you have obtained. A big part of this process is distinguishing relevant from irrelevant information and deciding which source contains the best and most credible information. This can be a daunting task for people who are relatively unfamiliar with scholarly publications. The purpose of the following section is to help you identify different types of scholarly publications and to give you some guidelines for determining their relative merit.

Types of Scholarly Publications

There are three basic types of scholarly publications—*books, non–peer-reviewed journals and professional magazines,* and *peer-reviewed journals.*

Books

Books can be focused on a single specialty topic (e.g., activity analysis) or they can be more general in nature (e.g., aging in Canadian society). Books may or may not be peer reviewed. The credibility of books may be judged by the credentials of the author(s), the reputation of the publisher, the reputation of the author of the preface, the reviews of the book from other reputable sources, the targeted audience (general public versus specific professionals), and the quality, currency, and the extent of the citations.

Non-Peer-Reviewed Journals and Professional Magazines

In non-peer-reviewed publications, an author submits a paper and it may or may not be reviewed by the editor and/or the editorial staff of the publication. While many non–peer-reviewed publications are of high quality, it is unwise to depend solely on these sources for the evidence to answer to your clinical question. Non–peer-reviewed publications tend to have faster turnover of papers (i.e., they get into print faster); therefore, while they can be useful for learning about current trends and controversies in your field of interest, they may not meet the same scientific scrutiny of peer-reviewed papers. Remember that non–peer-reviewed publications can be biased toward a targeted audience.

Peer-Reviewed Journals

Generally speaking, the articles published in peer-reviewed journals are considered more accurate and relevant. They are usually of a higher quality than those in non-peer-reviewed publications. All of the articles, usually with the exception of editorials, have been scrutinized by experts in the field for accuracy of content, quality of research, and relevance to the field. It should also be realized that some peer-reviewed journals are considered to be of higher quality than others.

Types of Articles in Peer-Reviewed Journals

- *Short reports:* Short reports tend to describe new or developing programs, projects, or treatment techniques. They are also used to present results of research pilot studies and preliminary results from ongoing research. These reports tend to provide the latest advances in a particular area.

- *Editorials:* In many peer-reviewed journals, editorials are invited papers written by experts in the field. They tend to raise important issues for the field, offer perspectives on controversial subjects, suggest gaps in current knowledge, or propose visionary directions for the future. Because editorials are usually written by an expert in the field, they tend to be useful when developing a background or rationale for proposals. However, these need to be assessed with great care since there are many editorials written that oppose each other even in the most prestigious journals.

- *Systematic reviews:* Generally speaking, systematic reviews are full-length articles that undergo full peer review. They can be critical reviews of the literature or meta-analyses of existing research. A systematic review is an overview of primary research studies that reach specific standards in terms of methodology. These reviews should be explicit about how the reviewers located the studies and which exclusion and inclusion criteria they used. A meta-analysis is a mathematical synthesis of the results of two or more primary studies that address the same research question and that use comparable methodologies. Systematic reviews usually provide broad background information and pre-appraised material for your question. This can be a very efficient and effective way to use systematic reviews to find an answer to your clinical question; however, you need to be aware of the limitations of systemic reviews (e.g., reviewer's bias, missing evidence). When there is any chance it may be available, clinicians should seek a high-quality systematic review rather than the primary studies addressing their clinical question. You can read more information about systematic reviews in Chapter 7.

- *Books and technology reviews:* Book and technology reviews are usually invited critiques of new resources that are available. Generally speaking, the authors have some degree of expertise in the field specific to the content of the reviewed resource. These reviews provide information on the newest resource materials in a particular area. However, like any review, even distinguished scholars may have opposing views.

- *Research articles:* There are many types of research articles and many topologies to describe them. Other chapters in this book provide details on the format of research articles and how to evaluate their quality. These articles provide information on the newest scientific findings and advances in a particular area.

Electronic Bibliographic Databases and the World Wide Web

It is very important to distinguish between electronic bibliographic database searches and general searches on the World Wide Web. Electronic bibliographic databases are compilations of published research, scholarly articles, books, government reports, newspaper articles, etc. There are different databases, and each database has a particular focus. For example, MEDLINE is an index of medical and biomedical publications, CINAHL focuses on publications from the allied health profession, ERIC focuses on materials from the field of education, AgeLine focuses on publications relating to older adults and aging, and SUMSearch provides a source of easy-to-read broad discussions of topics from multiple disciplines. It is important to know what databases are available and on what topics they focus. The information can usually be obtained from your local librarian or by reviewing the HELP section of the database. Most electronic bibliographic databases are international in scope, and as a result, will provide you with publications that are written in English as well as other languages.

In comparison to an electronic bibliographic database, the *World Wide Web* is made up of interconnected documents that are available through the Internet. The Internet contains a vast amount of information on just about any subject. Searching the World Wide Web will not limit you to published articles. Although you may find an article published on the Web, you will also find program descriptions, personal opinions, government documents, information on businesses, organizations, and agencies, etc.

There are many different types of information available on the Web, but most Web pages can be categorized into types such as news and current events, business and marketing, informational, advocacy, or personal. Table 5-1 provides the function and examples of different type Web sites. Remember that Web browsers such as Netscape and Internet Explorer simply go to Web addresses and are search engines that simply look for terms that you designate. It is crucial for you to understand that they do not evaluate the accuracy or value of the Web sites, and there are sites that contain inaccurate, out-of-date, or false information. You are responsible for determining the usefulness of the sites. Figure 5-2 presents three steps for evaluating Web sites. Many of the same criteria for judging library databases and resources can also be used for Web sites. *Relevancy* has been important in judging other kinds of information sources, and the relevance of Web sites accessed is also important when searching the Internet. Besides relevancy, you also need to evaluate the web site for its authority, accuracy, objectivity, currency, and commercialism. Table 5-2 provides a checklist of the questions you can ask yourself at each step as you evaluate a Web page.

You probably have noticed that the greatest advantage of the Internet is that some portion of the world's literature has been made conveniently available to you. You also need to keep in mind that a major disadvantage is that quality control simply does not exist. There are two major problems with searching the World Wide Web as part of a literature review. The first problem is narrowing your search enough to find useful information, and the second problem is identifying which sites are credible. Anyone can have a Web site or a Web page. Not all information that is taken off the World Wide Web can be considered credible, reliable, or even correct. As a result, it is important to have strict criteria for selecting sites to review. Generally speaking, it is a good idea to limit your searches initially to government, university, and professional association Web sites.

Google Scholar, located at http://scholar.google.com, is a free search engine that is useful for discovering, browsing, and quickly locating highly cited articles. For complete literature searches and literature reviews, you will obtain more current, comprehensive, and focused results using bibliographic citation databases.

CHOOSE THE BEST DATABASES OR PRINTED SOURCES: CONDUCTING A LITERATURE SEARCH

Ways of Searching

Once you have formulated a clinical question, you are ready to plan a literature search strategy to find specific information that will answer your question. After identifying your search sources, it is effective to identify your search terms (subject headings and keywords) before you begin to

Table 5-1

TYPES OF WEB SITES AND THEIR FUNCTIONS

Type of Sites	Function and Examples
News and current events	• Provide extremely up-to-date information • Include news centers, newspapers, and other periodicals • Examples include www.cbc.ca, www.cnn.com, and *The New York Times*
Business and marketing	• Usually are published by companies or other commercial enterprises • Primary purpose is to promote the company or to sell products • Often include a mixture of information, entertainment, and propaganda • For United States-based sites, the URL or Web address usually ends in .com • Examples include Microsoft (www.msn.com) and Indigo (www.indigo.ca)

Informational	• Often provided by government (.gov) or educational institutions (.edu)
	• Provide factual information on a particular topic
	• May include reference materials, research reports, databases, calendars of events, statistics, etc.
	• Examples include the following:
	  ◦ The National Institute of Health (www.nih.gov)
	  ◦ National Library of Medicine (www.nlm.nih.gov)
	  ◦ Canadian Occupational Therapy Association (www.caot.org)
	  ◦ Harvard University (www.harvard.edu)

Advocacy	• Usually are published by an organization with the purpose of influencing public opinion • Examples: Disabled Woman's Network (http://dawn.thot.net) and Advocacy Centre for Canadian Seniors (www.advocacycentreelderly.org)
Personal	• Are published by individuals who may or may not be part of a larger group or organization • May include almost any type of information, including biographical data, information on work, hobbies, etc. • For United States-based sites, the URL often includes a tilde (~) • Examples include individual or family home pages, individual faculty or students at a university, and member pages from an Internet service provider
Others	• Such as entertainment

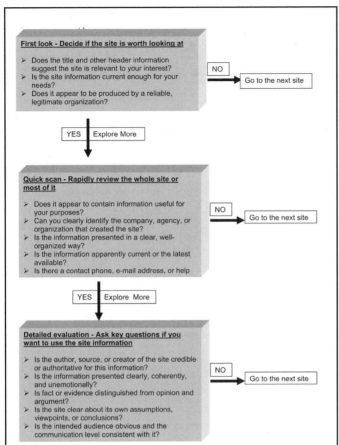

Figure 5-2. Three steps for evaluating Web sites.

search the bibliographic databases. Search terms can come from your clinical scenario and from background reading (e.g., books, Web sites, review articles). If necessary, you can use exclusion criteria or limiters to reduce the database search results to a small list of relevant citations. Evidence searching is done primarily by using the following methods/tools:

- Searching electronic bibliographic databases (e.g., MEDLINE, CINAHL, Healthstar, PsycINFO, ERIC, OTseeker, PEDro, etc.)
- Manually searching through specific journals (e.g., a journal that you know publishes materials in your areas of interest)
- Retrieving articles listed in the reference lists of articles that you already have on your topic of interest
- Searching the World Wide Web

A comprehensive literature search will probably use all of these methods/tools in an iterative fashion. There are two main goals to always keep in mind when you perform your searches:

- Increase the likelihood of retrieving relevant items—*sensitivity*
- Increase the likelihood of excluding irrelevant items—*specificity*

If you are doing a search and it yields an unmanageably large number of hits, you probably need to increase the specificity of your search. On the other hand, if you get too small a number of hits, you probably need to increase sensitivity or to broaden your search. Table 5-3 provides some tips on increasing specificity and sensitivity in your searches. Remember, an effective

Table 5-2

CHECKLIST OF QUESTIONS YOU CAN ASK YOURSELF AT EACH STEP AS YOU EVALUATE A WEB PAGE

Authority: Check who is responsible for the page and what their qualifications and associations are.

- Who is sponsoring the site? Authors and creators of Web sites should be clearly stated within the sites and means should be included for contacting them and/or the webmaster. Any commercial or organizational affiliations should also be included.
- What are the goals and/or values of the person/organization?
- What makes the author(s) an authority on this subject?
- Does the author(s) site his or her experience/credentials?
- Is he or she accredited or endorsed by a reputable organization?
- If the site contains articles, do they contain footnotes? If so, does material taken from other sources appear to be fully credited?

Accuracy: Try to determine the sources for the information at the site.

- Are the facts verifiable?
- Are the sources of information cited, and are individual articles signed and attributed?
- How is the information presented (i.e., fact, opinion, propaganda, etc.)? If presented as fact, is it accurate?

Objectivity: Look for the presence of bias and consider the impact of any stated affiliations on the possible attitudes about the topic.

- What is the purpose of the site? Consider the seven types of Web pages listed previously and consider whether the page is trying to entertain, inform, persuade, or advertise.
- Is there a bias (cultural, political, religious, etc.)? If so, is the bias clearly stated?

Currency: Consider how old the information is.

- Is the date of the last revision posted anywhere on the page?
- What is the date of the last revision?
- How frequently is it updated?
- Is some of the information out of date?

Scope, Coverage, and Relevance: Consider the scope of the site and its focus.

- What kind of information does it have and does this meet your needs? Who is the intended audience (general, specialized readership, scholars, etc.)?
- What is the level of the material (basic, advanced, etc.)?
- What time period is covered?
- What geographical area is covered?
- Is this information a subset of a more comprehensive source?

Commercialism

- Is the presenter selling something (i.e., a product, a philosophy, himself/herself)?
- Does the page have a corporate sponsor?
- Are there any hidden costs?
- Do you have to enter personal identification in order to proceed?

Table 5-3

STRATEGIES FOR EFFECTIVE SEARCHING ELECTRONIC DATABASES

Too many articles? You can increase specificity by narrowing or refining your search:

- Narrow your question.
- Use more specific search terms.
- Search using subject headings (controlled vocabulary) rather than keywords (free text/textword searching).
- Apply subheadings to subject headings to limit results to certain aspects of your topic.
- Combine terms using AND to represent other aspects of the question.
- Apply limiters such as English language, human subject, age group, publication type (e.g., review articles, RCTs, etc), country, or years of publication.

Too few articles? You can increase sensitivity by broadening your search:

- Broaden your question.
- Find more search terms from relevant records.
- Try different combinations of terms.
- Use truncation (* or $) in keyword searching to retrieve variant word endings.
- Add synonymous and related terms and combine them using OR.
- Use both subject heading and keywords as search terms.
- Use the Explode feature of subject heading searches.
- Apply all subheadings (or qualifiers) to subject headings.
- Search further back in time.
- Include all publication types.

Do not forget to use the Help function of the database to increase your searching effectiveness!

evidence search is not an aimless and tangential hunt with the hopes of finding something that might be useful—*systematic, explicit,* and *reproducible* are the guiding principles!

An effective search is:

- Guided by a specific answerable question or series of questions
- Completed in a systematic and methodological manner
- Documented explicitly
- Reproducible on subsequent days or by other people

Different Databases

There are numerous electronic bibliographic databases that can be used to conduct a search. Some are available on the "open Web" for free, while others are commercial and must be accessed through an institutional (library, university, hospital, professional association, etc.) or individual subscription.

MEDLINE

What Is MEDLINE?

MEDLINE is an electronic bibliographic database produced by the U.S. National Library of Medicine. Updated almost daily, it is widely recognized as the premier source for bibliographic and abstract coverage of a wide range of literature. MEDLINE encompasses the fields of medicine, nursing, rehabilitation therapy, allied health, dentistry, veterinary medicine, the health care system, and the preclinical sciences. More than 13 million records from more than 4,600 biomedical journals are indexed. Abstracts are included for more than 75% of the records. Although the majority of the records in MEDLINE relate to journal articles, the database also includes bibliographic details of systematic reviews, RCTs, and guidelines. Because the database is so large and comprehensive, MEDLINE is often a good place to start a search, as you will usually find something on your topic of interest.

MEDLINE can be accessed through the Web site of most medical libraries and coverage dates back to 1966. A separate database, OLDMEDLINE, indexes the period 1950 through 1965. The U.S. National Library of Medicine provides free access to MEDLINE through PubMed at www.ncbi.nlm.nih.gov. Because MEDLINE is sold to various database providers, you may find that the MEDLINE database looks different depending on where you use it as libraries offer different interfaces for database searching. Generally speaking, the information is the same and it is only the interface (i.e., the way you interact with the database) that differs.

How to Search MEDLINE

There are basically two ways of searching databases like MEDLINE: keyword or subject heading. Keyword searching, also known as text word or free text searching, is a method of searching by using words and phrases from the title, abstract, and keywords of references. There are some problems with this method of searching as the database will search for only exactly what you type in and does not automatically allow for variant spellings, plurals, and so on. In a keyword search, the database scans its records to see if any contain that exact term; therefore, if you enter the word therapy, you will retrieve citations containing the word therapy but not therapist or therapeutic. Compare the following book titles:

- *Motor control: Theory and practical applications*

- *Proprioception and neuromuscular control in joint stability*

- *Neurological rehabilitation: Optimizing motor performance*

These three books discuss the same general topic of motor function; however, the authors used different words to express this concept. Using a keyword search, you would need to search for these items using all the possible synonyms and word endings. On the other hand, using the Medical Subject Heading (MeSH) *motor skills* would retrieve all of these books regardless of the titles or authors' choice of wording. Similarly, the subject heading *musculoskeletal equilibrium* will retrieve citations containing the terms postural equilibrium or postural balance.

Most databases have some form of indexing system. MEDLINE's is called *MeSH*, short for Medical Subject Headings. This is a bit like the index at the back of a book. It attempts to solve the problems of different authors using different terms to describe the same concept or process. MeSH contains 23,000 subject headings. Each of these subject headings, or descriptors, represents a single concept appearing in the health care literature. A new MeSH is created as important new concepts appear. When a new citation is added to MEDLINE, indexers and subject specialists choose and apply the appropriate MeSH (usually 10 to 20) to represent the contents of the article.

You do not need to know the MeSH for your topic when you start a MEDLINE search. When you enter a keyword in Ovid MEDLINE, the interface will intuitively suggest appropriate MeSH. Another technique for finding MeSH is to look at what MeSH were assigned to relevant articles on your topic. Although using MeSH terms is a more precise and complete way of searching, there may be times when there is no MeSH available for the subject you are searching and you will need to search using keywords. For example, there is no MeSH that represents the concept of human occupation. However, there is a CINAHL (Cumulative Index to Nursing & Allied Health) subject heading: "occupation (human)."

MeSH are arranged into hierarchical structures called trees, starting with broad terms that branch off and become increasingly narrower with more specific terms. The tree structure of MeSH allows you to explode your search, which is less dangerous than it sounds! This means that you can search for a MeSH plus all its narrower terms simultaneously. For example, if you wanted to run a comprehensive search for citations relating to rehabilitation of the hearing impaired, you could explode the MeSH *rehabilitation of hearing impaired* to include all narrower terms:

- *Rehabilitation of Hearing Impaired*
  - *Communication Methods, Total*
  - *Lipreading*
  - *Manual Communication*

How to Refine Your Search

Some MEDLINE searches are very precise and neat. You may have a very specific MeSH term that retrieves a small and very well-focused set of about 20 citations that you can scan for applicability. Most of the time, it is not that simple and you will have to plan and execute a search strategy. To show that MEDLINE can become overwhelming, perform a MeSH search on Alzheimer's disease and see how many citations come up. Now try something different. Before you run the search, scroll down to the "Limits" tick boxes. There are a number of limiters, or filters, here that allow you to restrict the citations to those in English, those with an abstract, or those dealing with human subjects. How many of the articles on Alzheimer's disease that are in English *and* contain an abstract *and* deal with human studies now appear? You can also choose the years you wish to search, and you can restrict to certain age group (e.g., infants, adolescents, adults), language, date, male or female study participants, and publication types (e.g., review articles or randomized trials). By adding the limits, you are decreasing your search results. This can be especially useful if you are not doing a comprehensive literature review. Table 5-3 provides some tips on how to narrow or broaden your search. Aside from subject or topical searches, you can also search for specific authors, journal titles, or article titles.

CINAHL

The Cumulative Index to Nursing & Allied Health (CINAHL) database, which is located at www.cinahl.com or through institutional subscription, provides authoritative coverage of the literature related to nursing and allied health, including physical therapy, occupational therapy, and health education. More than 1,600 journals are regularly indexed, and online abstracts are available for more than 1,500 of these titles. New citations are added to the CINAHL database weekly. CINAHL uses CINAHL subject headings to index its literature, and over 70% of CINAHL subject headings are the same as MeSH. The other CINAHL headings were developed to reflect the terminology used by nursing and allied health professionals.

Ovid

Ovid, which is located at www.ovid.com, is a database provider for a collection of health and life sciences databases. Depending on your institution's subscription, it may include CINAHL (Cumulative Index to Nursing & Allied Health), EBM Reviews—Cochrane Database of

Systemic Reviews, EMBASE Drugs & Pharmacology, Health and Psychosocial Instruments (HAPI), HealthSTAR, MEDLINE, SPORTDiscus, and other databases.

Although you may simultaneously search several Ovid databases, it is unadvisable to do so because subject headings may differ between databases. For example, if you search CINAHL using the subject heading *assistive technology devices* and explode the term to include the more specific headings *ambulation aids, communication aids for disabled, limb prosthesis,* and *wheelchairs,* you will retrieve thousands of citations. If you search MEDLINE, a much larger database, using the same term, you will obtain zero results. MEDLINE does not recognize the CINAHL subject heading *assistive technology devices* because it uses the MeSH *self-help devices.* Later in this chapter there is a step-by-step search using Ovid for information that answers the question developed from Clinical Scenario #1.

The Cochrane Library

The Cochrane Library is a primary source for clinical effectiveness information. It contains four databases and several other useful sources of information. It is available through institutional subscription and may be offered at your institution on the Ovid interface.

Cochrane Database of Systematic Reviews

The Cochrane Database of Systematic Reviews (CDSR) contains the full text of systematic reviews undertaken by the Cochrane Collaboration, an international network of individuals and institutions committed to preparing, maintaining, and disseminating systematic reviews of the effects of health care. All reviews are updated as new studies are identified. CDSR contains completed reviews and protocols of reviews in progress.

Database of Abstracts of Reviews of Effectiveness

Database of Abstracts of Reviews of Effectiveness (DARE) is a full text database containing critical assessments of systematic reviews from a variety of medical journals. DARE records cover topics such as diagnosis, prevention, rehabilitation, screening, and treatment. Produced by the NHS (National Health Services) Centre for Reviews and Dissemination (CRD) at York, UK, the database includes structured abstracts of reviews identified and appraised by the CRD. DARE is also available on the World Wide Web, along with the CRD's NHS Economic Evaluations Database (NEED) at www.york.ac.uk/inst/crd/crddatabases.htm.

Cochrane Central Register of Controlled Trials

The Cochrane Central Register of Controlled Trials (CCTR) contains bibliographic references to over 300,000 controlled trials in health care. It is now the greatest single source of clinical trials.

Cochrane Review Methodology Database

This database contains references to articles and books on carrying out systematic reviews.

Other Useful Sources Of Information

The Cochrane Library includes additional information relevant to clinical effectiveness and EBP:

- *About the Cochrane Collaboration* at www.cochrane.org
  From here, you can access a range of information about the Cochrane Collaboration, including details of their Collaborative Review Groups, Methods Working Groups, networks, and centers.

- *Netting the Evidence* at www.shef.ac.uk/scharr/ir/netting
  This is a guide to sources of evidence on the Internet, compiled by Andrew Booth who is the Director of Information Resources at the School of Health and Related Research (ScHARR) at the University of Sheffield, UK.

- *INAHTA Technology Assessments*
  These are abstracts of technology assessments undertaken by members of the International Network of Agencies for Health Technology Assessment (INAHTA). This information is also available from the NHSCRD web site.

OTDBASE

OTDBASE, located at www.otdbase.org, is an occupational therapy journal literature search service that contains abstracts from 23 international occupational therapy journals dating back to 1970. It is accessible to individuals or institutions on an annual subscription basis.

OTSearch

OTSearch, formerly known as OT Bibsys, is an occupational therapy bibliographic database maintained by the American Occupational Therapy Association. It covers literature in occupational therapy and related subject areas such as rehabilitation, education, psychiatry or psychology, and health care delivery or administration. Author abstracts are included when available. OTSearch is only available through individual or institutional subscription.

OTSeeker

OTSeeker, located at www.otseeker.com, contains abstracts of systematic reviews and RCTs relevant to occupational therapy. Trials have been critically appraised and rated. It started in 2002 as collaboration between Australian universities and associations and is freely available on the Web.

PEDro

PEDro, located at www.pedro.fhs.usyd.edu.au/index.html, is intended to improve access to the results of physical therapy RCTs, systematic reviews, and evidence-based clinical practice guidelines. Most trials have been rated for quality. PEDro was created by the Centre for Evidence-Based Physiotherapy in Australia and is supported by various other organizations such as the Cochrane Collaboration. Updated monthly, it contains 6,000 records and is freely available on the Web.

RehabDATA

RehabData, located at www.naric.com/research, contains 70,000 abstracts of books, reports, articles, and audiovisual materials relating to disability and rehabilitation research. It is produced by the National Rehabilitation Information Center in Maryland and is freely available on the Web.

Center for International Rehabilitation Research Information & Exchange

The Center for International Rehabilitation Research Information & Exchange (CIRRIE) is located at http://cirrie.buffalo.edu. At the University at Buffalo, State University of New York, CIRRIE's mission is to facilitate the sharing of information and expertise in rehabilitation research between the United States and other countries. It maintains a bibliographic database of references to published reports of rehabilitation research published outside of the United States. CIRRIE is freely available on the Web.

OT CATS

OT CATs (Occupational Therapy Critically Appraised Topics) is located at www.otcats.com. Supported by the University of Western Sydney, the CATS (short, less rigorous versions of systematic reviews) have not been formally peer reviewed other than by the site developer, Dr. Annie McCluskey. It is freely available on the Web.

Critically Appraised Topics in Rehabilitation Therapy

Critically Appraised Topics in Rehabilitation Therapy, located at www.rehab.queensu.ca/cats, are mini versions of systematic reviews developed by students at Queen's University at Kingston, Canada. The site's aims are to illustrate the skills required for EBP and to communicate "bottom lines" for some clinical questions of interest to occupational therapists and physical therapists. It is freely available on the Web.

SUMSearch

SUMSearch, located at http://sumsearch.uthscsa.edu, is suitable for quickly but not necessarily accurately searching a variety of sources including PubMed, DARE, reviews, and guidelines. Developed at the University of Texas Health Sciences Center, it is freely available on the Web.

Combined Health Information Database

Combined Health Information database (CHID), located at http://chid.nih.gov, is a free bibliographic database produced by health-related agencies of the U.S. Federal Government. This database provides titles, abstracts, education resources, health promotion, and program descriptions that are not indexed elsewhere.

Turning Research Into Practice

Turning Research Into Practice (TRIP), located at www.tripdatabase.com, is a meta search tool that brings together evidence from systematic reviews, peer-reviewed journals, guidelines, textbooks, medical images, and patient information leaflets. It is available by subscription.

All About Outcomes

Developed at McMaster University, Hamilton, Ontario, Canada, *All About Outcomes* is not a citation database but rather computerized, multimedia software programs for practitioners working in rehabilitation with pediatrics, adults, and seniors. These two CD-ROMs enable the user to select the most appropriate outcome measure to use for an individual, client, service, and/or program evaluation. These programs guide the user through a protocol for making decisions about outcomes developed using a modified version of the International Classification of Impairment, Disability, and Handicap (ICIDH) framework. These software programs are linked to a database of critically appraised outcome measures. Users can select desired measurement criteria, and psychometric information (e.g., reliability, validity, sensitivity) on appropriate outcome measures will be provided. The interactive nature of these programs allows you to choose measures for specific clinical situations and compare measures for decision-making. There are over 139 outcomes measure in pediatrics, over 200 outcome measures in adults (ISBN 1-55642-325-X), and over 1,000 literature sources are included in *All About Outcomes*. The CD-ROMs are available from SLACK Incorporated.

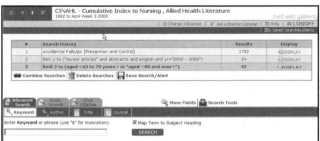

Figure 5-3. Subject heading search results.

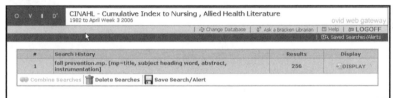

Figure 5-4. Keyword search results.

APPLY SEARCH STRATEGY USING SUBJECT TERMS, KEYWORDS, AND/OR INDEX ENTRIES

Step-by-Step Searching for Evidence for Clinical Scenario #1 Via Ovid

First, there are some questions you need to ask yourself at the beginning of your search:

- How far back in the literature do I wish to go?

- Which journals do I wish to review?

- Do I want only articles available either in online full text or in print at my library, or will I use an interlibrary loan service for articles not locally available?

- What sort of articles will be useful: recent research, overviews, systematic reviews?

- Are there any languages beyond my own that I would consider retrieving?

- Do I only want articles that have an online abstract?

Using the Ovid interface, we will search the CINAHL database for journal articles on fall prevention. Before we look for journal articles that address our specific research question, we may want to do some background reading in review articles to obtain a sense of the current state of research on fall prevention. Using the *accidental falls/prevention and control* heading/sub-heading combination, we retrieve 1,782 articles. This is obviously way too many to retrieve or review! Next, we will narrow our search on fall prevention to English-language review articles with abstracts published since the year 2000. This significantly reduces our search results to 54 citations. We can further limit our results to journal articles about the elderly using CINAHL's age group limiters, reducing our final set to 42 citations.

Although it may seem quicker to perform a database search using keywords rather than subject headings, you may get incomplete or irrelevant results. The subject heading search (Figure 5-3) retrieved 1,782 articles before limiters were applied. The keyword search (Figure 5-4) retrieved only 256 articles before limiters were applied, so a large body of evidence was overlooked.

The clinical question formulated earlier in this chapter asks whether patient education upon discharge from acute care is effective in preventing accidental falls in elderly clients who live

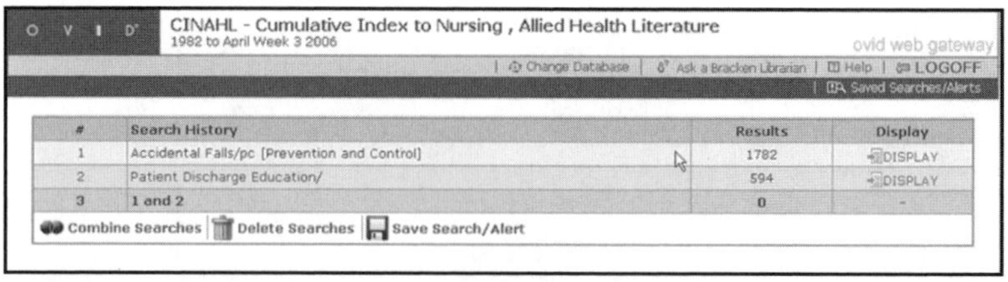

Figure 5-5. Combination search results.

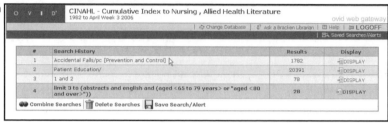

Figure 5-6. Refined search results.

independently at home. This time we will perform a database search that includes the intervention, patient education. When we combine the sets of results for accidental falls/prevention and control and for patient discharge education using AND, we are asking the database to retrieve citations that have been assigned both of those CINAHL subject headings (Figure 5-5).

Because this search yields no results, we will broaden our search term *patient discharge education* to *patient education*. This search yields 78 results. Note that it is more efficient to apply limiters to your results after sets are combined, rather than to each individual set (Figure 5-6).

We now have 28 articles that may answer the original clinical question. This is a manageable amount of evidence with which to start!

Our searches would be simple to reproduce because they contain few search terms and were performed in only one database, CINAHL. For research purposes, more complex multi-database searches should be documented so that others can reproduce them at a later date. When you need to do a comprehensive literature search, you may wish to ask a health sciences librarian to help you to plan and to document your searches. Systematic reviews in the Cochrane Database include a "search strategy for identification of studies." An example of a systematic review on physiotherapy interventions for shoulder pain contains many search terms, including both subject headings and keywords. However, because related terms are grouped together, the reader can quickly see which terms were searched to represent the patient group (sets 1 to 8), the interventions (sets 9 to 15), and the study design (sets 16 to 20). Using this search strategy, all the synonymous and related terms representing the concept of shoulder pain will be combined using OR; in other words, the database will retrieve either shoulder pain, shoulder impingement syndrome, rotator cuff, bursitis, etc. (Figure 5-7).

The next step is selecting the relevant articles from the search results.

Search strategy for identification of studies ⊞

MEDLINE, EMBASE, CINAHL (includes all major physiotherapy and occupational therapy journals from U.S.A., Canada, England, Australia and New Zealand), and Science Citation Index (SCISEARCH) were searched 1966 to June 2002.

1 Shoulder Pain/
2 Shoulder Impingement Syndrome/
3 Rotator Cuff/
4 exp Bursitis/
5 ((shoulder$ or rotator cuff) adj5 (bursitis or frozen or impinge$ or tendinitis or tendonitis or pain$)).mp.
6 rotator cuff.mp.
7 adhesive capulitis.mp.
8 or/1-7
9 exp Rehabilitation/
10 exp Physical Therapy Techniques/
11 exp Musculoskeletal Manipulations/
12 exp Exercise Movement Techniques/
13 exp Ultrasonography, Interventional/
14 (rehabilitat$ or physiotherap$ or physical therap$ or manual therap$ or exercis$ or ultrasound or ultrasonograph$ or TNS or TENS or shockwave or electrotherap$ or mobili$). mp.
15 or/9-14
16 Clinical trial.pt
17 random$.mp.
18 ((single or double) adj (blind$ or mask$)).mp.
19 placebo$.mp.
20 or/16-19
21 8 and 15 an 20

In addition, the Cochrane Controlled Trials Register (CCTR) Issue 2, 2002 was searched.

Figure 5-7. Example of search strategy for identification of studies.

Selecting Relevant Articles From the Literature Search: Modify Your Strategy to Achieve a More Efficient Search

Once you have obtained a copy of an article, you will want to see whether it is suitable for answering your question. You will want to judge its validity, reliability, and—most important of all—applicability. Here are the questions you need to ask yourself:

- Are the results of the article valid (validity)?
- What are the results (reliability)?
- Will the results help me in caring for my clients (applicability)?

You may find it helpful to use a checklist to assess whether it meets these three conditions. See Chapter 6 for more information about critically reviewing articles.

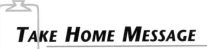

Take Home Message

Asking Questions

✔ A well-built question originates from professional practice, professional trends, existing published research, or existing theory.

✔ Answerable questions should include:
- specific client group or population
- intervention (assessment, treatment or other clinical issues)
- outcome interested in
- comparison.

✔ Good questions are relevant, direct, clear and focused.

Different Sources of Evidence

✔ Books: Important to judge their credibility.

✔ Non-peer reviewed journals or professional magazines: Good for learning about current trends, but do not carry absolute credibility.

✔ Peer-reviewed journals: Considered more accurate and relevant; usually of a higher quality.

Electronic Bibliographic Databases and the World Wide Web

✔ Electronic bibliographic databases are compilations of published research, scholarly articles books etc: each with a different focus (eg MEDLINE, CINAHL, Ovid).

✔ WWW - researcher is responsible for judging relevancy, authority, accuracy, objectivity, currency and commercialism; difficult to narrow search parameters to the degree needed to find relevant and useful information.

Conducting a Literature Search

✔ Adjust search parameters in accordance with sensitivity (to increase the likelihood of retrieving relevant items) and specificity (to increase the likelihood of excluding irrelevant items).

✔ All effective literature searches should be
- systematic
- explicit
- reproducible

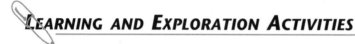

LEARNING AND EXPLORATION ACTIVITIES

Exercise 1: Developing an Answerable Question

Your Clinical Scenario

Write down a clinical scenario that you have encountered in your own experience.

Step 1: Identify the situation you are in.

P Patient/Population/ Problem			

Step 2: List the intervention—What do you wish to do?

P Patient/Population/ Problem	I Intervention		

Step 3: List the comparison, if any.

P Patient/Population/ Problem	I Intervention	C Comparison	

Step 4: Identify the outcome you wish to achieve.

P	I	C	O
Patient/Population/ Problem	Intervention	Comparison	Outcome

Step 5: Write out the question using the three key (or four) elements now.

P	I	C	O
Patient/Population/ Problem	Intervention	Comparison	Outcome
Question:			

Congratulations! You should have an answerable question now. Remember that your question should always be *relevant, direct and clear,* and *focused!*

Exercise 2: Searching for Evidence Question

List the key words in your question you developed from Exercise I. These key words should be grouped by P.I.C.O. concepts.

	P	I	C	O
	Patient/ Population/ Problem	Intervention	Comparison	Outcome
Keywords & Subject Headings				

Select databases (remember to use the ones you can access easily first).

Narrow or broaden your search by using some of the strategies in Table 5-3.

Set screening criteria to pick out the articles that are relevant to your original question.

As a tool to help you keep track of your searching a table, such as the one below, may be of assistance. Keeping track of searching terms over multiple databases, sessions or days can help in revealing searching patterns or keyword omissions.

Question:				
P:	I:	C:	O:	
Database	Keywords	Yield	Hits	Obtained

A completed chart may be:

Question: What are the issues regarding return to driving for people with spinal cord injuries (SCI)?				
P: Individuals with SCI	I: Adapted driving equipment	C: n/a		O: Return to driving
Database	**Keywords**	**Yield**	**Hits**	**Obtained**
Cochrane Central Register of Controlled Trials	SCI + automobile driving	0	0	0
CINAHL (1992-2005)	SCI + automobile driving	13	8	3
	SCI (mp) + driving (mp)	22	10	0 (3 rep)
	quadriplegia + automobile driving	3	3	0 (3 rep)
	paraplegia + automobile driving	1	1	0 (1 rep)
Medline (1996-2005)	SCI + driving	12	4	0 (4 rep)
	quadriplegia + driving	5	3	0 (3 rep)
	paraplegia + driving	1	0	0
EMBASE (1996-2005)	SCI + automobile driving	18	5	1 (3 rep, 1 French)
	quadriplegia + automobile driving	8	3	0 (3 rep)
	paraplegia + automobile driving	2	1	0

(rep) denotes repeat article

REFERENCE

Zemke, R., & Clark, F. (1996). *Occupational science: An evolving discipline*. Philadelphia, PA: F. A. Davis.

BIBLIOGRAPHY

Barber, G. (1995). Searching the therapy and rehabilitation literature. *British Journal of Therapeutic Rehabilitation, 2*, 203-208.

Booth, A. (1996). In search of the evidence: Informing effective practice. *Journal of Clinical Effect, 1*,25-29.

Centre for Evidence-Based Medicine. (2004). Formulating answerable clinical questions. Retrieved August 29, 2007, from http://www.cebm.utoronto.ca/practise/formulate

Finlayson, M., & Lou, JQ. (1999). *Practical steps to critical appraisal: A foundation for evidence-based practice*. Ft. Lauderdale, FL: Nova Southeastern University.

Giustini, D. (2005). How Google is changing medicine (Editorial). *British Medical Journal, 331*, 1487-1488.

Green, S., Buchbinder, R., & Hetrick, S. (2003). Physiotherapy interventions for shoulder pain. *Cochrane Database of Systematic Reviews, 2*. Art. No.: CD004258. DOI: 10.1002/14651858.CD004258.

Guyatt, G. H., & Rennie, D. (1993). Users' guides to the medical literature (Editorial). *Journal of the American Medical Association, 270*, 2096-2097.

Hunt, D. L., Jaeschke, R., & Mckibbon, K. A. (2000). Users' guides to the medical literature, XXI: Using electronic health information resources in EBP. *Journal of the American Medical Association, 283*, 1875-1879.

Oxman, A. D., Sackett, D. L., & Guyatt, G. H. (1993). Users' guides to the medical literature. I. How to get started. The Evidence-Based Medicine Working Group. *Journal of the American Medical Association. 270*, 2093-2095.

Richardson, W. S., Wilson, M. C., & Nishikawa, J. (1995). The well-built clinical question: A key to evidence-based decisions. *ACP Journal Club, 123*, A12-A13.

SECTION III:
ASSESSING THE EVIDENCE

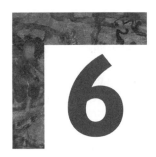

6

Evaluating the Evidence

Joy MacDermid, PT, PhD and Mary Law, PhD, OTReg(Ont), FCAOT

LEARNING OBJECTIVES

After reading this chapter, the student/practitioner will be able to:

- Define principles of quality in quantitative and qualitative approaches to research.
- Identify levels of evidence and variations in evidence-ranking systems.
- Find and select appropriate tools to critically appraise clinical evidence.
- Use critical appraisal tools to evaluate qualitative or quantitative evidence.
- Have a systematic process for selecting the best evidence to answer a clinical question.

Evaluating evidence is the foundation of evidence-based practice (EBP), as the confidence placed in evidence from clinical studies is dependent on the quality. Evaluating the quality of research evidence is important in becoming a successful evidence-based practitioner. After identifying a clinical question, formulating and completing a search of the literature, and reviewing the articles retrieved, the next step in the EBP process is evaluating the evidence. Evaluating the evidence means sifting through the articles and studies you have found in order to decide which are valid and clinically useful.

The importance of critical appraisal in EBP has led to the development of systems, processes, tools, and support systems for rating clinical research evidence. In this chapter, we will focus on how the practitioner can use research design principles, ranking systems, and appraisal tools to critically appraise and rank evidence according to its quality. In the next chapter, we will focus on processes and systems that support quality assessment.

Various study designs have different levels of rigor. When using quantitative information on treatment effectiveness, the "gold standard" of evidence—a randomized double-blinded controlled clinical trial—is considered the least susceptible to error because of the rigorous steps it requires researchers to follow. Its primary benefit is that, when properly conducted, it can control for known and unknown sources of bias and provide the strongest evidence that conclusions about the effects of interventions are valid. The caveat to this statement is that any study is still susceptible to unforeseen problems and contamination by bias. This may occur because of the way components of the study are designed or executed. Hence, even where type of study is clear, it is still important for the evidence-based consumer to be able to detect flaws in the study design, conduct, or interpretation. Ultimately, no evidence classification is absolutely "right" or "wrong," but the use of critical appraisal systems or tools can help therapists incorporate quality assessment into the process of using published evidence in clinical practice. As qualitative research becomes more prevalent in rehabilitation science, similar tools and processes are being developed for these studies. In these studies, the fit of design and methods to the research question being addressed are more important than the use of one particular design.

Critical appraisal can be performed using quick scales or classification systems, or in some cases using more detailed rating scales. Critical appraisal instruments range from very structured tools that contain specific questions and defined response categories to more open-ended scales in which the assessor makes guided subjective judgments on the quality of aspects of study design using a framework provided by the assessment tool. Clinicians can select different critical appraisal instruments depending on their clinical question/study design, their familiarity with critical appraisal, personal preferences, and the appropriate balance between time commitment and depth of analysis.

Different depths of critical appraisal are appropriate at different points in practice. For example, in some cases it is appropriate to do a quick scan of the literature and retrieve the single one or two papers that might provide the highest quality to obtain a quick but valid answer to an urgent clinical question. A five-"level" ordinal scale that classifies studies according to their basic study design will be useful for this purpose. In other cases, when planning to implement a new intervention, it would be important to delve more deeply into the study design to gain a more thorough understanding of issues that might affect the validity of the study conclusions, the clinical interpretability, or applicability to your patient. When practitioners conduct a thorough critical appraisal, this enhances their appraisal skills and appreciation of the issues that can compromise confidence in research studies. Quick rating scales or even pre-synthesized evidence ratings have the advantage of being less time consuming. It is important to realize that there are different ways to incorporate quality ratings into clinical decision-making and achieve the right fit for your practice.

This chapter will present several different critical appraisal tools, categorization schemes, and approaches that can be used to evaluate different types of evidence. We will discuss research using quantitative methods first.

HISTORICAL PERSPECTIVE

Important principles that are incorporated into EBP evolved from a variety of sources and across a time continuum. For example, the Scottish epidemiologist Archie Cochrane, who advocated the use of clinical evidence, was honoured for his significant contributions in the naming of the Cochrane Collaboration. The growth of the discipline of clinical epidemiology had much to do with the emergence of EBP. However, McMaster University is generally recognized as the birthplace of evidence-based medicine as evidenced by the following quote (Wikipedia, n.d.):

> *The explicit methodologies used to determine "best evidence" were largely established by the McMaster University research group led by David Sackett and Gordon Guyatt. The term "evidence-based medicine" first appeared in the medical literature in 1992 in a paper by Guyatt et al.*

A core group of McMaster clinical epidemiologists developed specific steps and approaches to evaluating the quality of evidence and disseminated these core concepts of EBP. From this historical perspective, it is apparent that rating the quality of clinical evidence is a fundamental feature of EBP. These concepts continue to evolve and experts have continued to improve the ratings (Atkins, Best, et al., 2004; Atkins, Eccles, et al., 2004) We refer to the levels of evidence developed by Sackett and colleagues as "the classic" levels of evidence to distinguish them from separate classification systems that evolved subsequently in other groups.

LEVELS OF EVIDENCE IN RESEARCH USING QUANTITATIVE METHODS

The concept of ranking levels of evidence is based on the principle that certain study types have more rigour and these higher quality study designs provide more confidence to associated clinical decision making. The "best" study design varies according to the type of study that is being conducted. For example, while the RCT is considered the best study design for detecting differences between intervention groups, a prospective cohort design with complete follow-up is the best design for studies in prognosis. Levels of evidence are important as they are a quick classification of evidence quality. In fact, systematic reviews of evidence often use these levels as cut-offs to determine which study types are included in evidence synthesis. For example, many evidence reviews performed by the Cochrane Collaboration include either only RCTs or the two highest levels of evidence when conducting a systematic review.

When the concept of levels of evidence was first introduced as a feature of EBP, it contained a novel concept. Although it might appear obvious and simplistic to us now, the concept that one's confidence in a clinical decision should be based on the extent to which rigorous clinical observations supported that decision was not universally accepted. It was common to assume that if effects were demonstrated in a laboratory situation, this provided sufficient evidence for implementing a similar course of action in clinical care. One of the striking elements of EBP is that clinical observations, even when not rigorously controlled, provide a more substantial basis for making clinical decisions than rigorously conducted laboratory observations—when these observations are not made on patients. This concept "turned the tables" so that bench research, expert opinion, and theoretical constructs were seen as low levels of evidence.

The true experiment that can establish that a specific intervention causes a specific treatment effect is the randomized controlled clinical trial conducted on patients. Early evidence rating systems ranked this at the top, or level 1 evidence. The number (and quality) of RCTs proliferated in part due to the emergence of EBP. It became necessary to have a mechanism to summarize multiple, sometimes conflicting, RCTs. Hence, the emergence of a new methodology: the systematic review. The original evidence rating scheme proposed by Sackett and colleagues was subsequently modified to reflect this new reality and include these in level 1. Systematic reviews will be covered in the following chapter.

The "Classic" Levels of Evidence For Treatment Effectiveness

The original levels of evidence developed at McMaster were subsequently updated and are clearly presented on the Web site for the Oxford Centre For Evidence-Based Medicine at www. cebm.net/levels_of_evidence.asp and Appendices E and F. The interested reader can download the levels, read or post questions, and access supplementary information and references on critical appraisal at this Web site. The importance of treatment effectiveness as an element of practice has placed significant emphasis on the role of the RCT, to the point that it sometimes overshadows that different research designs are matched to different study types. Five different types of studies are defined in the classic levels of evidence scheme.

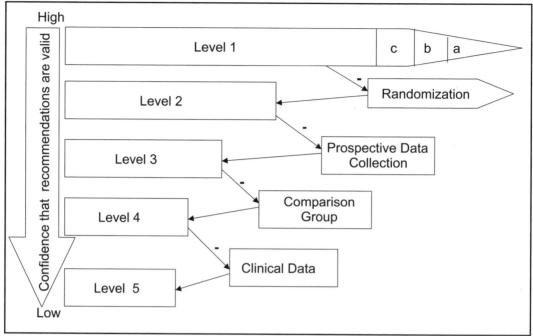

Figure 6-1. Levels of evidence.

Clinicians most commonly deal with the category where an RCT is the most rigorous study design. This would include studies on therapy, prevention, etiology, and harm. As previously discussed, the RCT has a major advantage; randomization of large numbers of patients will, by chance, tend to evenly distribute prognostic variables between comparison groups, removing their opportunity to bias conclusions. This means that difference observed between groups can be attributed to the manipulated variable—usually treatment. Three potential situations are considered to be sufficiently rigorous to be labelled as level 1. Level 1a would consist of a systematic review of a number of RCTs in which the studies substantially agree with each other in terms of the direction and approximate size of the effects observed. A level 1b study would be an individual RCT in which the size of the treatment effect was relatively precisely defined as indicated by a narrow confidence interval. A level 1C study is a very unusual circumstance in rehabilitation. This occurs when in the absence of a randomized study, an overwhelmingly dramatic change in outcomes can be demonstrated once a new treatment becomes available. For example, vaccination is widely accepted in practice although not originally based on RCT evidence. Cases where all patients die before an intervention is available and some patients survive following introduction of a new intervention can form overwhelming evidence on the effectiveness. Similarly, when some patients die before an intervention is available and following the intervention no one dies, this can provide similar confidence. Level 1 studies provide the highest internal validity, enhancing our confidence that if we select this intervention for our patients we will be able to achieve similar outcomes.

Figure 6-1 illustrates another way to think about levels of evidence. As we lose important elements of research design, we also lose confidence in the internal validity of the study conclusions and hence have lesser confidence that we might achieve the reported outcomes by selecting these interventions for our patients. Level 2 studies differ from RCTs in that we have lost randomization. The protection against potential biases and confounders is lessened (Mamdani et al., 2005). The most positive aspect of a prospective cohort study is that it identifies patients prior to having their outcome and follows them forward in time. This reduces some potential sources of bias. A number of additional elements of research design can be introduced to make this study design as rigorous as possible. Using either of the two critical appraisal forms and their associated guides provided in Appendices A, B, M, and N to assess effectiveness studies will provide more detail on these research design elements. However, these include the use of standardized outcome measures, adequate sampling, blinding of patients/evaluators/others involved in the study, rigorous follow-up, proper statistical analysis including adjusting for covariates and other design elements. In our classic levels of evidence, a level 2a study is a systematic review of cohort (prospective) studies that agree with each other in terms of the direction and approximate size of the effects obtained. A level 2b study is a single high-quality cohort study supporting a specific conclusion. In this case, high quality is indicated by greater than 80% follow-up of patients. The reason that such substantial emphasis is placed on follow-up in prospective cohort studies is that the greatest potential bias occurs when patients drop out of the study for different reasons. If patients that dropped out have overly favorable or unfavorable results compared to the remainder of the cohort, then estimates of the treatment effect will be biased.

Level 3 evidence for treatment effectiveness occurs when studies are case controlled. A case-control study design is one in which patients are identified for research after outcomes have been achieved. Data collection obtains information on patient exposures or interventions that have occurred in the past. The reason that we have dropped down another level of confidence at this point is because we have lost the potential protection against biases that result from collecting information on patients before their outcomes have been achieved. The primary threat to the internal validity of the case-control study is that the reasons or mechanisms by which patients are available for study after their outcomes have been achieved may introduce a bias into the sample and subsequent estimation of treatment effects. For example, in studying the effects of a rehabilitation program on total knee arthroplasty conducted in an outpatient setting, patients who died and were too unwell or immobile to participate in the study will be excluded. The sample of patients remaining to be studied may not be fully representative of all patients having a total knee arthroplasty. If we are studying the impact of an intervention on participation outcomes, the level of participation achieved may affect whether people volunteer for the study and this effect may be distributed differently across different intervention or exposure groups. For example, patients who resumed full participation may have busy work and leisure lives and be unwilling to participate in studies. Despite the potential for bias, there are specific techniques that can be used to maximize the potential internal validity of case-control studies, and these are covered in standard epidemiological textbooks. A level 3a study is a systematic review of case-control studies that agree with each other, whereas level 3b is a single individual case-control study.

To drop down another level of evidence, we again lose an important element of research design—our comparison group. Level 4 evidence for treatment effectiveness consists of case series. A case series evaluates the clinical outcomes of a single group of patients. No matter how rigorously we evaluate their outcomes, we remain uncertain what would have happened to these patients if an alternate intervention had been selected. While authors of these studies frequently try to compare the results to those reported in literature in other case series, these comparisons are tentative due to variations in study samples.

Finally, to drop down to our lowest level of evidence, we lose another critical component of research design in an EBP framework—observations made on patients. Level 5 consists of expert opinion without explicit critical appraisal, physiology, bench (lab) research, or first principles. In rehabilitation, it is not uncommon for expert opinion to be held in high regard. Some treatment approaches are even named for their developers, indicating the deference provided to the "expert." We also rely on numerous first principles or conceptual frameworks to support our interventions. While both experts and conceptual frameworks should be considered important in hypothesis generating, it is only through hypothesis testing that we are able to establish higher levels of confidence that expected treatment effects will occur in real patients. Similarly, although animal research has an important role in some circumstances, it is important to establish treatment effects in humans before we can have confidence that potential benefits of new interventions will be attainable in clinical situations.

One feature of this "classic" rating system is that it is possible to reduce the rating level assigned to an individual study if fundamental design flaws are detected. For example, low-quality RCTs would be level 2b, and a low quality cohort or case-control study is considered level 4.

The classic evidence rating system provides grades of recommendation ranging from an A to a D. A grade A recommendation is provided when there is consistent level 1 studies supporting a given conclusion. A grade B recommendation is provided when there are consistent level 2 or 3 studies supporting a given conclusion. When your clinical situation has substantial differences than reported in the literature, it is necessary to "extrapolate" the evidence. That is, you must generalize conclusions made in one (studied) circumstance to a potentially different clinical circumstance; naturally this lessens your confidence that the same treatment effect would be observed. A grade C recommendation is made from level 4 studies or extrapolations from level 2 or 3 studies. And finally, a grade D recommendation, the lowest grade, is provided when there is only level 5 evidence or at any time when the available studies are inconsistent and inconclusive.

THE CLASSIC RATING SYSTEM AS APPLIED TO OTHER STUDY DESIGNS

The importance placed on effectiveness sometimes overshadows the other types of clinical decisions for which evidence rating systems have been designed. These also are in Appendix E and on the Web site for the Oxford Centre for Evidence-Based Medicine. The other types of studies addressed include the following:

- Prognosis
- Diagnosis
- Differential diagnosis/symptom prevalence study
- Economic and decision analyses

The optical study design varies across these different types of clinical studies. For example, the optimal individual study (level 1b) for a prognosis study is an individual inception cohort study with greater than 80% follow-up, where a clinical decision rule has been validated in a single population. Clinical decision rules are algorithms or scoring systems that lead to a prognostic estimation or diagnostic category. Examples of these will be provided in Chapters 11 and 12. Conversely, the optimal study design for a diagnostic test study consists of a cohort study with good reference standards or a clinical decision rule tested within one clinical center. For differential diagnosis or symptom prevalence, a single prospective cohort study with good follow-up is considered to be a level 1b study. Finally, in economic and decision analyses, the estimates of effect should be based on clinically sensible costs/alternatives and systematic reviews of the evidence and include multi-way sensitivity analyses.

Despite differences in the optimal study design and hence the specifics of each level, certain consistencies are evident across different types of questions and their associated levels of evidence:

- A systematic review of high-quality studies always provides the highest level of rigor.
- An individual study using the optimal design for that type of clinical question is considered level 1.
- Prospective data collection indicates higher study quality than retrospective data collection.
- Expert opinion, bench research, and conceptual frameworks/theories/first principles are always considered the lowest (level 5) evidence.

OTHER RATING SYSTEMS

A number of authors have modified this classic rating system to try and accommodate additional study designs or types of evidence. It is interesting and potentially useful to be aware of some of these alternate rating systems. However, no single rating system addresses all study designs or covers all potential types of evidence. Many of the basic principles proposed by others retain key principles of the classic rating system.

OTHER LEVELS OF EVIDENCE CLASSIFICATION SYSTEMS

A system described by Greenhalgh (1997) is similar but includes other study designs:
- Systematic reviews and meta-analyses
- RCTs with definitive results
- RCTs with nondefinitive results
- Cohort studies
- Case-control studies
- Cross-sectional surveys
- Case reports

A second example of evidence classification comes from the *Canadian Medical Association Journal* (CMAJ) (Steering Committee, 1998). One important feature of the CMAJ classification is the mention of "false-positive" and "false-negative" results. False-positives (called type I errors in statistics) and false-negatives (type II errors) are important complications that the evidence-based practitioner must deal with, and they will be touched on in the chapter on meta-analysis. These levels of evidence are described as follows:

- **Level I**: Evidence is based on RCTs (or meta-analysis of such trials) of adequate size to ensure a low risk of incorporating false-positive or false-negative results.
- **Level II**: Evidence is based on RCTs that are too small to provide level I evidence. These may show either positive trends that are not statistically significant or no trends and are associated with a high risk of false-negative results.
- **Level III**: Evidence is based on non-randomized, controlled, or cohort studies; case series; case-controlled studies; or cross-sectional studies.
- **Level IV**: Evidence is based on the opinion of respected authorities or that of expert committees as indicated in published consensus conferences or guidelines.
- **Level V**: Evidence expresses the opinion of those individuals who have written and reviewed these guidelines, based on their experience, knowledge of the relevant literature, and discussion with their peers.

A third breakdown of the levels of evidence comes from the National Health Service (NHS) in the United Kingdom (2004).

The NHS system retains the same key features, although it sets up its classification somewhat differently. Here, the judgment of individual practitioners is incorporated. The difference between "a low risk of bias" and "a very low risk of bias" is left to the practitioner's judgement. As you use EBR and practice your critical appraisal skills, your skill at correctly identifying the biases and deficiencies of evidence will greatly improve.

- **1++**: High quality meta-analyses, systematic reviews of RCTs, or RCTs with a very low risk of bias
- **1+**: Well-conducted meta-analyses, systematic reviews of RCTs, or RCTs with a low risk of bias
- **1**: Meta-analyses, systematic reviews of RCTs, or RCTs with a high risk of bias
- **2++**: High quality systematic reviews of case-control or cohort studies; high quality case-control or cohort studies with a very low risk of confounding, bias, or chance; and a high probability that the relationship is causal
- **2+**: Well-conducted case-control or cohort studies with a low risk of confounding, bias, or chance and a moderate probability that the relationship is causal
- **2**: Case control or cohort studies with a high risk of confounding, bias, or chance and a significant risk that the relationship is not causal
- **3**: Nonanalytic studies (e.g., case reports, case series)
- **4**: Expert opinion

For our final example, we can look at the system proposed by U.S. Preventive Services Task Force (Current Methods, 2001). Advantages of this system are that it provides a common language framework for people to use, considers the balance between important health outcomes and potential harms, and provides a clear distinction for the situation where evidence is insufficient to make a recommendation. Rehabilitation practitioners might find this rating system useful as they often have to make clinical decisions in an environment of uncertainty. In fact, one of the authors (JM) modified these ratings as a means of providing consistent recommendations with CPGs (see Chapter 11).

Recommendation: A

Language: Recommends that clinicians routinely provide (the service) to eligible patients. There is found good evidence that (the service) improves important health outcomes and that benefits substantially outweigh harms

Recommendation: B

Language: Recommends that clinicians routinely provide (the service) to eligible patients. There is at least fair evidence that (the service) improves important health outcomes and that benefits outweigh harms.

Recommendation: C

Language: Makes no recommendation for or against routine provision of (the service). There is at least fair evidence that (the service) can improve health outcomes but the balance of the benefits and harms is too close to justify a general recommendation.

Recommendation: D

Language: recommends against routinely providing (the service) to asymptomatic patients. There is at least fair evidence that (the service) is ineffective or that harms outweigh benefits.

Recommendation: I

Language: Concludes that the evidence is insufficient to recommend for or against routinely providing [the service]. Evidence that (the service) is effective is lacking, of poor quality, or conflicting and the balance of benefits and harms cannot be determined.

Comparing the classification systems presented, there are, and should be, many similarities between evidence-ranking systems. In general, evidence rankings should have the same theme (i.e., moving from systematic reviews down to more individual assessments). Lower levels of evidence have less control over potential sources of bias. Although it is important to rank levels of evidence, it is also important to appreciate the role of different forms and levels of evidence to the ongoing development and refinement of clinical knowledge. Knowledge in any profession is built piece by piece, often beginning with a case report and proceeding to further and larger studies (as discussed in Chapter 2). It is important to integrate qualitative and quantitative information, although classification systems do not provide guidance on how this might be done. Similarly, it is unclear where clinical practice guidelines and algorithms rank in these systems. Complex integration of evidence can be assisted by formal processes but is rarely a simple linear process. We have included examples in Table 6-1 of where we might fit other types of rehabilitation literature into the five-level framework. Figure 6-2 is an algorithm that practitioners might use to find the best levels of evidence for a treatment approach using an EBR approach. We recognize that developing rehabilitation knowledge is an ongoing process and that each piece in the puzzle is important.

APPRECIATION FOR OTHER RESEARCH DESIGN ISSUES

Within all quantitative studies, there are a range of research design issues that work together to form overall quality of the study. We summarize these in Table 6-2.

CRITICAL APPRAISAL TOOLS

While it is important to understand the basic principles involved in critical appraisal, the use of tools to provide structure to the process can be invaluable. In this section we provide critical appraisal tools developed by the chapter authors and provide Web sites where additional forms can be obtained. Critical appraisal forms developed by Law and colleagues in 1998 appear in Appendices A and B. These can be downloaded from the CanChild Centre for Childhood Disability Research at McMaster University Web site at www.fhs.mcmaster.ca/canchild. Hard copies are in Appendices A, B, C, and D. These tools have been used to teach and perform critical appraisal in a variety of rehabilitation and educational contexts. The forms provide a structure for recording study type and potential sources of bias. The accompanying guidelines describe the process as well as key features that should be considered when assessing each element of research design. One tool addresses quantitative research (Appendices A and B) and the other qualitative research (Appendices C and D).

A second set of forms was developed by MacDermid in 2004. These tools have been used to teach and perform critical appraisal and to conduct systematic reviews in rehabilitation. Appendices M and N provide significant structure by posing specific questions on research

Table 6-1

EXAMPLES OF WHERE OTHER TYPES OF REHABILITATION LITERATURE FIT INTO THE FIVE-LEVEL FRAMEWORK

Level	Classic "Levels of Evidence" for Therapy/Prevention, Etiology/Harm	Placement of Additional Types of Clinical Evidence* Used in Rehabilitation for Therapy/Prevention, Etiology/Harm
1a	Systematic review (with homogeneity) of RCTs	CPGs where recommendations are based on systematic reviews that contain multiple RCTs and the development includes supplemental data or expert opinion to make recommendations only where evidence is lacking
1b	Individual RCT (with narrow Confidence Interval)	
1c	All or none	
2a	Systematic review (with homogeneity) of cohort studies	Lower quality CPGs that are based on informal evidence review and expert consensus, where few RCTs are identified
2b	Individual cohort study (including low quality RCT; e.g., <80% follow-up)	
2c	"Outcomes" research; ecological studies	
3a	Systematic review (with homogeneity) of case-control studies	Structured consensus processes based on quantitative ratings of agreement and formal consensus processes using qualified experts
3b	Individual case-control study	
4	Case-series (and poor quality cohort and case-control studies)	Unstructured quantitative or qualitative expert consensus; large descriptive practice analysis/survey that defines common ground; critical appraisal/comprehensive systematic review or synthesis of biologic studies, qualitative studies, or first principles
5	Expert opinion without explicit critical appraisal, or based on physiology, bench research, or "first principles"	CPGs that are not based on the use of evidence review or quantitative data; clinic protocols, rehabilitation theory, behavioral, social, or cognitive theory, treatment approach theories (e.g., MacKenzie, Bobath, manual therapy, constrained movement)

These classic levels are described in the text. The right column places additional forms of evidence commonly used in rehabilitation along this spectrum.

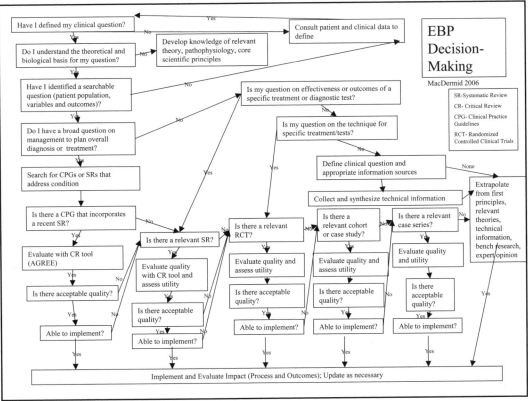

Figure 6-2. EBP decision making.

Table 6-2			
RESEARCH DESIGN ISSUES IN QUANTITATIVE RESEARCH			
Research Design Issue	*Objective*	*Optimal Design*	*Threats to Internal Validity*
Sampling of subjects	A sample that represents the target population	A random sample selected from the population	Differential sampling between groups will affect internal validity; convenience sampling may affect external validity
Sample size	The optimal number of subjects is large enough to detect important treatment effects small enough to conduct the study in a timely, efficient manner	The correct number of subjects is determined by an accurate sample size calculation	Small sample sizes

continued

Table 6-2, continued

RESEARCH DESIGN ISSUES IN QUANTITATIVE RESEARCH

Research Design Issue	Objective	Optimal Design	Threats to Internal Validity
Allocation of treatment	Unbiased	Random allocation	Nonrandom (observational)
Blinding (to treatment allocation and/or outcomes)	To minimize sources of bias introduced by study personnel or participants	Ideally everyone involved in the study would be blinded to the fullest extent possible, including study coordinators, participants, evaluators and providers, and data analysts	Blinding is difficult in rehabilitation and may result in bias from differential diagnosis, outcome assessments, attention, and follow-up procedures
Outcome ascertainment	To accurately determine pretreatment status and reflect all important changes in outcome following treatment	Outcomes are measured at all likely relevant time points using reliable, valid, and responsive measures according to a standardized protocol	Outcome measures that reflect only certain domains may be biased toward specific treatments; important effects will be missed if relevant time points are not assessed or outcome measures are not responsive; poor reliability and validity may invalidate conclusions
Follow-up	To accurately portray the treatment effects obtained by all participants	100% follow-up	Differential loss to follow-up can introduce bias in estimates of effects
Statistical analysis	To provide accurate estimates of the size and significance of the observed effects	Accurate and appropriate analysis of all data	Inappropriate analysis may lead to faulty conclusions

design that must be answered on a three-point rating scale. Specific scoring criteria for each item is provided in an accompanying interpretation guide. In general, score of 2 is provided for optimal study design, a score of one is assigned if only some elements were appropriate, and a score of zero is recorded when inappropriate methods were used or none described. The forms for effectiveness studies can be used across all levels of evidence—not just RCTs. A separate tool and guide are provided for psychometric outcome measure (Appendix G) and diagnostic test studies (Appendix H).

Other potential critical appraisal tools can be used. The newer version of the classic textbook *Evidence-Based Medicine: How to Practice and Teach EBM* now comes with a CD containing a variety of examples from different types of articles and different disciplines (Sackett, Straus, Richardson, Rosenberg, & Haynes, 2000). The items used in the Pedro scale are sometimes used for critical appraisal in other circumstances including systematic reviews (www.pedro.fhs.usyd. edu.au/scale_item.html). Table 6-3 highlights other resources.

A systematic review addressed 120 different critical appraisal tools appearing in the literature (Katrak, Bialocerkowski, Massy-Westropp, Kumar, & Grimmer, 2004). This review found substantial variation between instruments in scope, structure, and scoring. Table 6-2 provides additional Web sites that provide access to a variety of critical appraisal forms, and outline their purpose and number of items. Rehabilitation practitioners should avoid scales designed only for use with RCTs (especially those that focus on blinding issues) as these will have limited usefulness in rehabilitation literature.

LEARNING BIOSTATISTICS AND CRITICAL APPRAISAL

Lack of confidence in performing critical appraisal is a frequently reported barrier to EBP (Bryar et al., 2003). A variety of strategies can be used to enhance skill and confidence. It has been demonstrated that improved performance in critical appraisal is obtained using a variety of strategies; however, not all strategies result in changes in clinician behavior (Bennett et al., 1987; Coomarasamy & Khan, 2004; Coomarasamy, Taylor, & Khan, 2003).

In order to comprehend, analyze, and put into practice evidence from clinical journals and other sources, one will need to have a working knowledge of biostatistics. The CMAJ has published a series of basic statistics for clinicians—articles that can be found in the references and are helpful when reviewing research articles (Guyatt, Jaeschke, et al., 1995a, 1995b; Guyatt, Walter, et al., 1995). A number of online statistical texts and critical appraisal Web sites are listed at the end of this chapter.

Critical appraisal is most useful and most interesting when conducted in a group situation. Evidence-based journal clubs are useful means of encouraging clinicians to read, appraise, and make action-based decisions about clinical evidence emerging in the literature. The use of journal clubs in physiotherapy has been studied and indicates substantial variability in the use of problems and evidence, as well as staff enthusiasm (Turner & Mjolne, 2001). Strategies for success include regular meeting times, access to evidence-based resources, a commitment to critical appraisal of all articles, the use of patient-based cases or scenarios to bring meaning to the evidence, a process to institute change and ongoing evaluation.

THE CRITICAL REVIEW OF RESEARCH USING QUALITATIVE METHODS

In research, there often exists a perceived hierarchy of research design and methods that quantitative methods are of higher quality than qualitative methods. In fact, the generation

Table 6-3

ONLINE CRITICAL APPRAISAL TOOLS

Web Site	Type of Studies Evaluated	Number of Items
Aggressive Research Intelligence Facility* www.arif.bham.ac.uk/casp/caprocess.htm	Systematic review	14
Appraisal of Guidelines for Research and Evaluation* www.agreecollaboration.org	Clinical practice guidelines	23
Best Evidence Topics www.bestbets.org/cgi-bin/public_pdf.pl	Diagnostic test Economic analysis Prognosis Systematic review Qualitative research Clinical practice guidelines	29 34 37 33 40 32
Center for Evidence-Based Emergency Medicine www.ebem.org/analyse.html	Treatment effectiveness Prognosis Diagnostic test Systematic review	13 10 11 12 to 15
Centre for Evidence-Based Medicine, Oxford www.cebm.net/critical_appraisal.asp	Treatment effectiveness Prognosis Diagnostic test Economic analysis Systematic review Clinical practice guidelines	11 10 8 14 10 18
Centre for Evidence-Based Medicine, Oxford CATmaker www.cebm.net/catmaker.asp	Treatment effectiveness Prognosis Diagnostic test Systematic review	
Centre for Evidence-Based Medicine, Toronto www.cebm.utoronto.ca/teach/materials/ caworksheets.htm	Treatment effectiveness Prognosis Diagnostic test Systematic review	14 10 9 10
Centre for Evidence-Based Mental Health http://cebmh.warne.ox.ac.uk/cebmh/edu-cation_critical_appraisal.htm www.cebmh.com	Treatment effectiveness Prognosis Diagnostic test Systematic review	9 9 8 9

*Has guide to interpretation.

continued

Table 6-3, continued

ONLINE CRITICAL APPRAISAL TOOLS

Web Site	Type of Studies Evaluated	Number of Items
Centre for Health Evidence*	Treatment effectiveness	12
www.cche.net/usersguides/main.asp	Diagnostic test	9
	Prognosis	9
	Clinical practice guideline	10
	Economic analysis	10
	Qualitative research	8
Critical Appraisal Skills Programme*	Diagnostic test	12
www.phru.nhs.uk/Pages/PHD/CASP.htm	Qualitative study	10
	Economic analysis	10
	Systematic review	10
Evidence-Based Medicine, Alberta*	Treatment effectiveness	11
www.ebm.med.ualberta.ca	Prognosis	10
	Diagnostic test	10
	Economic analysis	10
	Systematic review	11
	Clinical practice guidelines	11
Evidence-Based Medicine, Duke	Treatment effectiveness	12
www.mclibrary.duke.edu/subject/ebm?tab =appraising&extra=worksheets	Prognosis	9
	Diagnostic test	9
	Qualitative study	7
	Economic analysis	10
	Systematic review	10
	Clinical practice guidelines	4
Glasgow	Systematic review	10
http://ssrc.tums.ac.ir/SystematicReview/ Glasgow.asp		
Health Care Practice Research and Development Unit	Treatment effectiveness	51
	Qualitative study	44
www.fhsc.salford.ac.uk/hcprdu/critical- appraisal.htm	Economic analysis	68
Journal Club, Evidence-Based Medicine	Prognosis	8
www.geh.nhs.uk/services/edu/Library/ Jclub/appraisal_tools.asp	Systematic review	13
McMaster—Occupational Therapy*	Treatment effectiveness	15
www.fhs.mcmaster.ca/rehab/ebp	Qualitative study	27

*Has guide to interpretation.

continued

Table 6-3, continued

ONLINE CRITICAL APPRAISAL TOOLS

Web Site	Type of Studies Evaluated	Number of Items
Quality of Reporting of Meta-Analyses www.consort-statement.org/QUOROM.pdf	Systematic review	17
School of Health and Related Research (ScHARR), University of Sheffield* www.shef.ac.uk/scharr/sections/ir/links	Systematic review Qualitative study	10 10

*Has guide to interpretation.

of knowledge from both types of designs is important and often complementary. The most appropriate design to be used in a specific study depends more on the research question and the knowledge required than on a priori ideas of best methods. For example, the final testing of a drug is best accomplished using a RCT because one wants to ensure that the results are causal in nature and applicable to the broad population. Equally, the experience of living in the community with a newly acquired disability is best studied using a qualitative method such as ethnography or biography. The use of qualitative methods in rehabilitation research is increasing and has generated much knowledge about the experience of illness and disability as well as other issues important to persons involved in rehabilitation.

Increasingly, mixed-methods are being used in rehabilitation. This combination of two different research designs can be very informative. Take for example a clinical trial looking at access to a self-referral mobility clinic to help seniors live at home and participate in their community. Moderate and statistically significant quantitative outcomes might be established for this intervention by measuring patient satisfaction, FIM scores, and scores on a relevant participation measure. However, it might also be useful to use qualitative methods to define why some seniors did not use the intervention, what aspects were valued by participants who achieved successful outcomes, and what features accounted for failures within the trial. Selecting subgroups of participants from these categories and performing qualitative analyses might provide a deeper understanding of the intervention and how its effect might be maximized or customized to achieve better outcomes.

With the proliferation of qualitative research in rehabilitation, there is increased awareness of the aspects of quality that pertain to this form of inquiry. Rigorous quality is equally important in this study design but manifests itself in different ways. Appraisal guides for qualitative methods are now available (see Table 6-2) and the online versions listed at the end of this chapter (Appendix C). Issues to pay particular attention to when evaluating qualitative research follow.

Study Design

In constructing qualitative research, there are many different types of research approaches or designs. Creswell (1998) has outlined five major approaches or designs used in qualitative research and these include biography, ethnography, phenomenology, grounded theory, and case study. Of these approaches, ethnography, phenomenology, and grounded theory are most often seen in the rehabilitation literature and will be discussed in more detail here.

Ethnography

Ethnography is a qualitative research approach that traces its history to development in the field of anthropology. In this research design, the purpose is to study a particular culture or group of people to identify their daily life patterns, meanings, and beliefs. Ethnography has been used to study cultural groups as well as groups of people with health problems or disabilities.

Phenomenology

A research study using this approach or design focuses on the lived experience of the person or a group of people. The purpose of this research is to understand lived experience, interpret that experience, and thus provide information that can be shared with and used by others.

Grounded Theory

Grounded theory design is very common in rehabilitation and nursing research literature. The primary purpose of this approach is theory construction and verification. Using grounded theory, researchers seek to understand and identify theoretical processes in the real world. Themes that emerge from research are used to develop an understanding and theoretical explanation of the social world of the people being studied.

Methods

There are a variety of methods used by qualitative researchers, including participant observation, interviews, focus groups, and review of documents or other material. The methods chosen for particular study should be the most appropriate in collecting research data for that study. Commonly, qualitative researchers use multiple methods to enhance the trustworthiness of their findings. The use of multiple methods is one type of triangulation, a group of strategies used to ensure the rigor of a qualitative research study.

Sampling

The purpose of sampling in qualitative research is quite different from quantitative methods. In qualitative research, participants are selected for a specific purpose; random selection is not used. For example, participants may be chosen because they are of a certain age or culture or have experienced specific events better important to the study. The sampling strategies used in a study should be well described and justified by the authors. Sample size of qualitative studies is generally smaller than quantitative studies and there are no specific formulae to calculate appropriate sample size. Rather, sampling in a qualitative study is continued until sampling redundancy or theoretical saturation of the data is achieved.

Data Collection

Achieving descriptive clarity is a very important characteristic for a qualitative research study. Authors of qualitative studies should include clear descriptive information about the participants, the study site, and the researcher so that readers develop an excellent understanding of the context of the research. All data collection procedures should be explicitly described, including specific methods, training of data gatherers, the length of time for the study and the data collected. Procedures to enhance the rigor of the study, such as triangulation, member checking, and consistency of coding themes should be described.

TAKE-HOME MESSAGES

Evaluating the Evidence

✔ EBP requires the researcher to search through the evidence and evaluate different study designs as a means of defining the confidence to be placed in study conclusions.

✔ Different levels of evidence for effectiveness include (in order) systematic reviews, RCTs, cohort studies, case-control studies, case series, and finally, expert opinion, bench research, or theoretical principles.

✔ A variety of structured and semistructured appraisal tools are available to assist with critical appraisal.

✔ Critical review of different studies must be done using criteria specific for that type of methodology

✔ Critical appraisal is a skill that improves with practice. Evidence-based journal clubs provide a useful mechanism to achieve this.

LEARNING AND EXPLORATION ACTIVITIES

The purpose of this chapter is to introduce students to various types of evidence and the different means of classifying this evidence. The following practical exercises are intended to allow the student to become comfortable with the different means of evaluating the evidence.

1. Decide upon a treatment of interest (perhaps one you have been studying in class) and perform a search of the literature for articles or studies relating to that treatment. When you find one, attempt to place it in one of the "levels of evidence" system cited in this chapter. What are the greatest strengths of the study? The greatest weaknesses? Why did you place it where you did in the hierarchy? Justify your answers. Did one system work better than another for this study?

2. Obtain the following article from the library—Friedman, R., & Tappen, R. M. (1991). The effect of planned walking on communication in Alzheimer's Disease. *Journal of American Geriatrics Society, 39,* 650-654. Using the Quantitative Critical Review Form and Guidelines (Appendices A and B), critically review this study and complete the review form. Use this as a basis for discussion of the rigor of this study with your fellow students.

3. Select a rehabilitation outcome measure that you are currently studying or are interested in learning. Perform a literature review to identify research on the measure. Obtain the measure's manual if there is one. Using Appendices E and F, complete a critical review of this measure. Some suggested measures to review include the Functional Independence Measure (FIM), Barthel Index, Medical Outcomes Study (MOS) SF-36, Oswestry Low Back Pain Disability Questionnaire.

4. Obtain the following article from the library—Borell, L., Gustavsson, A., Sandman, P. O., Kielhofner, G. (1994). Occupational programming in a day hospital for patients with dementia. *The Occupational Therapy Journal of Research, 14*(4), 219-238. Using the Qualitative Critical Review Form and Guidelines (Appendices C and D), critically review this study and complete the review form. Use this as a basis for discussion of the rigor of this study with your fellow students.

5. Choose a quantitative and/or qualitative article that focuses on a rehabilitation intervention of your choice. Use Appendices A, B, C, and D to critically review these articles.

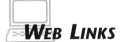
WEB LINKS

- *McMaster's Centre for Evidence-Based Rehabilitation critical appraisal Web page*
  www.fhs.mcmaster.ca/rehab/research/appraisevidence.html

- *The CONSORT Statement*
  www.consort-statement.org
  The CONSORT statement lays out a number of guidelines for conducting good RCTs, which are essential for sound SRs. The homepage has more detailed information and updates on current work.

- *Centre for Evidence-Based Medicine Levels of Evidence Classification*
  www.cebm.net/levels_of_evidence.asp
  This "levels of evidence" system is an updated version of the original description of levels of evidence, as described by Sackett, Haynes, and others.

- *Guide to Research Methods: The Evidence Pyramid*
  http://library.downstate.edu/EBM2/2100.htm
  The Evidence Pyramid was prepared by the Suny Downstate Medical Center. The evidence-based tutorial provides basic definitions and examples of clinical research designs to help the medical student or new clinician understand how the design of a research study may affect whether or not to accept its findings in caring for a patient.

- *University of Illinois at Chicago: Is All Evidence Created Equal?*
  www.uic.edu/depts/lib/lhsp/resources/levels.shtml
  This site, compiled by the University of Chicago Library, takes an open-ended approach to the topic. Students will likely find the bottom of the page the most useful, as it discusses the characteristics of specific types of evidence and where to find them.

- *A New View of Statistics*
  www.sportsci.org/resource/stats/index.html
  An excellent primer or refresher to many aspects of statistics, complied and created by New Zealander William Hopkins.

- *The Research Advocacy Network*
  www.researchadvocacy.org/advocateInstitute/pdf/RAN_ShortcutLevelsOfEvidence.pdf.
  This shortcut sheet was developed by Research Advocacy Network to assist advocates in understanding Levels of Evidence and how these concepts apply to clinical practice.

- http://davidmlane.com/hyperstat/index.html
  Free online stats textbook

- http://statpages.org
  Free online stats calculations

- http://nilesonline.com/stats
  Easy reading stats textbook

- *PEDro.*
  www.pedro.fhs.usyd.edu.au
  This is a searchable physiotherapy evidence database that provides bibliographic details, abstracts, and ratings of RCTs, systematic reviews, and evidence-based clinical practice guidelines in physiotherapy.

- *OTseeker*
  www.otseeker.com

This is a searchable database that provides abstracts and ratings of randomized controlled trials and systematic reviews relevant to occupational therapy.

- *Evidence-Based Medicine Tool Kit*
  www.med.ualberta.ca/ebm/ebm.htm
  This site provides critical appraisal tools.

- *Aggressive Research Intelligence Facility*
  www.arif.bham.ac.uk/casp/caindex.htm
  This site provides information on the critical appraisal process.

- *Appraisal of Guidelines for Research & Evaluation*
  www.agreecollaboration.org
  This site provides critical appraisal tools for CPGs (see Chapter 13).

- *Best Evidence Topics*
  www.bestbets.org/cgi-bin/public_pdf.pl
  This site provides a database of critically appraised topics and tools.

- *Center for Evidence-Based Emergency Medicine*
  www.ebem.org/analyse.html
  This site provides critical appraisal tools.

- *Centre for Evidence-Based Medicine, Oxford*
  www.cebm.net/critical_appraisal.asp
  This site provides a database of critically appraised topics and tools.

- *Centre for Evidence-Based Medicine, Oxford CATmaker*
  www.cebm.net/catmaker.asp
  This site provides a software tool to help create critically appraised topics.

- *Centre for Evidence-Based Medicine, Toronto*
  www.cebm.utoronto.ca/teach/materials/caworksheets.htm
  This site provides critical appraisal tools.

- *Centre for Evidence-Based Mental Health*
  www.cebmh.com
  This site provides critical appraisal tools.

- *Centre for Health Evidence*
  www.cche.net/usersguides/main.asp
  This site provides critical appraisal tools.

- *Critical Appraisal Skills Programme*
  www.phru.nhs.uk/casp/critical_appraisal_tools.htm
  This site provides critical appraisal tools.

- *Evidence-Based Medicine, Duke*
  www.mclibrary.duke.edu/subject/ebm?tab=appraising&extra=worksheets
  This site provides critical appraisal tools.

- *Glasgow Appraisal Tool*
  http://ssrc.tums.ac.ir/SystematicReview/Glasgow.asp
  This site provides critical appraisal tools.

- *Health Care Practice Research & Development Unit*
  www.fhsc.salford.ac.uk/hcprdu/critical-appraisal.htm
  This site provides critical appraisal tools.

- *Journal Club, Evidence-Based Medicine*
  www.geh.nhs.uk/services/edu/Library/Jclub/appraisal_tools.asp
  This site provides a list of completed appraisals and critical appraisal tools.

- *McMaster University—Occupational Therapy*
  www.fhs.mcmaster.ca/rehab/ebp
  This site provides critical appraisal tools.

- *Quality of Reporting of Meta-Analyses*
  www.consort-statement.org/QUOROM.pdf
  This is a checklist for evaluating meta-analyses and RCTs.

- *School of Health and Related Research (ScHARR), University of Sheffield*
  www.shef.ac.uk/scharr/sections/ir/links
  This site provides critical appraisal tools.

REFERENCES

Atkins, D., Best, D., Briss, P. A., Eccles, M., Falck-Ytter, Y., Flottorp, S., et al. (2004). Grading quality of evidence and strength of recommendations. *British Medical Journal, 328,* 1490.

Atkins, D., Eccles, M., Flottorp, S., Guyatt, G. H., Henry, D., Hill, S., et al. (2004). Systems for grading the quality of evidence and the strength of recommendations I: critical appraisal of existing approaches. The GRADE Working Group. *BMC Health Services Research, 4,* 38.

Bennett, K. J., Sackett, D. L., Haynes, R. B., Neufeld, V. R., Tugwell, P., & Roberts, R. (1987). A controlled trial of teaching critical appraisal of the clinical literature to medical students. *Journal of the American Medical Association, 257,* 2451-2454.

Bryar, R. M., Closs, S. J., Baum, G., Cooke, J., Griffiths, J., Hostick, T., et al. (2003). The Yorkshire BARRIERS project: Diagnostic analysis of barriers to research utilisation. *International Journal of Nursing Studies, 40,* 73-84.

Coomarasamy, A., & Khan, K. S. (2004). What is the evidence that postgraduate teaching in Evidence-Based medicine changes anything? A systematic review. *British Medical Journal, 329,* 1017.

Coomarasamy, A., Taylor, R., & Khan, K. S. (2003). A systematic review of postgraduate teaching in evidence-based medicine and critical appraisal. *Medical Teacher, 25,* 77-81.

Creswell, J. W. (1998). *Qualitative inquiry and research design: Choosing among five traditions.* Thousand Oaks, CA: Sage.

Current Methods of the U.S. Preventive Services Task Force: A Review of the Process [Electronic version]. (2001). *American Journal of Preventive Medicine, 20*(35) 21-34

Greenhalgh, T. (1997). Assessing the methodological quality of published papers. *British Medical Journal, 315,* 305-308.

Guyatt, G., Jaeschke, R., Heddle, N., Cook, D., Shannon, H., & Walter, S. (1995a). Basic statistics for clinicians: 1. Hypothesis testing. *Canadian Medical Association Journal, 152,* 27-32.

Guyatt, G., Jaeschke, R., Heddle, N., Cook, D., Shannon, H., & Walter, S. (1995b). Basic statistics for clinicians: 2. Interpreting study results: Confidence intervals. *Canadian Medical Association Journal, 152,* 169-173.

Guyatt, G., Walter, S., Shannon, H., Cook, D., Jaeschke, R., & Heddle, N. (1995c). Basic statistics for clinicians: 4. Correlation and regression. *Canadian Medical Association Journal, 152,* 497-504.

Katrak, P., Bialocerkowski, A. E., Massy-Westropp, N., Kumar, V. S., & Grimmer, K. (2004). A systematic review of the content of critical appraisal tools. *BMC Medical Research Methodology., 4,* 22.

Mamdani, M., Sykora, K., Li, P., Normand, S. L., Streiner, D. L., Austin, P. C., et al. (2005). Reader's guide to critical appraisal of cohort studies: 2. Assessing potential for confounding. *British Medical Journal, 330,* 960-962.

National Health Service (NHS) in the United Kingdom. (2004). Section 6: Forming guideline recommendations. Retrieved October 22, 2007, from http://www.sign.ac.uk/guidelines/fulltext/50/section6.html

Sackett, D. L., Straus, S. E., Richardson, W. S., Rosenberg, W., & Haynes, R. B. (2000). *Evidence-based medicine. How to practice and teach EBM* (2nd ed.). Toronto, ON: Churchill Livingstone.

Steering Committee on Clinical Practice Guidelines for the Care and Treatment of Breast Cancer. (1998). Clinical practice guidelines for the care and treatment of breast cancer. Retrieved October 22, 2007, from http://www.cmaj.ca/cgi/content/full/158/3/DC1

Turner, P., & Mjolne, I. (2001). Journal provision and the prevalence of journal clubs: A survey of physiotherapy departments in England and Australia. *Physiotherapy Research International, 6,* 157-169.

Wikipedia. (n.d.). Evidence-based medicine. Retrieved August 29, 2007, from http://en.wikipedia.org/wiki/Evidence-Based_Medicine.

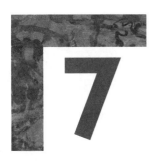

Systematically
Reviewing the Evidence

Laura Bradley, MSc OT, OTReg(Ont) and Mary Law, PhD, OTReg(Ont), FCAOT

LEARNING OBJECTIVES

After reading this chapter, the student/practitioner will be able to:
- Understand the difference between narrative reviews, systematic reviews, meta-analyses, and metasynthesis.
- Understand the method for conducting a systematic review or metasynthesis..
- Understand the best method for critically appraising a systematic review
- Understand the best method for critically appraising a metasynthesis.

You are now well on your way to developing the art and science of evidence-based rehabilitation. You have been increasing your skills in finding, assessing, and using the evidence in everyday practice. You are experienced at asking relevant questions, and you have an understanding of where to find the information you need. You recognize the importance of reviewing several sources of information, including journals, colleagues, and client choice with your own clinical experience to arrive at clinical decisions. The process is becoming second nature, but you are still left wondering, "Did I get it all?"

With constant demands on the time and resources available to clinicians, the expectation of appraising and understanding all research pertaining to a specific subject matter can be daunting. High-quality literature is being published at too great a rate to be thoroughly analyzed by each practitioner. In order to keep current in any given field, a practitioner would need to read, on average, 19 original articles each day (Klassen, Jadad, & Moher, 1998). Furthermore, it is difficult for a clinician to remain unbiased in the evaluation of literature surrounding his or her question. There is a tendency to appraise or find articles that support what was originally being sought. To address these issues, critical reviews have arisen. A review sets out to analyze and summarize a specific subset of research information and come to a conclusion based on the information included in the review. There are two main categories of quantitative review: narrative and systematic (Table 7-1). A qualitative review, or metasynthesis, will be further explored later in the chapter.

Table 7-1

DIFFERENCES BETWEEN NARRATIVE AND SYSTEMATIC REVIEWS

Feature	Narrative Review	Systematic Review
Question	Often broad in scope	Often a focused clinical question
Sources and search	Not usually specified, potentially biased	Comprehensive sources and explicit search strategy
Selection	Not usually specified, potentially biased	Criterion-based selection, uniformly applied
Appraisal	Variable	Rigorous critical appraisal
Synthesis	Often a qualitative summary	Quantitative* summary
Inferences	Sometimes evidence-based	Usually evidence-based

*A quantitative summary that includes a statistical synthesis is a meta-analysis.

Reprinted from Cook, M.D., Mulrow, C.D., & Haynes, R.B. (1997). Systematic reviews: Synthesis of best evidence for clinical decisions. *Annals of Internal Medicine, 126*(5), 376-380 with permission of BMJ Publishing Group.

A narrative review is a gathering of information by an individual who may be considered an expert in the field (Klassen et al., 1998). This type of review can also be considered an unsystematic review as it sets out to answer a research question but lacks the explicit description of an organized approach to gathering the literature (Duffy, 2005). This facet of the narrative review becomes its chief limitation; the decision tree to include or exclude articles is not provided for the reader, making it difficult to evaluate the quality of the information contained within the publication.

A systematic review, by contrast, is a summary of the literature that uses clear methods to perform a thorough search and critical appraisal of individual studies (The Cochrane Collaboration, n.d.). The goal of this summary is to investigate a specific research question in ways that minimize bias and random error. Such a review will include clear inclusion and exclusion criteria, with only some if the pool of literature is included. In essence, a systematic review will critically appraise relevant studies for you and provide you with a conclusion that you can then apply to practice. Quantitative systematic reviews, or meta-analyses, contain a statistical summary of at least one outcome in two or more trials.

The completion of a systematic review is time consuming and can be very costly. Various schools of thought on systematic reviews have produced slightly different methodologies for conducting reviews. Although these differences exist, they generally follow along the same path. The path presented, adapted from Duffy (2005), outlines a general process that this may take:

Formulating a review question
↓
Conducting a comprehensive search of the literature
↓
Critically appraising each of the studies
↓

Table 7-2

LEVELS OF EVIDENCE IN SYSTEMATIC REVIEWS

Review Type	*Level of Best Evidence*
Treatment and/or prevention	Randomized controlled trials
Diagnostic tests	Comparison to a gold standard
Prognosis	Cohort studies
Review of risk factors	Cohort, case/control, or ecologic studies

Adapted from Counsell, C. (1997). Formulating questions and locating primary studies for inclusion in systematic reviews. *Annals of Internal Medicine, 127*(5), 380-387.

Synthesizing the findings
↓
Reporting the results

STEP 1: FORMULATING A REVIEW QUESTION

As systematic reviews set out to answer a specific clinical question, the development and clarity of that question is paramount. Ask a poor question, and you are likely to have a systematic review of limited use. Ask a clear and specific question, and you are likely to have a systematic review that can potentially be applied to clinical practice (Klassen et al., 1998). Questions generally arise from a gap in the literature, clinical encounters, clinician or patient queries, or clinical trends (Akonbeng, 2005; Counsell, 1997; Lapier, 2003). At times, questions result from the introduction of a new treatment or technique, which must be compared to the standard. Alternately, different clinics, professionals, or even countries may approach the same situations in different ways. These too must be compared to ensure best practice. Finally, different elements of treatment can have different costs associated with them. Questions can set out to examine which treatment is most cost effective for a particular situation.

Questions for systematic review classically focus on one of the following areas: diagnosis, etiology, prognosis, treatment, or prevention (Mulrow & Cook, 1997). As discussed in earlier chapters, clinical research can be defined on the basis of four elements: population, intervention, comparison, and outcome. A good systematic review question will use these to define inclusion and exclusion criteria that direct which articles are retrieved for the review. More recently, we have started to see more innovative applications of the systematic review process. For example, using a systematic review process to classify outcome measures used by clinical research into conceptual frameworks like health models. Regardless of the review, the process should find and extract conclusions and make recommendations on the basis of the best possible evidence. To this end, there are types of publications that lend themselves better to answering different review questions (Table 7-2). In the absence of the best levels of evidence, other types of evidence, or lower levels of evidence, may be included.

STEP 2: CONDUCTING A COMPREHENSIVE SEARCH OF THE LITERATURE

After the question has been posed and the inclusion and exclusion criteria have been outlined, the reviewers begin the process of combing the literature for relevant articles. This process of searching the evidence is presented in detail in Chapter 5. The systems used to search the evidence should be clearly indicated by the reviewers, as well as the search terms used.

The most common place to begin searching for information is through electronic databases such as CINAHL or EMBASE. Although this seems a fairly straightforward process, it often becomes quite complicated. As you may remember, many of the different databases use different headings and subheadings for the same information. For example, the term *cancer*, which is common in most databases, has the heading neoplasms in MEDLINE. Similarly, one databases hyperlink may not exist in another. For example, in CINAHL, the term *occupational therapy* can be exploded and searched independently. In MEDLINE, it can only be searched as a keyword. These differences make it vital for the reviewers to include terms that they have searched in order to ensure that relevant articles have not been missed. See Chapter 5 for more details.

After all electronic databases have been exhaustively searched, other techniques can be used to gather relevant sources of information. Reviewers can opt to hand search the reference lists in relevant journals or conference proceedings. Similarly, reviewers can manually search the reference lists of articles already identified for inclusion. Caution in this technique must be used, however, as reference bias can result in more favorable results being referenced more often (Counsell, 1997).

Regardless of the method of choosing articles, the reviewers should state clearly what that method was, as well as relevant search terms used, and the inclusion and exclusion criteria that began the search.

STEP 3: CRITICALLY APPRAISING EACH STUDY

As in primary research studies, flaws in the data can affect the results of a systematic review. For this reason, each article must be appraised for its relevance to the inclusion criteria, methodological strengths, and potential sources of bias. Publication bias is one area in which reviewers often face difficulty (Akobeng, 2005; Moher, Jadad, & Klassen, 1998). On one hand, articles included for publication in peer-reviewed journals can be viewed as a strong source of evidence. On the other hand, articles with favorable results may be published more often than those with unfavorable results, hence the term *publication bias*. These unpublished papers often provide valuable information but are not included for appraisal by the general public. Some reviewers include these unpublished studies even though they have not been peer reviewed to attempt to minimize this source of potential bias.

Appraising each article for the review should be undertaken by at least two reviewers with a predetermined set of criteria. In most cases, the reviewers appraise the articles independently, often assigning a score to each article. Common criteria include the level of methodology, the use of blinding, the reporting and treatment of missing data, and the way that subjects who were lost to follow-up were included in the final result (Whitney, 2004). These were addressed in more detail in the previous chapter. The reviewers then get together to compare results. Any discrepancies are discussed and a common ground is found. In some cases, disputed articles are brought to an outside reviewer for appraisal.

As with the previous step, regardless of the way the articles were appraised, the method and appraisal criteria should be clearly explained for the reader.

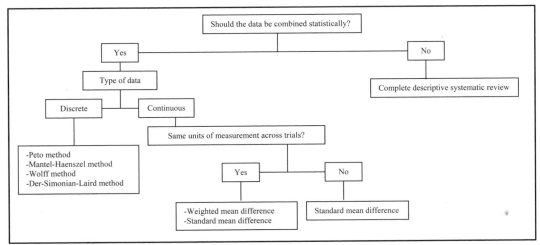

Figure 7-1. Statistical choices available to systematic reviewers. (Reprinted with permission from Moher, D., Jadad, A., & Klassen., T. (1998). Guides for reading and interpreting systematic reviews. *Archives of Pediatric and Adolescent Medicine, 152,* 915-920. © 1998 American Medical Association. All rights reserved.)

STEP 4: SYNTHESIZING THE FINDINGS

There is presently no agreed upon method that items should be synthesized in a qualitative systematic review. Clinical judgment should be used to determine the appropriate combination of the reviewed studies. Were the included studies, in fact, similar enough in methodology, population, or outcome measure to have their findings pooled? Often the reviewers make a statement to this fact before presenting the summary results.

A quantitative systematic review, or meta-analysis, offers a different picture. As you recall, the goal of a meta-analysis is to reach a conclusion through statistical means. At this point, the reviewers have several options available to them. Figure 7-1, taken from Moher, Jadad, and Klassen (1998), outlines some of these choices.

STEP 5: REPORTING THE RESULTS

The final process, reporting the findings, is also the most important to the reader. In this step, all of the work that has been put into the systematic review can be shared with potential readers. The entire process, not just the end result, must be written up. All of the variables and choices made along the way affect how the final outcome emerges. The reviewers must cite any and all possibilities for bias that could have existed both in the original trials and in the secondary work of the systematic review. For an example of a completed systematic review, see Chapter 8.

META-ANALYSIS

The quantitative approach of a meta-analysis, as mentioned earlier, contains a statistical summary of at least one outcome in two or more trials. These results are presented statistically in graphic form. The graphic form, or forest plot, is well known in the EBP world, most commonly as the logo of the Cochrane Collaboration (Figure 7-2). A forest plot shows the reader "information from the individual studies that went into the meta-analysis and an estimate of the overall

Figure 7-2. Cochrane Collaboration logo. (This logo has been reproduced with kind permission of the Cochrane Collaboration.)

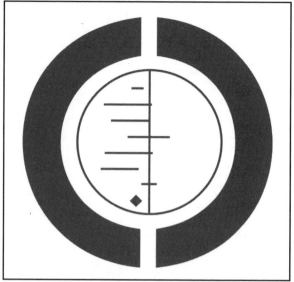

results" (Akonbeng, 2005, p. 846). Visually, it is a vertical line with a number of horizontal lines running across it. During meta-analysis, each study involved is distilled down to a confidence interval, which states with 95% certainty what the effects of that study were. Thus, a forest plot represents the pooled odds ratios of all the studies in the review. If a (horizontal) confidence interval of a result crosses the (vertical) line of no effect, it means either that a significant difference does not exist between the treatment and the control or that the sample size was too small to allow us to be confident where the true result lies. The diamond represents the pooled data from all the studies in question. In the example of the Cochrane logo, the diamond is to the left of the line of no effect. If this were a true forest plot, we could say that the meta-analysis has showed the treatment in question has had no effect. For an example of a forest plot related to a rehabilitation intervention, see Chapter 8. Although potentially very useful, there are advantages and disadvantages of using the meta-analysis as a source of information (Table 7-3).

The goal of a systematic review, aside from offering a summary of original articles, is to be published. Much in the same way as original articles, systematic reviews can also suffer from publication biases. Many people think that a systematic review finding no significant results from a group of trials is not useful. The truth could not be more to the contrary. Many clinical misjudgments are made daily because of the negative publication bias, or the tendency for journals to only publish results that are positive. If practitioners knew about the negative results coming from some systematic reviews, they may change their practice habits. However, negative results are not as interesting as positive ones, and therefore get less coverage. Publishing both positive and negative systematic reviews is the only way in which a more complete knowledge of which interventions or treatments are beneficial can be garnered. Through the publication of all research, the health sciences and rehabilitation community can find out which currently practiced treatments deserve to be altered or abandoned.

Using systematic reviews in clinical practice, although in many cases preferable, still contains some inherent risks. Just as in individual studies, there are high and low quality systematic reviews. Systematic reviews presenting results of poor quality studies with questionable methods or an unclear question will still not be of clinical use. The existence of a systematic review on a topic does not replace your ability to look at literature with a critical eye (Klassen, Jadad, &

Table 7-3

ADVANTAGES AND DISADVANTAGES OF META-ANALYSIS

Advantages	Disadvantages
Produces a single, precise estimate of benefits and harm	The "numerical bottom line" can be distracting and overlook important sources of bias and diversity between individual trials.
Can be applied (with caution) to cohort and case control studies as well as RCTs	Conclusions expressed as recommendations for the average or typical patient may be unhelpful in practice.
	Few interventions have been adequately addressed by meta-analysis, and the method, while theoretically sound, "often fails in ways that are invisible to the analyst."

Adapted from www.shef.ac.uk/scharr/ir/units/systrev/advdis.htm

Moher, 1998). How then can a practitioner know if a systematic review is of use or good enough quality to apply to clinical practice?

CRITICALLY APPRAISING SYSTEMATIC REVIEWS

Critically appraising systematic reviews should be considered an art as well as a science. A clinician appraising a systematic review needs to rely as much on clinical judgment as preset review forms. Many methods of evaluating systematic reviews have been proposed; however, it is ultimately a clinician's choice as to which method is most useful. One method, developed by Oxman & Guyatt (1991), has been shown to distinguish between systematic reviews of good and poor quality. This method, outlined in Table 7-4, asks the reader to rate specific elements of a systematic review. The scoring, presented in Table 7-5, distinguishes between a systematic review that has minimal (a score of 7), minor (a score of 5 to 6), major (a score of 3 to 4), or extensive (a score of 1 to 2) flaws. Ultimately, the clinical user will decide what this score will mean (Peach, 2002). For example, a systematic review with a lower score may be used in the absence of other higher quality research. Similarly, a systematic review with a very high score may not be of clinical use if it cannot be applied to the specific population of interest.

Another system of critically appraising systematic reviews is presented in the Centre for Evidence-Based Medicine in the University of Alberta. These researchers have compiled a list of questions and a worksheet to help guide you through appraising a systematic review. The information can be found at www.ebm.med.ualberta.ca/sysrev.htm (questions) and www.ebm.med. ualberta.ca/sysrevworksheet.htm (worksheets). The following sections go through this method of appraisal in more detail. The more questions that receive a "yes" response, the higher the quality of the review (Duffy, 2005). Throughout this section, statistical concepts will be briefly explained. As the goal of this chapter is not to teach statistics, further information—should it be needed—can be found in and good quality statistical text. All statistical definitions in this section (indicated in bold) have been taken from the University of Toronto's Center for Evidence-Based Medicine, found at www.cebm.utoronto.ca/glossary/index.htm#c.

Table 7-4

GUIDE TO APPRAISING SYSTEMATIC REVIEWS

Question	Answer		
Were the methods used to find primary research studies reported?	No	Partially	Yes
Was the search comprehensive?	No	Cannot tell	Yes
Were the criteria used for deciding which studies to include in the review reported?	No	Partially	Yes
Was bias in the selection of studies avoided?	No	Cannot tell	Yes
Were the criteria used for assessing validity of the studies reported?	No	Partially	Yes
Was the validity of all studies assessed using appropriate criteria?	No	Cannot tell	Yes
Were the methods used to combine findings of the studies to reach a conclusion reported?	No	Cannot tell	Yes
Were the methods appropriate?	No	Partially	Yes
Was the conclusion supported by the data and/or analysis?	No	Partially	Yes
What was the overall scientific quality of the review?	Extensive/major/minor/minimal flaws		

Adapted from Oxman, A., & Guyatt, G. (1991). Validation of an index of the quality of review articles. *Journal of Clinical Epidemiology, 44,* 1271-1278.

SECTION 1: ARE THE RESULTS VALID?

1. *Did the overview address a focused clinical question?* As with any research, reviews that ask a poor question will have a lower quality. Each element of P.I.C.O. should be present in the reviewer's question.

2. *Were the criteria used to select articles for inclusion appropriate?* It is important to note if the inclusion and exclusion criteria for the review are appropriate and will serve to answer the question. Without strong, clear, and appropriate inclusion criteria, it is possible that the overall results will be weakened by studies that are not valid to the original question.

3. *Is it unlikely that important, relevant studies were missed?* What were the reviewers searching methods? Have they been presented in a way that will allow you to decide if there are any gaps? The greater the rigor of the original search, the less likely that the final review will suffer from random error and publication bias (Counsell, 1997; Whitney, 2004). Appropriate search strategies have been discussed earlier in this chapter.

4. *Was the validity of the included studies appraised?* Validity refers to the study's level of truth, or potential freedom from bias. The higher the validity of each included study, the greater the overall validity of the final review.

Table 7-5		
SCORING OF A SYSTEMATIC REVIEW		
Step 1	Is the "no" option used for one or more of questions 2, 4, 6, or 8?	No: Go to step 3
		Yes: Go to step 2
Step 2	How often is the "no" option used for questions 2, 4, 6, and 8?	4 times: review scores a 1
		2 to 3 times: review scores a 2
		1 time: review scores a 3
Step 3	Is the "cannot tell" option used for one or more of questions 2, 4, 6, or 8?	No: review scores a 7
		Yes: review scores a 4

Adapted from Oxman, A., & Guyatt, G. (1991). Validation of an index of the quality of review articles. *Journal of Clinical Epidemiology, 44,* 1271-1278.

5. *Were assessments of studies reproducible?* There should be some explanation as to how the reviewing team came to include each of the studies. For example, evidence that the reviewers were blinded or that there was a system in place should the reviewers disagree will add strength to the final product.

6. *Were the results similar from study to study?* This can be examined through tests for homogeneity. Homogeneity means that the results of each individual trial are mathematically compatible with the results of any of the others (Greenhalgh, 1997). Reviewers should not be comparing studies that are too different in either population or outcome.

SECTION 2: WHAT ARE THE RESULTS?

1. *What are the overall results of the review?* The results of the review need to be clearly stated in order for you to determine if it is useful to your situation or may be applied to your practice. If the overall results were not statistically significant, review some of the reasons why this may be so in order to determine if the review is still of clinical significance. A meta-analysis may report the results in terms of an odds ratio (OR) or relative risk (RR), defined below. The OR and RR are reported in relation to 1: greater than 1 indicates an increased likelihood of the outcome found in the treatment group and less than 1 indicates the decreased likelihood of the outcome found in the treatment group. An OR or RR of 1 indicates no difference.

   • **Odds ratio:** The ratio of the odds of having the target disorder in the experimental group relative to the odds in favor of having the target disorder in the control group (in cohort studies or systematic reviews) or the odds in favor of being exposed in subjects with the target disorder divided by the odds in favor of being exposed in control subjects (without the target disorder).

   • **Relative risk:** The ratio of risk in the treated group to the risk in the control group.

2. *How precise were the results?* The investigator should present his or her results in terms of how precise they are. This is termed a *confidence interval*, defined below, which quantifies the uncertainty of the measurement.

- **Confidence intervals**: It is usually reported as a 95% CI, which is the range of values within which we can be 95% sure that the true value for the whole population lies. For example, for a numbers needed to treat (NNT) of 10 with a 95% CI of 5 to 15, we would have 95% confidence that the true NNT value lies between 5 and 15.

SECTION 3: WILL THE RESULTS HELP ME IN CARING FOR MY PATIENTS?

1. *Can the results be applied to my patient care?* In order for the results of the review to be useful, the results must deal with patients, demographics, and conditions similar to a particular clinical practice or question. If a clinician had a question about the benefit of a particular intervention with their geriatric population, a review dealing with a pediatric population may be of limited use. Similarly, there should be no obvious reason (such as poor methodology or indications of potential harm) why the results of this review should not be applied.

2. *Were all clinically important outcomes considered?* Are the outcomes provided in the review the most appropriate target outcomes for the treatment? For example, if you are interested in the community reintegration of youth after brain injury, a systematic review focused on the outcome of memory would not be an appropriate indicator.

3. *Are the likely treatment benefits worth the potential harms and costs?* Every treatment is associated with costs and the potential for benefit in relation to harm. It is up to the discretion of individual clinicians (working within potential institutional guidelines) if the treatment benefits to clients presented within the review are worth the potential harms and costs associated with that treatment. NNT, defined below, is often included in reviews. This will help a clinician make that choice.

- **NNT**: The number of patients who need to be treated in order to prevent one additional (poor) outcome.

FINDING SYSTEMATIC REVIEWS

Although systematic reviews are being completed at an increased rate (Duffy, 2005), there is still planning involved to find them. Thankfully, a clinician in search of systematic reviews has several options available to them.

First, the American National Library of Medicine (NLM) offers an electronic text-based search and retrieval system that contains many databases, including PubMed. This site, found at www.ncbi.nlm.nih.gov/entrez, allows you to search full text and abstracts using keywords. As an addition to narrow down your searching, the keyword systematic reviews can be added. Although not all articles are full text, this is a good place to begin your searching.

Systematic reviews can also be found while searching databases such as OVID and MEDLINE. Similar to searching for primary studies and original articles, systematic reviews can be found by entering keywords about the topic you are searching for. As a strategy to narrow down your search, these databases (and others) allow you to limit your results to only systematic reviews.

Both OTSeeker and the physiotherapy evidence database (PEDro) can be sources of information specific to rehabilitation professionals. OTSeeker, found at www.otseeker.com, is a database that contains abstracts of systematic reviews and randomized controlled trials relevant to occupational therapy. PEDro, found at http://www.pedro.fhs.usyd.edu.au, offers bibliographic details and abstracts of randomized controlled trials, systematic reviews, and evidence-based clinical practice guidelines in physiotherapy. Both of these sites, although not directly linking to full texts, offer an option to select only systematic reviews. Searching these databases provides a method for rehabilitation professionals to see what research has been done in order to have a more specific search strategy in the other databases.

Finally, systematic reviews can be accessed through a central location, discussed in more detail below.

THE COCHRANE COLLABORATION

What should practitioners do with systematic reviews and meta-analyses once they have been completed? Of course each reviewer will hold on to completed studies, but that number represents only a handful of reviews potentially completed on the same topic. Could the results of systematic reviews and meta-analyses from around the world somehow be brought together?

It was this question that inspired the creation of the Cochrane Collaboration. The Collaboration is named after the British epidemiologist Archie Cochrane, who strongly advocated for the widespread use of systematic reviews to guide practice. It was Dr. Cochrane's belief that we need to change the way we provide health care because of the outpouring of health care information created each year. To resolve this problem, Dr. Cochrane proposed creating an organization that would conduct systematic reviews in all aspects of health care and would act as a clearinghouse, distributing them worldwide. The creation of the Cochrane Collaboration was also spurred on by the realization that a medical failure can result from the lack of systematic reviews.

As such, the Collaboration itself is based around the following 10 founding principles, which all members attempt to uphold in their work:

1. Collaboration
2. Building on the enthusiasm of individuals
3. Avoiding duplication
4. Minimizing bias
5. Keeping up to date
6. Ensuring relevance
7. Ensuring access
8. Continually improving the quality of its work
9. Continuity
10. Enabling wide participation (Source: www.cochrane.org/docs/tenprinciples.htm)

There are a number of tasks that the Cochrane Collaboration undertakes, but the main output of the Cochrane Collaboration is systematic reviews.

The Cochrane Library itself is the mainstay of the Cochrane Collaboration and is composed of a number of parts. Firstly, The Cochrane Controlled Trials Register (CCTR) contains a collection of nearly 300,000 randomized controlled trials, which supply high-quality evidence for systematic reviews. A second part of the library is the Cochrane Database of Systematic Reviews (CDSR), which lists the Cochrane Collaboration's completed reviews and outlines of its reviews in progress. It currently holds approximately 4,500 entries. The Database of Abstracts of Reviews of Effectiveness (DARE) also lists systematic reviews, but those that were undertaken and published outside of the Cochrane Collaboration. Finally, the Cochrane Review Methodology Database (CRMD) provides information on the procedures, methods, and processes of EBP. The Cochrane Library is available through Wiley interscience at www3.interscience.wiley.com/cgi-bin/mrwhome/106568753/AccessCochraneLibrary.html.

To find the Cochrane Centre in your area, consult the list of regional Cochrane Centre Web sites at www.cochrane.org/cochrane/crgs.htm#CENTRES. The Cochrane Collaboration Brochure, from which much of the above information was found, is also online at www.cochrane.org.

The Cochrane Collaboration represents a vast worldwide effort toward EBP, which will become more and more necessary as the volume of health care information grows while budgets shrink. The Collaboration itself is a first step toward creating a more integrated, evidence-based network for drawing on the vast resources of the entire medical profession to serve clients.

THE CAMPBELL COLLABORATION

A second source for randomized controlled trial and systematic reviews is the Campbell Collaboration, which is available at www.campbellcollaboration.org. Their objective is to help people make evidence-based decisions regarding interventions through the preparation, maintenance, and dissemination of systematic reviews. The Campbell Collaboration (C2) library houses two databases. The first, C2 Social, Psychological, Education, and Criminological Trials Registry (C2-SPECTR), contains approximately 12,000 entries in education, social welfare, and criminal justice. This registry serves as a starting point for researchers in the collaboration completing systematic reviews. The second, C2 Reviews of Interventions and Policy Evaluations (C2-RIPE) offers researchers, practitioners, and the public access to systematic reviews free of charge.

METASYNTHESIS

As discussed earlier in the chapter, qualitative research can be reviewed for much the same reasons as quantitative research. In qualitative research, the investigator sets out to "understand the thoughts, feelings and experiences of individuals, focusing on direct, face-to-face knowledge of patients as human beings coping with their treatment in a given social setting" (Polgar & Thomas, 2000, p.91). The results from qualitative literature offer a holistic picture of the participants in their natural setting and can be used to provide an in-depth understanding of a particular phenomenon or experience from the participant's point of view (Polgar & Thomas, 2000; Spencer, Ritchie, Lewis, & Dillon, 2003). To the uninitiated reader, qualitative research is very different, as it relies on language-based data rather than the numerical statistics found in quantitative research (Eakin & Mykhalovskiy, 2003).

To date, however, many valuable qualitative research studies have remained isolated from each other, with fewer attempts to put the results together than has been seen in the quantitative world (Sandelowski, Docherty, & Emden, 1997). However, to make these findings more useful and accessible to clinicians, researchers, and policy makers, the pooling together of results has become an increasing need (Finfgeld, 2003). From this need came the metasynthesis (also labeled meta-ethnography). As Sandelowski and Barroso (2003, pp. 784-785) say, a metasynthesis is a:

> study of the processes and results of previous studies in a target domain that moves beyond those studies to situate historically, define for the present, and chart future

directions in that domain. In meta-studies, the researcher seeks not only to combine the results from previous studies but also to reflect on them

This characteristic is the main difference between the meta-analysis and the metasynthesis; the researcher in the metasynthesis offers an interpretive product as well as an analytic process from the findings of primary authors rather than raw data (Sandelowski & Barroso, 2003). The goal of a metasynthesis is to "produce a new and integrative interpretation of findings that is more substantive than those resulting from individual investigations" (Finfgeld, 2003, p. 893).

Metasyntheses can also generate new models and theories, determine the existence of different "schools of thought and complement the findings of a systematic review" (Booth, 2001). The completion of metasyntheses, however, is not without controversy. In fact, due to the subjective nature of qualitative research and the potential for different methodological approaches, some authors have suggested that it may not be appropriate to synthesize it at all (Barbour, 1998; Sandelowski, 2006). Despite this controversy, metasyntheses remain an important contribution to health care literature and qualitative research as a whole (Sandelowski & Barroso, 2003).

Finfgeld (2003) has proposed three types of metasynthesis: theory building, theory explication, and descriptive metasynthesis. The first type, theory building, sets out to investigate a number of studies in order to move forward a given theory beyond what is possible in a single study. Syntheses within this category include grounded formal theory and the metastudy. Grounded formal theory uses substantive grounded theory findings to create formal theories. A metastudy brings about three types of formal qualitative analysis to create new theoretical interpretation. The second type, or theory explanation, examines abstract concepts within the original findings and expands upon them, resulting in a new understanding of that particular phenomenon. The final type, descriptive metasynthesis, involves the broad translation of findings across studies dealing with a particular phenomenon. The reader should be aware that other types of metasyntheses may exist, and a single metasynthesis may provide information in more than one category.

Similar to meta-analysis, there is no single accepted method for conducting a metasynthesis. Presented below is a method for conducting metasyntheses proposed by Finfgeld (2003), although the reader should be aware that other variations have been proposed (Finfgeld, 2003).

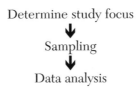

Determine study focus
↓
Sampling
↓
Data analysis

Step 1: Determine Study Focus

Similar to systematic reviews, a metasynthesis must have a clear focus in order to offer more precise results (Mays, Pope, & Popay, 2005). On one hand, the question should be broad enough to encompass all aspects of the phenomenon in question, but it should also be specific enough to be useful for policy makers, readers, and clinicians (Finfgeld, 2003). In setting out to ask a research question, it is important for the investigator to reflect on how the completion of this metasynthesis might be used to "answer existing clinical questions, build theory, [or] inform public policy" (Finfgeld, 2003, p. 898). This may be a more difficult task than first thought, as the investigators must examine their topic of interest and then determine how study findings can be compared. This can be a problem, as it may be difficult to conclude which studies are examining the same phenomenon or aspect of human experience (Sandelowski et al., 1997). For example, within one phenomenon, studies may examine a specific time period, feelings surrounding that experience, or the day-to-day management that the phenomenon entails (Sandelowski, Docherty, & Emden, 1997).

Step 2: Sampling

Once the question has been proposed, the investigators must begin the process of sampling current research that sets out to answer that question. No consensus exists on the best method for searching; however, many of the same principles that are found in selecting articles for systematic reviews apply for metasynthesis. Setting inclusion criteria is important as this will guide the investigators' choice. Sampling should then occur across disciplines, Internet, conferences, databases, and demographic elements (such as gender and ethnicity) to ensure that no relevant studies have been missed and assist in the generalizability of findings (Booth, 2001; Finfgeld, 2003, Mays et al., 2005). Sandelowski et al. (1997) suggest that studies should not be excluded for reasons of quality as there are many variations within the standards of qualitative research, and valuable information may be missed due to methodological weaknesses. They suggest that although quality should not be a reason for exclusion, it should remain an element within analysis, and it may take a true qualitative artist to distinguish between "surface errors and mistakes fatal enough to discount findings" (Sandelowski et al., 1997).

Searching the databases for qualitative literature can also be challenging as there is no central location for qualitative research similar to the Cochrane library. Investigators may also come up against poor indexing within databases, as well as variations within indexing terms. For example, CINAHL uses many different indexing terms for qualitative research, while MEDLINE does not index qualitative studies at all (Mays et al., 2005). Ensuring that all relevant research has been included may involve explicit strategies other than searching databases (e.g., hand searching reference lists and contacting researchers in the field of interest) (Booth, 2001; Mays et al., 2005).

Questions have been proposed as to how many articles should be included in a metasynthesis. Answers have ranged from 3 (Finfgeld, 2003), to no more than 10 (Sandelowski et al., 1997), to 292 (Patterson, Thorne, Canam, & Jillings, 2001). These variations may be due to topic breadth or the type of metasynthesis offered (Finfgeld, 2003). It has been cautioned that although no set limit has been accepted, overly large sample sizes may make deep analysis difficult (Sandelowski et al., 1997). If there are too many primary studies to include, the investigator may choose to narrow his or her focus (or question) to produce more manageable results (Dixon-Woods, Agarwal, Jones, Young, & Sutton, 2005).

Step 3: Data Analysis

At this stage, the investigators have a list of primary studies to be included in the metasynthesis. The next step is to determine if these studies can be compared as well as the similarities and differences between them. Qualitative research offers several methodologies from which to choose (e.g., ethnography, phenomenology, or grounded theory) (Creswell, 1998). Investigators must remember, however, that one researcher's grounded theory may be another's ethnography (Sandelowski et al., 1997). Each individual study includes the voice of the initial researcher; as such, it must be detected to assist in the methodological comparability and relationship to the metasynthesis as a whole (Sandelowski et al., 1997). Differences may exist not only between studies, but "also among lives-as-lived, lives-as-experienced, and lives-as-told" (Sandelowski & Boshamer, 2006). Once the comparability of original studies has been established, the investigators can begin to identify common or recurring concepts in each of these studies. These concepts are laid out in a table, from which second- and third-order interpretations can be made, leading to larger narratives or general theories derived from all studies (Mays et al., 2005; Sandelowski et al., 1997). The key lies in the investigator's ability to synthesize findings in an understandable way while maintaining the "integrity of individual studies" (Booth, 2001, p.8).

The following are examples of metasyntheses to further illustrate their construction and use as a clinical tool:

1. Britten, N., Campbell, R., Pope, C., Donovan, J., Morgan, M., & Pill, R. (2002). Using meta-ethnography to synthesize qualitative research: A worked example. *Journal of Health Services Research & Policy, 7*(4), 209-215.

2. Duggan, F., and Banwell, L. (2004). Constructing a model of effective information dissemination in a crisis. *Information Research, 9*(3) paper 178 [Available at http://InformationR. net/ir/9-3/paper178.html]

CRITICALLY APPRAISING METASYNTHESES

The conduct of metasyntheses is still in its early stages so there is no agreed-upon method to critically reviewing these works. In general, readers should pay close attention to the following characteristics:

- Did the reviewers ask a clear question that is relevant to your clinical practice?
- What was the rigor of the included studies?
- Were the reviewers clear about their methods for analyzing data?
- Was there a clear description of the similarities and differences between the primary studies?
- Did the reviewer synthesize the studies in an understandable way?

CONCLUSION

The need to critically evaluate the evidence available constitutes an integral aspect to EBP. Through an understanding of the details of different types of studies and the corresponding factors, one can better address the search for evidence to incorporate into practice. Although different methodologies exist for both the completion and appraisal of systematic reviews and metasynthesis, the production of these will allow a clinician to build a better EBP. The efficient finding and use of systematically reviewed qualitative and quantitative evidence can be a valuable tool in a busy clinician's toolbox; one that can contribute to quality client care.

TAKE HOME MESSAGES

Systematic Reviews

✔ Use scientific strategies to incorporate clinical trials done by different researchers on the same topic.

✔ There are various methodologies for preparing systematic reviews.

✔ Analyze Randomized Controlled Trials with respect to methodological quality, precision and external validity.

✔ All randomized controlled trials within the study will have some small error, but those studies with significant error should be rejected.

✔ CONSORT statement consists of checklists and flowcharts to help standardize the researcher report Randomized Controlled Trials and to guard against methodological error.

✔ Even without positive results systematic reviews should still be published.

Meta-Analysis

✔ Analysis of analyses; integrate findings from a large variety of individual studies to achieve a systematic review.

✔ Result portrayed in a forest plot with a diagram using confidence intervals.

✔ Meta-analysis often critiqued for publication bias and missing data.

Cochrane Collaboration

✔ Database of systematic reviews and meta-analyses from around the world.

✔ Main output is systematic reviews; groups and databases to address different practice areas.

✔ Represents an integrated evidence-based network

LEARNING AND EXPLORATION ACTIVITIES

The purpose of this chapter is to introduce students to different methods for systematically reviewing the evidence as well as demonstrating some of the appropriate tools with which to perform these evaluations.

1. Systematic Reviews

a. Read through the systematic review methodologies listed and explore them until you feel you have a good sense of the commonalities between all of them. Now, write a simple methodology in your own words. Compare this with those your fellow students have prepared. Where do they differ? Where are they similar? If possible, attempt as a group to merge all of your individual methodologies by consensus and produce a methodological statement that is distinctly your own. This will be helpful for understanding why reviews are structured as they are.

b. Look briefly at the CONSORT statement (listed in Weblinks). What are the important factors that an RCT must have? What makes a good RCT? What makes a poor RCT? Write a short paragraph answering these questions. Now, search for RCTs on a topic of interest (your best bet is to use MEDLINE) and find two or more. Examine each and assess its strengths and weaknesses. Which of the two is better? Why? Justify your answer.

2. Meta-Analysis

Search on MEDLINE for meta-analyses on a topic of your choosing. Attempt to find more than one and compare the results. Did they both reach the same conclusion? Why? Why not? What does this say about meta-analysis?

3. The Cochrane Collaboration

Go online and find your local Cochrane Centre. Browse through the page and become familiar with its layout. Go to your local Health Sciences library and find out how to log onto the Cochrane Library from their computers. Search for systematic reviews on a topic of interest and find out how to retrieve them. Continue working until you understand how the software functions and you are comfortable with its features.

4. Reviews of Evidence

Compare and contrast the methods of qualitative and quantitative reviews. What is each trying to discover? In what instances can one be considered of more use than the other?

REFERENCES

Akobeng, A. (2005). Understanding systematic reviews and meta-analysis. *Archives of Disability and Childhood, 90*, 845-848.

Barbour, S. (1998). Mixing qualitative methods: Quality assurance or qualitative quagmire? *Qualitative Health Research, 8*(3), 352-361.

Booth, A. (2001). *Cochrane or cock-eyed? How should we conduct systematic reviews of qualitative research?* Paper presented at the Qualitative Evidence-based Practice Conference, Taking a Critical Stance, Coventry University Coventry, UK.

Cochrane collaboration. (n.d.). Guide to the format of a Cochrane review. Retrieved June 20, 2007, from: http://www.cochrane.uk.cochrane/handbook/hbookAPPENDIX_2A_GUIDE_TO_THE_FORMAT_.htm.

Counsell, C. (1997). Formulating questions and locating primary studies for inclusion in systematic reviews. *Annals of Internal Medicine, 127*(5), 380-7.

Creswell, J. (1998). *Qualitative inquiry and research design: Choosing among five traditions.* Thousand Oaks, CA: Sage.

Dixon-Woods, M., Agarwal, S., Jones, D., Young, B., & Sutton, A. (2005). Synthesizing qualitative and quantitative evidence: A review of possible methods. *Journal of Health Services Research & Policy, 10*(1), 45-53b.

Duffy, M. (2005). Systematic reviews: Their role and contribution to evidence-based practice. *Clinical Nurse Specialist, 19*(1), 15-17.

Eakin, J., & Mykhalovskiy, E. (2003). Reframing the evaluation of qualitative health research: Reflections on a review of appraisal guidelines in the health sciences. *Journal of Evaluation in Clinical Practice, 9*(2), 187-194.

Finfgeld, D. (2003). Metasynthesis: The state of the art—So far. *Qualitative Health Research, 13*(7), 893-904.

Greenhalgh T. (1997). Assessing the methodological quality of published papers. *British Medical Journal, 315*(7013), 305-308.

Klassen, T., Jadad, A., & Moher, D. (1998). Guides for reading and interpreting systematic reviews. *Archives of Pediatric and Adolescent Medicine, 152*, 700-704.

Lapier, T. (2003). Methods for finding systematic reviews relevant to physical therapy: Bridging research and clinical practice. *Cardiopulmonary Physical Therapy Journal, 14*(1), 9-12.

Mays, N., Pope, C., & Popay, J. (2005). Systematically reviewing qualitative and quantitative evidence to inform management and policy making in the health field. *Journal of Health Services Research & Policy, 10*(1), 6-20.

Moher, D., Jadad, A., & Klassen., T. (1998). Guides for reading and interpreting systematic reviews. *Archives of Pediatric and Adolescent Medicine, 152*, 915-920.

Mulrow, C., & Cook, D. (1997). Formulating questions and locating primary studies for inclusion in systematic reviews. *Annals of Internal Medicine, 127*(5), 380-387.

Oxman, A., & Guyatt, G. (1991). Validation of an index of the quality of review articles. *Journal of Clinical Epidemiology, 44*, 1271-1278.

Patterson, B., Thorne, S., Canam, C., & Jillings, C. (2001). *Meta-study of qualitative health research.* Thousand Oaks, CA: Sage.

Peach, H. (2002). Reading systematic reviews. *Australian Family Physician, 31*(8), 1-5.

Polgar, S., & Thomas, S. (Eds.). (2000). *Qualitative field research. In Introduction to research in the health sciences* (4th ed., pp. 91-103). Toronto, ON: Churchill Livingstone.

Sandelowski, M. (2006). "Meta-jeopardy": The crisis of representation in qualitative metasynthesis. *Nursing Outlook, 54*(1), 10-16.

Sandelowski, M., & Barroso, J. (2003). Writing the proposal for a qualitative research methodology project. *Qualitative Health Research, 13*(6), 781-790.

Sandelowski, M., & Boshamer, C. C. (2006). Divide and conquer: Avoiding duplication in the reporting of qualitative research. *Research Nursing & Health, 29*(5), 371-373.

Sandelowski, M., Docherty, S., & Emden, C. (1997). Qualitative metasynthesis: Issues and techniques. *Research in Nursing & Health, 20*, 365-371.

Spencer, L., Ritchie, J., Lewis, J., & Dillon, L. (2003). *Quality in qualitative evaluation: A framework for assessing research evidence*. Government Chief Social Researcher's Office, London: Cabinet Office.

Whitney, J. (2004). Reading and using systematic reviews. T*he Journal of Wound, Ostomy and Continence Nursing, 31*(1), 14-17.

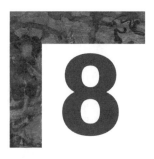

8

Comparison of Forms of Evidence

Systematic Reviews Versus Clinical Practice
Guidelines, Algorithms, and Clinical Pathways

Joy MacDermid, PT, PhD

LEARNING OBJECTIVES

After reading this chapter, the student/practitioner will be able to:

- Provide examples of clinical practice guidelines (CPGs), algorithms, and clinical pathways (CPs).

- Compare evidence in published systematic reviews to each of the clinical support tools above.

- Contrast and compare the form and content of systematic reviews as compared to CPGs, algorithms, and CPs addressing rehabilitation topics..

This chapter provides an opportunity to look at examples of some of the different types of evidence-based tools discussed in this book. For each of the exemplar topics below, we searched for systematic reviews that had been conducted on the topic and followed this with an alternative form of evidence syntheses that focused on application of the evidence. For successive problems, the alternate form is either an algorithm, CPG, or CP that has been developed to address this issue. We are not recommending any specific systematic review or CPG but are taking examples from different developers and topic areas within rehabilitation to provide practical exposure to a spectrum of these different evidence resources.

We suggest you use these as an opportunity to explore the benefits and drawbacks of different forms of evidence. At each step compare the knowledge available in published systematic reviews with these other forms of evidence. Think about scope, content, quality, and clinical usefulness.

In the case of CPGs, we have decided to present two examples that exemplify different types of CPGs. Broad problem- or condition-based CPGs are common in rehabilitation literature and focus on how to manage specific conditions or clinical populations. In other cases, a narrower approach can be used to focus on how a specific intervention might be used. We provide examples of each below.

EXAMPLE 1—LOW BACK PAIN:
SYSTEMATIC REVIEWS AND AN ALGORITHM

For our example of a situation in which one might use a clinical algorithm, we take the common case of management of occupational back pain. We conducted a literature search to identify systematic reviews that addressed low back pain, or were specifically related occupational disability. We present this list, which indicates that there is a large number of systematic reviews on this topic, below.

- Search #1: Lumbar or low back or back pain AND systematic review

Inclusion criteria:

1. Studied predictors of low pain or return to work of occupational injury, including low back pain.
2. Studied effectiveness of rehabilitation intervention for low back pain in terms of disorder or occupational outcomes.

Exclusion criteria: Medical management only addressed.

Relevant Systematic Reviews

Ammendolia, C., Kerr, M. S., & Bombardier, C. (2005). Back belt use for prevention of occupational low back pain: A systematic review. *Journal of Manipulative and Physiological Therapeutics, 28,* 128-134.

Assendelft, W. J., Koes, B. W., van der Heijden, G. J., Bouter, L. M. (1996). The effectiveness of chiropractic for treatment of low back pain: An update and attempt at statistical pooling. *Journal of Manipulative and Physiological Therapeutics, 19,* 499-507.

Borge, J. A., Leboeuf-Yde, C., & Lothe, J. (2001). Prognostic values of physical examination findings in patients with chronic low back pain treated conservatively: A systematic literature review. *Journal of Manipulative and Physiological Therapeutics, 24,* 292-295.

Boswell, M. V., Shah, R. V., Everett, C. R., Sehgal, N., Brown, A. M., Abdi, S., et al. (2005). Interventional techniques in the management of chronic spinal pain: evidence-based practice guidelines. *Pain Physician, 8,* 1-47.

Bressler, H. B., Keyes, W. J., Rochon, P. A., & Badley, E. (1999). The prevalence of low back pain in the elderly. A systematic review of the literature. *Spine, 24,* 1813-1819.

Bronfort, G., Haas, M., Evans, R. L., & Bouter, L. M. (2004). Efficacy of spinal manipulation and mobilization for low back pain and neck pain: A systematic review and best evidence synthesis. *The Spine Journal, 4,* 335-356.

Brox, J. I., Hagen, K. B., Juel, N. G., & Storheim, K. (1999). Is exercise therapy and manipulation effective in low back pain?. *Tidsskr Nor Laegeforen, 119,* 2042-2050.

Carnes, D., Ashby, D., & Underwood, M. (2006). A systematic review of pain drawing literature: Should pain drawings be used for psychologic screening? *The Clinical Journal of Pain, 22,* 449-457.

Cieza, A., Stucki, G., Weigl, M., Disler, P., Jackel, W., van der, L. S., et al. (2004). ICF core sets for low back pain. *Journal of Rehabilitation Medicine, Suppl. 44,* 69-74.

Clare, H. A., Adams, R., & Maher, C. G. (2004). A systematic review of efficacy of McKenzie therapy for spinal pain. *The Australian Journal of Physiotherapy, 50,* 209-216.

Clarke, J., van Tulder, M., Blomberg, S., de Vet, H., van der, H. G., & Bronfort, G. (2006). Traction for low back pain with or without sciatica: An updated systematic review within the framework of the Cochrane collaboration. *Spine, 31,* 1591-1599.

Cooperstein, R., Perle, S. M., Gatterman, M. I., Lantz, C., & Schneider, M. J. (2001). Chiropractic technique procedures for specific low back conditions: Characterizing the literature. *Journal of Manipulative and Physiological Therapeutics, 24,* 407-424.

den Boer, J. J., Oostendorp, R. A., Beems, T., Munneke, M., Oerlemans, M., & Evers, A. W. (2006). A systematic review of bio-psychosocial risk factors for an unfavourable outcome after lumbar disc surgery. *European Spine Journal, 15,* 527-536.

Deville, W. L., van der Windt, D. A., Dzaferagic, A., Bezemer, P. D., & Bouter, L. M. (2000). The test of Lasegue: Systematic review of the accuracy in diagnosing herniated discs. *Spine, 25,* 1140-1147.

Ernst, E., &Canter, P. H. (2006). A systematic review of systematic reviews of spinal manipulation. *Journal of the Royal Society of Medicine, 99,* 192-196.

Ernst, E. (1999). Massage therapy for low back pain: A systematic review. *Journal of Pain and Symptom Management, 17,* 65-69.

Fayad, F., Lefevre-Colau, M. M., Poiraudeau, S., Fermanian, J., Rannou, F., Wlodyka, D. S., et al. (2004). Chronicity, recurrence, and return to work in low back pain: common prognostic factors. *Annales de Readaptation et de Medecine Physique, 47,* 179-189.

Ferreira, M. L., Ferreira, P. H., Latimer, J., Herbert, R., & Maher, C. G. (2002). Does spinal manipulative therapy help people with chronic low back pain? *The Australian Journal of Physiotherapy, 48,* 277-284.

Ferreira, P. H., Ferreira, M. L., Maher, C. G., Herbert, R. D., & Refshauge, K. (2006). Specific stabilisation exercise for spinal and pelvic pain: A systematic review. *The Australian Journal of Physiotherapy, 52,* 79-88.

French, S. D., Cameron, M., Walker, B. F., Reggars, J. W., & Esterman, A. J. (2006). A Cochrane review of superficial heat or cold for low back pain. *Spine, 31,* 998-1006.

Furlan, A. D., Clarke, J., Esmail, R., Sinclair, S., Irvin, E., & Bombardier, C. (2001). A critical review of reviews on the treatment of chronic low back pain. *Spine, 26,* E155-E162.

Furlan, A. D., van Tulder, M., Cherkin, D., Tsukayama, H., Lao, L., Koes, B., et al. (2005). Acupuncture and dry-needling for low back pain: An updated systematic review within the framework of the Cochrane collaboration. *Spine, 30,* 944-963.

Furlan, A. D., Brosseau, L., Imamura, M., & Irvin, E. (2002). Massage for low-back pain: A systematic review within the framework of the Cochrane Collaboration Back Review Group. *Spine, 27,* 1896-1910.

Gagnier, J. J., van Tulder, M. W., Berman, B., & Bombardier, C. (2007). Herbal medicine for low back pain: A Cochrane review. *Spine, 32,* 82-92.

Grotle, M., Brox, J. I., & Vollestad, N. K. (2005). Functional status and disability questionnaires: What do they assess? A systematic review of back-specific outcome questionnaires. *Spine, 30,* 130-140.

Guzman, J., Esmail, R., Karjalainen, K., Malmivaara, A., Irvin, E., & Bombardier, C. (2001). Multidisciplinary rehabilitation for chronic low back pain: Systematic review. *British Medical Journal, 322,* 1511-1516.

Hagen, K. B., Hilde, G., Jamtvedt, G., & Winnem, M. F. (2000). The Cochrane review of bed rest for acute low back pain and sciatica. *Spine, 25,* 2932-2939.

Hagen, K. B., Hilde, G., Jamtvedt, G., & Winnem, M. F. (2002). The Cochrane review of advice to stay active as a single treatment for low back pain and sciatica. *Spine, 27,* 1736-1741.

Hagen, K. B., Jamtvedt, G., Hilde, G., & Winnem, M. F. (2005). The updated Cochrane review of bed rest for low back pain and sciatica. *Spine, 30,* 542-546.

Harte, A. A., Baxter, G. D., & Gracey, J. H. (2003). The efficacy of traction for back pain: A systematic review of randomized controlled trials. *Archives of Physical Medicine and Rehabilitation, 84,* 1542-1553.

Hayden, J. A., van Tulder, M. W., & Tomlinson, G. (2005). Systematic review: strategies for using exercise therapy to improve outcomes in chronic low back pain. *Annals of Internal Medicine, 142,* 776-785.

Henderson, H. (2002). Acupuncture: Evidence for its use in chronic low back pain. *British Journal of Nursing, 11,* 1395-1403.

Henrotin, Y. E., Cedraschi, C., Duplan, B., Bazin, T., & Duquesnoy, B. (2006). Information and low back pain management: A systematic review. *Spine, 31,* E326-E334.

Heymans, M. W., van Tulder, M. W., Esmail, R., Bombardier, C., & Koes, B. W. (2005). Back schools for nonspecific low back pain: A systematic review within the framework of the Cochrane Collaboration Back Review Group. *Spine, 30,* 2153-2163.

Hunt, D. G., Zuberbier, O. A., Kozlowski, A. J., Berkowitz, J., Schultz, I. Z., Milner, R. A., et al. (2002). Are components of a comprehensive medical assessment predictive of work disability after an episode of occupational low back trouble? *Spine, 27,* 2715-2719.

Hunter, J. (2001). Physical symptoms and signs and chronic pain. *The Clinical Journal of Pain, 17,* S26-S32.

Huppe, A., & Raspe, H. (2003). Efficacy of inpatient rehabilitation for chronic back pain in Germany: A systematic review 1980-2001]. *Rehabilitation* (Stuttg), *42,* 143-154.

Hurwitz, E. L., Aker, P. D., Adams, A. H., Meeker, W. C., & Shekelle, P. G. (1996). Manipulation and mobilization of the cervical spine: A systematic review of the literature. *Spine, 21,* 1746-1759.

Jellema, P., van Tulder, M. W., van Poppel, M. N., Nachemson, A. L., & Bouter, L. M. (2001). Lumbar supports for prevention and treatment of low back pain: A systematic review within the framework of the Cochrane Back Review Group. *Spine, 26,* 377-386.

Karjalainen, K., Malmivaara, A., van Tulder, M., Roine, R., Jauhiainen, M., Hurri, H., et al. (2000). Multidisciplinary biopsychosocial rehabilitation for subacute low back pain among working age adults. *Cochrane Database of Systematic Reviews,* CD002193.

Karjalainen, K., Malmivaara, A., van Tulder, M., Roine, R., Jauhiainen, M., Hurri, H., et al. (2001). Multidisciplinary biopsychosocial rehabilitation for subacute low back pain in working-age adults: A systematic review within the framework of the Cochrane Collaboration Back Review Group. *Spine, 26,* 262-269.

Karjalainen, K., Malmivaara, A., van Tulder, M., Roine, R., Jauhiainen, M., Hurri, H., et al. (2003). Multidisciplinary biopsychosocial rehabilitation for subacute low back pain among working age adults. *Cochrane Database of Systematic Reviews,* CD002193.

Khadilkar, A., Milne, S., Brosseau, L., Wells, G., Tugwell, P., Robinson, V., et al. (2005). Transcutaneous electrical nerve stimulation for the treatment of chronic low back pain: A systematic review. *Spine, 30,* 2657-2666.

Koes, B. W., Assendelft, W. J., van der Heijden, G. J., & Bouter, L. M. (1996). Spinal manipulation for low back pain: An updated systematic review of randomized clinical trials. *Spine, 21,* 2860-2871.

Kuijer, W., Groothoff, J. W., Brouwer, S., Geertzen, J. H., & Dijkstra, P. U. (2006). Prediction of sickness absence in patients with chronic low back pain: A systematic review. *Journal of Occupational Rehabilitation, 16,* 430-458.

Leboeuf-Yde, C. (1999). Smoking and low back pain. A systematic literature review of 41 journal articles reporting 47 epidemiologic studies. *Spine, 24,* 1463-1470.

Leboeuf-Yde, C. (2000). Body weight and low back pain. A systematic literature review of 56 journal articles reporting on 65 epidemiologic studies. *Spine, 25,* 226-237.

Leboeuf-Yde, C., & Lauritsen, J. M. (1995). The prevalence of low back pain in the literature: A structured review of 26 Nordic studies from 1954 to 1993. *Spine, 20,* 2112-2118.

Li, L., Irvin, E., Guzman, J., & Bombardier, C. (2001). Surfing for back pain patients: The nature and quality of back pain information on the Internet. *Spine, 26,* 545-557.

Licciardone, J. C., Brimhall, .A K., & King, L. N. (2005). Osteopathic manipulative treatment for low back pain: A systematic review and meta-analysis of randomized controlled trials. *BMC Musculoskeletal Disorders, 6,* 43.

Loney, P. L., & Stratford, P. W. (1999). The prevalence of low back pain in adults: A methodological review of the literature. *Physical Therapy, 79,* 384-396.

Machado, L. A., de Souza, M. S., Ferreira, P. H., & Ferreira, M. L. (2006). The McKenzie method for low back pain: A systematic review of the literature with a meta-analysis approach. *Spine, 31,* E254-E262.

May, S. (2000). Re: Exercise therapy for low back pain: A systematic review within the framework of the Cochrane Collaboration Back Review Group. *Spine, 25,* 2784-2796.

May, S., Littlewood, C., & Bishop, A. (2006). Reliability of procedures used in the physical examination of non-specific low back pain: a systematic review. *Australian Journal of Physiotherapy, 52,* 91-102.

McKenzie-Brown, A. M., Shah, R. V., Sehgal, N., & Everett, C. R. (2005). A systematic review of sacroiliac joint interventions. *Pain Physician, 8,* 115-125.

McNeely, M. L., Torrance, G., & Magee, D. J. (2003). A systematic review of physiotherapy for spondyloly-sis and spondylolisthesis. *Manual Therapy, 8*, 80-91.

Meijer, E. M., Sluiter, J. K., & Frings-Dresen, M. H. (2005). Evaluation of effective return-to-work treat-ment programs for sick-listed patients with non-specific musculoskeletal complaints: A systematic review. *International Archives of Occupational and Environmental Health, 78*, 523-532.

Milne, S., Welch, V., Brosseau, L., Saginur, M., Shea,B., Tugwell, P., et al. (2001). Transcutaneous electri-cal nerve stimulation (TENS) for chronic low back pain. *Cochrane Database of Systematic Reviews*, CD003008.

Mior, S. (2001). Exercise in the treatment of chronic pain. *The Clinical Journal of Pain, 17*, S77-S85.

Oliphant, D. (2004). Safety of spinal manipulation in the treatment of lumbar disk herniations: A systematic review and risk assessment. *Journal of Manipulative and Physiological Therapeutics, 27*, 197-210.

Ostelo, R. W., de Vet, H. C., Waddell, G., Kerckhoffs, M. R., Leffers, P., & van Tulder, M. (2003). Rehabilitation following first-time lumbar disc surgery: A systematic review within the framework of the Cochrane collaboration. *Spine, 28*, 209-218.

Pengel, H. M., Maher, C. G., & Refshauge, K. M. (2002). Systematic review of conservative interventions for subacute low back pain. *Clinical Rehabilitation, 16*, 811-820.

Pengel, L. H., Herbert, R. D., Maher, C. G., & Refshauge, K. M. (2003). Acute low back pain: Systematic review of its prognosis. *British Medical Journal, 327*, 323.

Pincus, T., Burton, A. K., Vogel, S., & Field, A. P. A systematic review of psychological factors as predictors of chronicity/disability in prospective cohorts of low back pain. *Spine, 27*, E109-E120.

Pincus, T., Vlaeyen, J. W., Kendall, N. A., Von Korff, M. R, Kalauokalani, D. A., & Reis, S. (2002). Cognitive-behavioral therapy and psychosocial factors in low back pain: Directions for the future. *Spine, 27*, E133-E138.

Pincus, T., Vogel, S., Burton, A. K., Santos, R, & Field, A. P. (2006). Fear avoidance and prognosis in back pain: A systematic review and synthesis of current evidence. *Arthritis and Rheumatism, 54*, 3999-4010.

Pittler, M. H., Karagulle, M. Z., Karagulle, M., & Ernst, E. (2006). Spa therapy and balneotherapy for treat-ing low back pain: Meta-analysis of randomized trials. *Rheumatology* (Oxford), *45*, 880-884.

Rabago, D., Best, T. M., Beamsley, M., & Patterson, J. (2005). A systematic review of prolotherapy for chronic musculoskeletal pain. *Clinical Journal of Sports Medicine, 15*, 376-380.

Rackwitz, B., de Bie, R., Limm, H, von Garnier, K., Ewert, T., & Stucki, G. (2006). Segmental stabilizing exercises and low back pain. What is the evidence? A systematic review of randomized controlled trials. *Clinical Rehabilitation, 20*, 553-567.

Raine, R., Haines, A., Sensky, T, Hutchings, A., Larkin, K., & Black, N. (2002). Systematic review of mental health interventions for patients with common somatic symptoms: Can research evidence from second-ary care be extrapolated to primary care? *British Medical Journal, 325*, 1082.

Rebain, R., Baxter, G. D., & McDonough, S. (2002). A systematic review of the passive straight leg raising test as a diagnostic aid for low back pain (1989 to 2000). *Spine, 27*, E388-E395.

Schonstein, E., Kenny, D., Keating, J., Koes, B., & Herbert, R. D. (2003). Physical conditioning programs for workers with back and neck pain: A Cochrane systematic review. *Spine, 28*, E391-E395.

Sehgal, N., Shah, R. V., McKenzie-Brown, A. M., & Everett, C. R. (2005). Diagnostic utility of facet (zyg-apophysial) joint injections in chronic spinal pain: a systematic review of evidence. *Pain Physician, 8*, 211-224.

Slade, S. C., & Keating, J. L. (2006). Trunk-strengthening exercises for chronic low back pain: A systematic review. *Journal of Manipulative and Physiological Therapeutics, 29*, 163-173.

Smeets, R. J, Wade, D., Hidding, A., Van Leeuwen, P. J., Vlaeyen, J. W., & Knottnerus, J. A. (2006). The association of physical deconditioning and chronic low back pain: A hypothesis-oriented systematic review. *Disability and Rehabilitation, 28*, 673-693.

Steele, E. J., Dawson, A. P., & Hiller, J. E. (2006). School-based interventions for spinal pain: A systematic review. *Spine, 31*, 226-233.

Steenstra, I. A., Verbeek, J. H., Heymans, M. W., & Bongers, P. M. (2005). Prognostic factors for duration of sick leave in patients sick listed with acute low back pain: A systematic review of the literature. *Occupational and Environmental Medicine, 62,* 851-860.

Urrutia, G., Burton, K., Morral, A., Bonfill, X., & Zanoli, G. (2005). Neuroreflexotherapy for nonspecific low back pain: A systematic review. *Spine, 30,* E148-E153.

van der, H. M., Vollenbroek-Hutten, M. M., & Ijzerman, M. J. (2005). A systematic review of sociodemographic, physical, and psychological predictors of multidisciplinary rehabilitation-or, back school treatment outcome in patients with chronic low back pain. *Spine, 30,* 813-825.

van der, R. N., Goossen, M. E., Evers, S. M., & van Tulder, M. W. (2005). What is the most cost-effective treatment for patients with low back pain? A systematic review. Best Practice & Research. *Clinical Rheumatology, 19,* 671-684.

van Poppel, M. N., Hooftman, W. E., & Koes, B. W. (2004). An update of a systematic review of controlled clinical trials on the primary prevention of back pain at the workplace. *Occupational Medicine* (Oxford, England), *54,* 345-352.

van Poppel, M. N., de Looze, M. P., Koes, B. W., Smid, T., & Bouter, L. M. (2000). Mechanisms of action of lumbar supports: A systematic review. *Spine, 25,* 2103-2113.

van Trijffel, E., Anderegg, Q., Bossuyt, P. M.,& Lucas, C. Inter-examiner reliability of passive assessment of intervertebral motion in the cervical and lumbar spine: A systematic review. *Manual Therapy, 10,* 256-269.

van Tulder, M., Malmivaara, A, Esmail, R., & Koes, B. (2000). Exercise therapy for low back pain: A systematic review within the framework of the Cochrane collaboration back review group. *Spine, 25,* 2784-2796.

van Tulder, M. W., Esmail, R., Bombardier, C., & Koes, B. W. (2000). Back schools for non-specific low back pain. *Cochrane Database of Systematic Reviews,* CD000261.

van Tulder, M. W., Ostelo, R, Vlaeyen, J. W., Linton, S. J., Morley, S. J., & Assendelft, W. J. (2000). Behavioral treatment for chronic low back pain: A systematic review within the framework of the Cochrane Back Review Group. *Spine, 25,* 2688-2699.

van Tulde, M. W., Ostelo, R., Vlaeyen, J. W., Linton, S. J., Morley, S. J., & Assendelft, W. J. (2001). Behavioral treatment for chronic low back pain: A systematic review within the framework of the Cochrane Back Review Group. *Spine, 26,* 270-281.

van Tulder, M. W., Ostelo, R. W., Vlaeyen, J. W., Linton, S. J., Morley, S. J., & Assendelft, W. J. (2000). Behavioural treatment for chronic low back pain. *Cochrane Database of Systematic Reviews,* CD002014.

van Tulder, M. W., Koes, B. W., & Bouter, L. M. Conservative treatment of acute and chronic nonspecific low back pain. A systematic review of randomized controlled trials of the most common interventions. *Spine, 22,* 2128-2156.

van Tulder, M. W., Jellema, P., van Poppel, M. N., Nachemson, A. L., & Bouter, L. M. (2000). Lumbar supports for prevention and treatment of low back pain. *Cochrane Database of Systematic Reviews,* CD001823.

van Tulder, M. W., Touray, T., Furlan, A. D., Solway, S, & Bouter, L. M. (2003). Muscle relaxants for nonspecific low back pain: A systematic review within the framework of the Cochrane collaboration. *Spine, 28,* 1978-1992.

van Tulder, M. W., Scholten, R. J., Koes, B. W., & Deyo, R. A. (2000). Non-steroidal anti-inflammatory drugs for low back pain. *Cochrane Database of Systematic Reviews,* CD000396.

van Tulder, M. W., Scholten, R. J., Koes, B. W., & Deyo, R. A. (2000). Nonsteroidal anti-inflammatory drugs for low back pain: A systematic review within the framework of the Cochrane Collaboration Back Review Group. *Spine, 25,* 2501-2513.

van Tulder, M. W., Assendelft, W. J., Koes, B. W., & Bouter, L. M. (1997). Spinal radiographic findings and nonspecific low back pain: A systematic review of observational studies. *Spine, 22,* 427-434.

van Tulder, M. W., Cherkin, D. C, Berman, B., Lao, L., & Koes, B. W. (1999). The effectiveness of acupuncture in the management of acute and chronic low back pain: A systematic review within the framework of the Cochrane Collaboration Back Review Group. *Spine, 24,* 1113-1123.

Verbeek, J., Sengers, M. J., Riemens, L., & Haafkens, J. (2004). Patient expectations of treatment for back pain: A systematic review of qualitative and quantitative studies. *Spine, 29*, 2309-2318.

Waddell, G., Feder, G., & Lewis, M. (1997). Systematic reviews of bed rest and advice to stay active for acute low back pain. *British Journal of General Practice, 47*, 647-652.

Walker, B. F. (1999). The prevalence of low back pain in Australian adults. A systematic review of the literature from 1966-1998. *Asia-Pacific Journal of Public Health, 11*, 45-51.

Walker, B. F. (2000). The prevalence of low back pain: A systematic review of the literature from 1966 to 1998. *Journal of Spine Disorders, 13*, 205-217.

Weevers, H. J., van der Beek, A. J., Anema, J. R., van der, W. G., & van Mechelen, W. (2005). Work-related disease in general practice: A systematic review. *Family Practice, 22*, 197-204.

Weiner, D. K., & Ernst, E. (2004). Complementary and alternative approaches to the treatment of persistent musculoskeletal pain. *Clinical Journal of Pain, 20*, 244-255.

Wessels, T., van Tulder, M., Sigl, T., Ewert, T., Limm, H., & Stucki, G. (2006). What predicts outcome in non-operative treatments of chronic low back pain? A systematic review. *European Spine Journal, 15*, 1633-1644.

An Algorithm for Managing Back Pain

The sheer number of systematic reviews may overwhelm clinicians. Now we provide an example algorithm developed by The Alberta Workers Compensation Board to direct management of occupational low back pain using evidence reviews and stakeholder input to develop the following algorithm. Recommendations for the management of occupational back pain include an executive summary of the literature, and the algorithms are below. These were developed on the basis of the CPG produced by the Agency for Health Care Policy and Research, U.S. Department of Health and Human Services, December, 1994 and are available at www.wcb.ab.ca (Alberta WCB). This document is used with their permission (Figure 8-1).

EXAMPLE 2—CLINICAL PRACTICE GUIDELINES FOR POPULATIONS OR INTERVENTIONS

In this section we provide excerpts from a CPG that was designed to focus on another common problem in rehabilitation (stroke) and one design to focus on provision of a specific treatment (cervical manipulation). There are reasons why many CPGs are broad in nature; they are often intended to provide direction or policy statements on how to best manage a clinical population that shares a common diagnosis or disorder. Conversely, in some cases the point of a CPG is to promote optimal use of a specific intervention. This is particularly relevant in our example of cervical manipulation, which is a controversial intervention in rehabilitation. Given the small potential for serious complications, it is important that practitioners who use this type of intervention are clear about the evidence so they can obtain adequate informed consent. Of course policy makers, patients, and those considering using this intervention would also need this information.

You may choose to look at one or both scenarios below or contrast the format of these two.

- Search #1: Stroke AND rehabilitation AND systematic review (62 references retrieved [see p. 173]).

continued on page 173

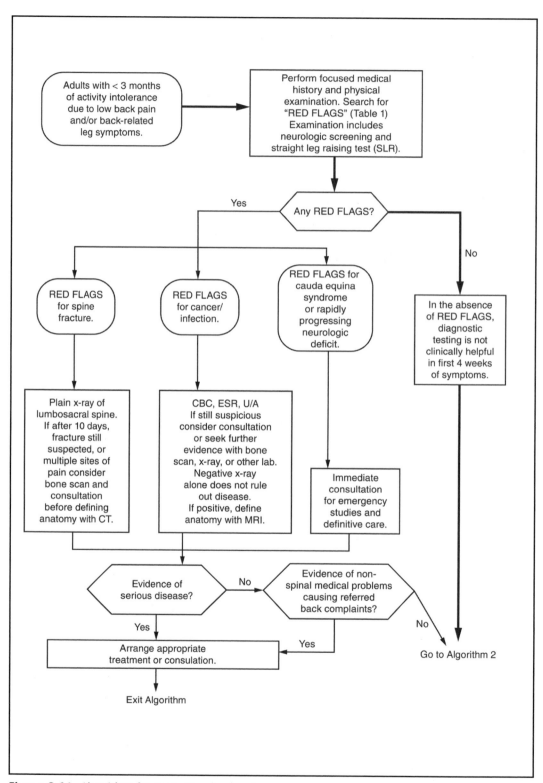

Figure 8-1A. Algorithm for managing back pain.

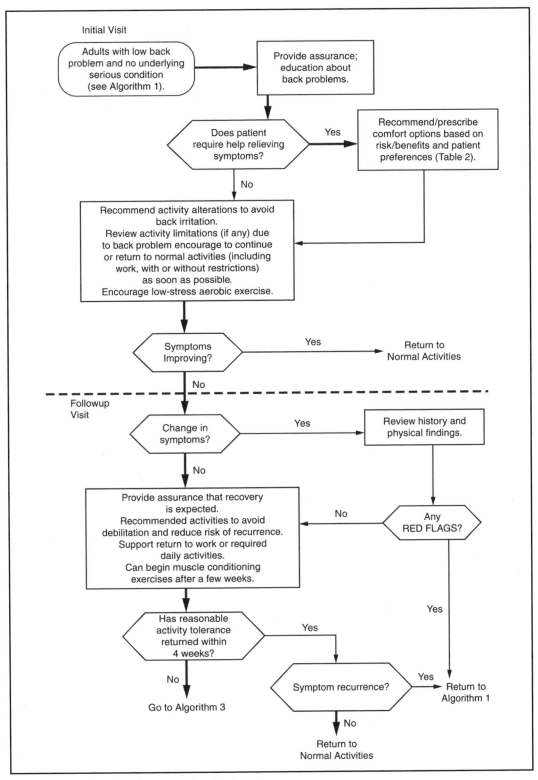

Figure 8-1B. Algorithm for managing back pain.

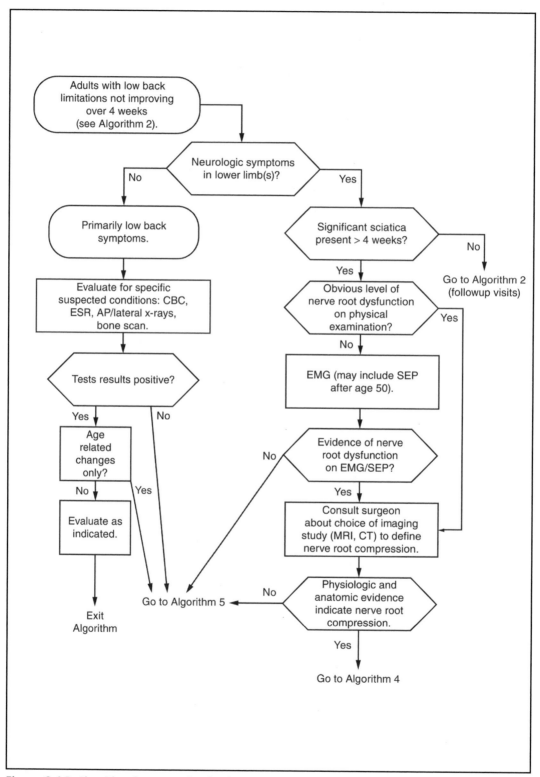

Figure 8-1C. Algorithm for managing back pain.

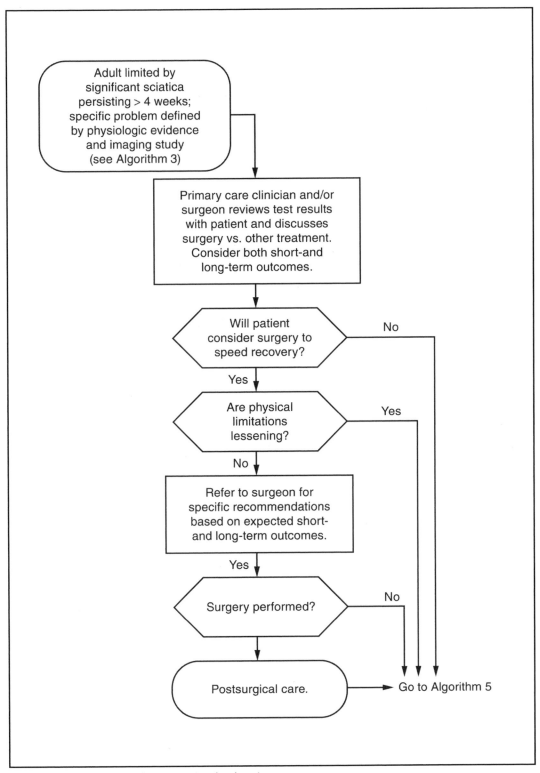

Figure 8-1D. Algorithm for managing back pain.

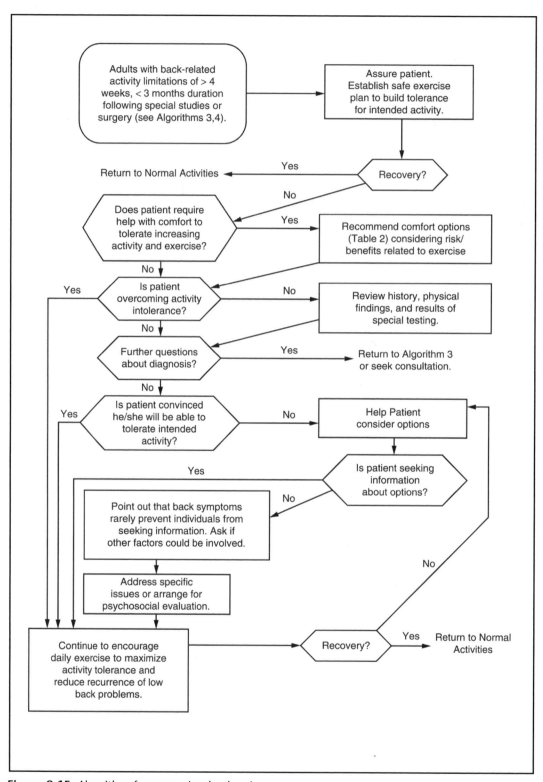

Figure 8-1E. Algorithm for managing back pain.

Stroke Rehabilitation Relevant Systematic Reviews

Anderson, C., Ni, M. C., Brown, P. M., & Carter, K. (2002). Stroke rehabilitation services to accelerate hospital discharge and provide home-based care: An overview and cost analysis. *Pharmacoeconomics, 20*(8), 537-552.

Barreca, S., Wolf, S. L., Fasoli, S., & Bohannon, R. (2003). Treatment interventions for the paretic upper limb of stroke survivors: A critical review. *Neurorehabilitation and Neural Repair, 17*(4), 220-226.

Bhogal, S. K., Teasell, R. W., Foley, N. C., & Speechley, M. R. (2003). Community reintegration after stroke. *Topics in Stroke Rehabilitation, 10*(2), 107-129.

Bowen, A., McKenna, K., & Tallis, R. C. (1999). Reasons for variability in the reported rate of occurrence of unilateral spatial neglect after stroke. *Stroke, 30*(6), 1196-1202.

Brady, B. K., McGahan, L., & Skidmore, B. (2005). Systematic review of economic evidence on stroke rehabilitation services. *International Journal of Technology Assessment in Health Care, 21*(1), 15-21.

Braun, S. M., Beurskens, A. J., Borm, P. J., Schack, T., & Wade, D. T. (2006). The effects of mental practice in stroke rehabilitation: A systematic review. *Archives of Physical Medicine and Rehabilitation, 87*(6), 842-852.

Carson, S., McDonagh, M., Russman, B., & Helfand, M. (2005). Hyperbaric oxygen therapy for stroke: a systematic review of the evidence. *Clinical Rehabilitation, 19*(8), 819-833.

Cicerone, K. D., Dahlber, C., Malec, J. F., Langenbahn, D. M., Felicetti, T., Kneipp, S., et al. (2005). Evidence-based cognitive rehabilitation: Updated review of the literature from 1998 through 2002. *Archives of Physical Medicine and Rehabilitation, 86*(8), 1681-1692.

Cole, M. G., Elie, L. M., McCusker, J., Bellavance, F., & Mansour, A. (2001). Feasibility and effectiveness of treatments for post-stroke depression in elderly inpatients: Systematic review. *Journal of Geriatric Psychiatry and Neurology, 14*(1), 37-41.

de Kroon, J. R., van der Lee, J. H., Ijzerman, M. J., & Lankhorst, G. J. (2002). Therapeutic electrical stimulation to improve motor control and functional abilities of the upper extremity after stroke: A systematic review. *Clinical Rehabilitation, 16*(4), 350-360.

Dumoulin, C., Korner-Bitensky, N., & Tannenbaum, C. (2005). Urinary incontinence after stroke: Does rehabilitation make a difference? A systematic review of the effectiveness of behavioral therapy. *Topics in Stroke Rehabilitation, 12*(3), 66-76.

Duncan, P. W., Jorgensen, H. S., & Wade, D. T. (2000). Outcome measures in acute stroke trials: A systematic review and some recommendations to improve practice. *Stroke, 31*(6), 1429-1438.

Foley, N. C., Teasell, R. W., Bhogal, S. K., Doherty, T., & Speechley, M. R. (2003). The efficacy of stroke rehabilitation: A qualitative review. *Topics in Stroke Rehabilitation, 10*(2), 1-18.

Gensini, G. F., & Gusinu, R. (2006). The systematic review of organised stroke care: A model for an unbiased assessment of trials on the effects of service organisation. The clinician's point of view. *Internal and Emergency Medicine, 1*(1), 77-78.

Geyh, S., Cieza, A., Schouten, J., Dickson, H., Frommelt, P., Omar, Z., et al. (2004). ICF core sets for stroke. *Journal of Rehabilitation Medicine, 44*(Suppl.), 135-141.

Greener, J., Enderby, P., Whurr, R., & Grant, A. (1998). Treatment for aphasia following stroke: Evidence for effectiveness. *International Journal of Language & Communication Disorders, 33*(Suppl.), 158-161.

Hackett, M. L., & Anderson, C. S. (2005). Predictors of depression after stroke: A systematic review of observational studies. *Stroke, 36*(10), 2296-2301.

Hakkennes, S., & Keating, J. L. (2005). Constraint-induced movement therapy following stroke: A systematic review of randomised controlled trials. *The Australian Journal of Physiotherapy, 51*(4), 221-231.

Hendricks, H. T., van Limbeek, J., Geurts, A. C., & Zwarts, M. J. (2002). Motor recovery after stroke: A systematic review of the literature. *Archives of Physical Medicine and Rehabilitation, 83*(11), 1629-1637.

Hendricks, H. T., Zwarts, M. J., Plat, E. F., & van Limbeek, J. (2002). Systematic review for the early prediction of motor and functional outcome after stroke by using motor-evoked potentials. *Archives of Physical Medicine and Rehabilitation, 83*(9), 1303-1308.

Hopwood, V., & Lewith, G. T. (2005). Does acupuncture help stroke patients become more independent? *Journal of Alternativew and Complementary Medicine, 11*(1), 175-177.

Jolliffe, J. A., Rees, K., Taylor, R. S., Thompson, D., Oldridge, N., & Ebrahim, S. (2000). Exercise-based rehabilitation for coronary heart disease. *Cochrane Database of Systematic Reviews, 4,* CD001800.

Kottink, A. I., Oostendorp, L. J., Buurke, J. H., Nene, A. V., Hermens, H. J., & Ijzerman, M. J. (2004). The orthotic effect of functional electrical stimulation on the improvement of walking in stroke patients with a dropped foot: A systematic review. *Artificial Organs, 28*(6), 577-586.

Kwakkel, G., van Peppen, R., Wagenaar, R. C., Wood, D. S., Richards, C., Ashburn, A., et al. (2004). Effects of augmented exercise therapy time after stroke: A meta-analysis. *Stroke, 35*(11), 2529-2539.

Langhorne P, Duncan P. (2001). Does the organization of postacute stroke care really matter? *Stroke, 32*(1), 268-274.

Langhorne, P., & Pollock, A. (2002). What are the components of effective stroke unit care? *Age and Ageing, 31*(5), 365-371.

Langhorne, P., Wagenaar, R., & Partridge, C. (1996). Physiotherapy after stroke: more is better? *Physiotherapy Research International, 1*(2), 75-88.

Lannin, N. A., & Herbert, R. D. (2003). Is hand splinting effective for adults following stroke? A systematic review and methodologic critique of published research. *Clinical Rehabilitation, 17*(8), 807-816.

Liberati, A., Gensini, G. F., & Gusinu, R. (2006). The systematic review of organised stroke care: A model for an unbiased assessment of trials on the effects of service organisation. *Internal and Emergency Medicine, 1*(1), 76-77.

Luaute, J., Halligan, P., Rode, G., Rossetti, Y., & Boisson, D. (2006). Visuo-spatial neglect: a systematic review of current interventions and their effectiveness. *Neuroscience and Biobehavioral Reviews, 30*(7), 961-982.

Legg, L., & Langhorne, P. Rehabilitation therapy services for stroke patients living at home: Systematic review of randomised trials. *Lancet, 363*(9406), 352-356.

MacHale, S. M., O'Rourke, S. J., Wardlaw, J. M., & Dennis, M. S. (1998). Depression and its relation to lesion location after stroke. *Journal of Neurology Neurosurg Psychiatry, 64*(3), 371-374.

McKevitt, C., Redfern, J., Mold, F., & Wolfe, C. (2004). Qualitative studies of stroke: A systematic review. *Stroke, 35*(6), 1499-1505.

Meek, C., Pollock, A., Potter, J., & Langhorne, P. (2003). A systematic review of exercise trials post stroke. *Clinical Rehabilitation, 17*(1), 6-13.

Meijer, R., Ihnenfeldt, D. S., de Groot, I. J., van Limbeek, J., Vermeulen, M., & de Haan, R. J. (2003). Prognostic factors for ambulation and activities of daily living in the subacute phase after stroke. A systematic review of the literature. *Clinical Rehabilitation, 17*(2), 119-129.

Meijer, R., Ihnenfeldt, D. S., van Limbeek, J., Vermeulen, M., & de Haan, R. J. (2003). Prognostic factors in the subacute phase after stroke for the future residence after six months to one year: A systematic review of the literature. *Clinical Rehabilitation, 17*(5), 512-520.

Meijer, R., van Limbeek, J., Kriek, B., Ihnenfeldt, D., Vermeulen, M., & de Haan, R. (2004). Prognostic social factors in the subacute phase after a stroke for the discharge destination from the hospital stroke-unit: A systematic review of the literature. *Disability and Rehabilitation, 26*(4), 191-197.

Morris, S. L., Dodd, K. J., & Morris, M. E. (2004). Outcomes of progressive resistance strength training following stroke: a systematic review. *Clinical Rehabilitation, 18*(1), 27-39.

Moseley, A. M., Stark, A., Cameron, I. D., & Pollock, A. (2003). Treadmill training and body weight support for walking after stroke. *Cochrane Database of Systematic Reviews, 3,* CD002840.

Moseley, A. M., Stark, A., Cameron, I. D., & Pollock, A. (2005). Treadmill training and body weight support for walking after stroke. *Cochrane Database of Systematic Reviews, 4,* CD002840.

Ouimet, M. A., Primeau, F., & Cole, M. G. (2001). Psychosocial risk factors in poststroke depression: A systematic review. *Canadian Journal of Psychiatry, 46*(9), 819-828.

Pang, M. Y., Eng, J. J., Dawson, A. S., & Gylfadottir, S. (2006). The use of aerobic exercise training in improving aerobic capacity in individuals with stroke: A meta-analysis. *Clinical Rehabilitation, 20*(2), 97-111.

Park, J., Hopwood, V., White, A. R., & Ernst, E. (2001). Effectiveness of acupuncture for stroke: A systematic review. *Journal of Neurology, 248*(7), 558-563.

Parker, G., Bhakta, P., Katbamna, S., Lovett, C., Paisley, S., Parker, S., et al. (2000). Best place of care for older people after acute and during subacute illness: a systematic review. *Journal of Health Services Research and Policy, 5*(3), 76-189.

Platz, T. (2003). Evidence-based arm rehabilitation—A systematic review of the literature. *Nervenarzt, 74*(10), 841-849.

Prange, G. B., Jannink, M. J., Groothuis-Oudshoorn, C. G., Hermens, H. J., & Ijzerman, M. J. (2006). Systematic review of the effect of robot-aided therapy on recovery of the hemiparetic arm after stroke. *Journal of Rehabilitation Research and Development, 43*(2), 171-184.

Sellars, C., Hughes, T., & Langhorne, P. (2002). Speech and language therapy for dysarthria due to nonprogressive brain damage: A systematic Cochrane review. *Clinical Rehabilitation, 16*(1), 61-68.

Steultjens, E. M., Dekker, J., Bouter, L. M., van de Nes, J. C., Cup, E. H., & van den Ende, C. H. (2003). Occupational therapy for stroke patients: A systematic review. *Stroke, 34*(3), 676-687.

Stewart, K. C., Cauraugh, J. H., & Summers, J. J. (2006). Bilateral movement training and stroke rehabilitation: a systematic review and meta-analysis. *Journal of Neurological Sciences, 244*(1-2), 89-95.

Stroke Unit Trialists' Collaboration. (1997). Collaborative systematic review of the randomised trials of organised inpatient (stroke unit) care after stroke. *British Medical Journal, 314*(7088), 1151-1159.

Stroke Unit Trialists Collaboration. (1997). How do stroke units improve patient outcomes? A collaborative systematic review of the randomized trials. *Stroke, 28*(11), 2139-2144.

Teasell, R. W., Foley, N. C., Bhogal, S. K., & Speechley, M. R. (2003). Early supported discharge in stroke rehabilitation. *Topics in Stroke Rehabilitation, 10*(2), 19-33.

Turner-Stokes, L., & Hassan, N. (2002). Depression after stroke: A review of the evidence base to inform the development of an integrated care pathway. Part 1: Diagnosis, frequency and impact. *Clinical Rehabilitation, 16*(3), 231-247.

Turner-Stokes, L., & Hassan, N. (2002). Depression after stroke: Areview of the evidence base to inform the development of an integrated care pathway. Part 2: Treatment alternatives. *Clinical Rehabilitation, 16*(3), 248-260.

Turner-Stokes, L., & Jackson, D. (2002). Shoulder pain after stroke: A review of the evidence base to inform the development of an integrated care pathway. *Clinical Rehabilitation, 16*(3), 276-298.

van der Lee, J. H., Snels, I. A., Beckerman, H., Lankhorst, G. J., Wagenaar, R. C., & Bouter, L. M. (2001). Exercise therapy for arm function in stroke patients: A systematic review of randomized controlled trials. *Clinical Rehabilitation, 15*(1), 20-31.

van Kuijk, A. A., Geurts, A. C., Bevaart, B. J., & van Limbeek, J. (2002). Treatment of upper extremity spasticity in stroke patients by focal neuronal or neuromuscular blockade: A systematic review of the literature. *Journal of Rehabilitation Medicine, 34*(2), 51-61.

Van Peppen, R. P., Kortsmit, M., Lindeman, E., & Kwakkel, G. (2006). Effects of visual feedback therapy on postural control in bilateral standing after stroke: A systematic review. *Journal of Rehabilitation Medicine, 38*(1), 3-9.

Van Peppen, R. P., Kwakkel, G., Wood-Dauphinee, S., Hendriks, H. J., Van der Wees, P. J., & Dekker, J. (2004). The impact of physical therapy on functional outcomes after stroke: What's the evidence? *Clinical Rehabilitation, 18*(8), 833-862.

Wells, J. L., Seabrook, J. A., Stolee, P., Borrie, M. J., & Knoefel, F. (2003). State of the art in geriatric rehabilitation. Part I: review of frailty and comprehensive geriatric assessment. *Archives of Physical Medicine and Rehabilitation, 84*(6), 890-897.

Wells, J. L., Seabrook, J. A., Stolee, P., Borrie, M. J., & Knoefel, F. (2003). State of the art in geriatric rehabilitation. Part II: Clinical challenges. *Archives of Physical Medicine and Rehabilitation, 84*(6), 898-903.

Clinical Practice Guidelines on Stroke Rehabilitation

We obtained a CPG that is in progress, but the developers have shared the draft format (Figure 8-2A) of two specific areas of recommendation arising from the Canadian Stroke Strategy.

Canadian Stroke Strategy Recommendations

20. Components of Inpatient Stroke Rehabilitation

Best Practice Recommendation 20: Components of Inpatient Stroke Rehabilitation

All patients with stroke should begin rehabilitation therapy as early as possible once medical stability is reached. (AHS/ASA; Evidence Level I)

- ♦ Patients should undergo as much therapy appropriate to their needs as they are willing and able to tolerate. (RCP; Evidence Level A)
- ♦ The team should promote the practice of skills gained in therapy into the patient's daily routine in a consistent manner. (RCP; Evidence Level A)
- ♦ Therapy should include repetitive and intense use of novel tasks that challenge the patient to acquire necessary motor skills to use the involved limb during functional tasks and activities. (SCORE; Evidence Level A)
- ♦ Stroke unit teams should conduct at least one formal interdisciplinary meeting per week at which patient problems are identified, rehabilitation goals set, progress monitored, and support after discharge planned. (SIGN 64; Evidence Level B)

Rationale

To obtain the benefits of inpatient stroke rehabilitation units, a number of important components must be present. Both animal and human research suggests that the earlier rehabilitation starts the better the outcome. In fact, people who start rehabilitation later may never recover as much as those who start early. Early and enhanced intensive rehabilitation care for both acute or subacute stroke survivors improves arm and leg motor recovery, walking mobility, and functional status, including independence in self-care and participation in leisure activities. It is important that the rehabilitation be tailored to the tasks that need to be retrained; it is not adequate to focus on muscle strengthening alone.

Another vital component is that all the professionals involved work together as a coordinated specialized team, meeting regularly to discuss the rehabilitation goals and progress. This ensures the whole team takes advantage of the opportunity to work on goals throughout the day, and makes it easier to identify potential barriers to discharge.

System Implications

- ➤ Organized stroke care available including stroke units with critical mass of trained staff, interdisciplinary team during the rehabilitation period following stroke.
- ➤ Initial assessment performed by clinicians experienced in stroke and stroke rehabilitation.
- ➤ Timely access to specialized, interdisciplinary stroke rehabilitation services.
- ➤ Timely access to appropriate type and intensity of rehabilitation for stroke survivors.
- ➤ Optimization of strategies to prevent the recurrence of stroke.
- ➤ Stroke rehabilitation support provided to caregivers
- ➤ Long term rehabilitation services widely available in nursing and continuing care facilities, and in outpatient and community programs
- ➤ Definition, dissemination, and implementation of best practices for stroke rehabilitation across the continuum of care.
- ➤ Mechanisms for ongoing monitoring and evaluation, with a feedback loop for interpretation of findings and opportunities for quality improvement.

Performance Measures

- i. **Length of time from stroke admission in an acute care hospital to assessment of rehabilitation potential by a rehabilitation healthcare professional.**
- ii. **Length of time between stroke onset and admission to stroke inpatient rehabilitation.**
- iii. **Number/percentage of patients admitted to a coordinated stroke unit – either a combined acute care and rehabilitation unit, or a rehabilitation stroke unit in an inpatient rehabilitation facility at any time during their hospital stay (acute and/or rehabilitation). [c]**

DRAFT   08/11/2006

Figure 8-2A1. Example of CPG on stroke rehabilitation.

Canadian Stroke Strategy Recommendations

iv.	**Final discharge disposition for stroke survivors following inpatient rehabilitation: percentage discharged to their original place of residence; percentage discharged to a long term care facility or nursing home; percentage of patients requiring readmission to an acute care hospital for stroke related causes.** [c]
v.	Median length of time spent on a stroke unit during inpatient rehabilitation.
vi.	Median number of days in spent as 'alternate level of care' in an acute care setting prior to arrival in inpatient rehabilitation setting.
vii.	Change (improvement) in functional status scores using a standardized assessment tool from admission to an inpatient rehabilitation program to discharge.
viii.	Total length of time (days) spent in inpatient rehabilitation, by stroke type.
ix.	Number of patients screened for cognitive impairment using valid screening tool during inpatient rehabilitation.
x.	Time from stroke onset to mobilization: a) sitting; b) standing upright; c) walking with/without assistance.

Measurement Notes:

a. Some acute care hospitals provide combined acute and rehabilitation stroke units, where patients progress to 'rehabilitation status' and may not actually move or change locations. This information could be found in patient records through primary chart audit.

b. Many performance measures require primary chart audit of inpatient rehabilitation records. Documentation quality by rehabilitation staff may create data availability and data quality concerns.

c. The Canadian Institute for Health Information has a database known as the National Rehabilitation System (NRS). The NRS includes data on all inpatient rehabilitation encounters to designated rehabilitation beds. It is mandated in some provinces to submit data to the NRS; others are optional. Currently seven provinces contribute to the NRS and two more are expected to join by 2008. The NRS has information on approximately 75% of all inpatient rehabilitation encounters in Canada, and can distinguish stroke cases by diagnosis from other rehabilitation patients.

d. Duration/intensity of services by rehabilitation professionals requires a chart review or consistent use of reliable workload measurement tools that are implemented locally/regionally.

Summary of the Evidence

Early onset of Rehabilitation: In their review, Cifu and Stewart (1999) report that there were four studies of moderate quality that demonstrated a positive correlation between early onset of rehabilitation interventions following stroke and improved functional outcomes. They note that: "Overall, the available literature demonstrates that early onset of rehabilitation interventions – within 3 to 30 days post stroke – is strongly associated with improved functional outcome".

Ottenbacher and Jannell (1993) conducted a meta-analysis including 36 studies with 3,717 stroke survivors, and demonstrated a positive correlation between early intervention of rehabilitation and improved functional outcome. (Reference SREBR)

According to the Ottawa Panel CPGs, which include a recent systematic review (2006):

♦ early care for patients with acute stroke versus standard customary care in stroke unit, Level I (RCT), (one RCT, n=30) (Hayes 1986) a clinically important benefit with statistical significance (Grade A) was shown for length of stay (days).

♦ six days/week of rehabilitation for patients with post-acute stroke versus seven days/week treatment, Level I (RCT), one RCT (n=113) (Ruff 1999) showed clinically important benefits without statistical significance for mobility (ambulation section of Functional Recovery Scale) at end of treatment, 3 weeks (19% RD).

♦ enhanced upper-limb treatment for patients with sub-acute stroke versus interdisciplinary treatment, Level I (RCT), (one RCT, n=626) (Rodgers 2003) showed a clinically important

DRAFT   08/11/2006

Figure 8-2A2. Example of CPG on stroke rehabilitation.

Canadian Stroke Strategy Recommendations

benefit with statistical significance (Grade A) for motor function (Frenchay Arm test) and functional status (Barthel index) at follow-up, 18 weeks.

♦ Enhanced occupational therapy for patients with sub-acute stroke versus standard customary occupational therapy, Level I (RCT), (five RCTs, n=492) (Gibson 1997, Gilbertson 2000, Drummond 1996b, 1995, Logan 1997), clinically important benefits with statistical significance (Grade A) were demonstrated for functional status (# of patients improved in ADL) at end of treatment, 8 weeks and 6 months (23-18% RD), life habit/leisure (overall leisure score) at end of treatment, 3 and 6 months (15-24%), life habit/leisure (total leisure activity score) at end of treatment, 6 months (23%), mobility (Nottingham EADL score for mobility) at end of treatment, 3 and 6 months (56%-58%) and functional status (Nottingham EADL score) at end of treatment, 8 weeks, 3 months and 6 months (16%, 91% and 28% respectively). Clinically important benefits without statistical significance (Grade C+) were demonstrated for quality of life (# of patients living independently) at end of treatment, 3 weeks (28%), functional status (FIM for UE and LE dressing) (41 and 50% respectively) at end of treatment, 3 weeks (28%) and functional status (EADL total score) at follow-up 3 months (28%).

♦ enhanced occupational therapy for patients with sub-acute stroke versus no therapy, Level I (RCT), (five RCTs, n=481) (Jongbloed 1991, Drummond 1996b, 1995, Gilbertson 2000, Corr 1995) clinically important benefits with statistical significance (Grade A) were demonstrated for mobility (NHP for mobility and EADL for mobility) at end of treatment, 3 months and 6 months (49-62% and 39-40% RD respectively), life habit/leisure (Overall Leisure score and Total Leisure activity) at end of treatment, 3 and 6 months (24-30% and 20-30% respectively), functional status (number of patients improved in ADL) at follow-up, 6 months (19%). Clinically important benefits were demonstrated without statistical significance (Grade C+) for activity involvement (Katz adjustment index: # of patients satisfied with their walking) at follow-up, 13 weeks (20%), for activity involvement (# of patients satisfied with their work in the yard) at end of treatment, 5 weeks (15%) and functional status (EADL) at follow-up, 1 year (40%).

♦ enhanced physiotherapy for patients with sub-acute stroke versus standard customary physiotherapy, Level I (RCT), (two RCTs, n=564) (Parry 1999, Lincoln 1999), clinically important benefits with statistical significance (Grade A) were demonstrated for motor function (Action Research Arm test) at follow-up, 21 weeks (18% RD). A clinically important benefit was demonstrated without statistical significance (Grade C+) for functional status (Barthel index) at follow-up, 3 and 16 weeks (15%).

Figure 8-2A3. Example of CPG on stroke rehabilitation.

Canadian Stroke Strategy Recommendations

23. Community-Based Rehabilitation

Best Practice Recommendation 23: Community-Based Rehabilitation

Stroke survivors should continue to have access to specialized stroke care and rehabilitation after leaving hospital (acute and/or inpatient rehabilitation). (RCP; Evidence Level A)

♦ Early supported discharge services provided by a well resourced, coordinated specialist interdisciplinary team are an acceptable alternative to more prolonged hospital stroke unit care and can reduce the length of hospital stay for selected patients. (SIGN 64; Evidence Level A) In addition, early supported discharge services to generic (non-specific) community services should not be undertaken. (RCP; Evidence Level A) See rationale below for explanation of early supported discharge.

♦ People who have difficulty in activities of daily living (ADL) should receive Occupational Therapy or multi-disciplinary interventions targeting ADL. (Australian; Evidence Level 1)

♦ Multifactorial interventions provided in the community including an individually prescribed exercise program, may be provided for people who are at risk of falling, in order to prevent or reduce the number and severity of falls. (Australian; Evidence Level 1)

Rationale

Community based rehabilitation may be defined as care received in the community once the patient has past the acute stage and has transitioned back to their home and community environment. Options for specialized stroke care and rehabilitation may include outpatient services, day hospital programs, home-based rehabilitation services or other alternative services. While there are several options for ongoing rehabilitation environments, location should be based on clients' "medical status, function, social support, and access to care (Duncan, 2005, e137)".

Community based stroke rehabilitation may be characterized by:

▪ A case coordination approach,
▪ An inter-disciplinary team of specialists in stroke care and rehabilitation,
▪ Services that are delivered in the most suited environment based on client issues and strengths
▪ Emphasis on client and family centered practice,
▪ Focus on clients' re-engagement in and attainment of their desired life activities and roles,
▪ Enhancing clients' quality of life after stroke, and,
▪ Provision of intensive rehabilitation services where indicated to promote/ assist in the achievement of client goals.

Early supported discharge (ESD) links inpatient care with community services. It enables stroke survivors to go home earlier than might otherwise be possible, with the support of rehabilitation (Occupational Therapy, Physiotherapy, Speech Language Pathology) and nursing services in the home, while reducing disability and need for long-term institutional care. ESD programs can reduce hospital lengths of stay for high-level (higher functioning) stroke patients by approximately one week. (Teasell et al, 2005) ESD services also reduce adverse events (e.g. readmission rates), and increase the likelihood of being independent and living at home. To work effectively, ESD services must have similar elements to those of organized stroke teams. ESD services should target stroke survivors with mild to moderate disability and should only be considered where there are adequate community services for rehabilitation and caregiver support. Stroke survivors have reported greater satisfaction following ESD than conventional care.

For patients with moderate to severe strokes, specialized stroke care and rehabilitation result in improved functional outcomes. Enhanced stroke rehabilitation for these patients reduces length of hospital stay and increases the likelihood of discharge home (Teasell et al, page 32, 2005). Community based stroke rehabilitation services can enhance mobility and fitness, reduce or prevent the number and severity of falls (Langhorne 2005), and enable clients to access relevant information about community

DRAFT   08/11/2006

Figure 8-2A4. Example of CPG on stroke rehabilitation.

Canadian Stroke Strategy Recommendations

programs and resources. In addition, occupational therapy can improve function in ADL and extended activities of daily living (Langhorne 2005). Such interventions may reduce the potential for hospital readmission as well as reducing health care and caregiver burden. Approximately 1 in 15 stroke patients are spared a poor outcome when receiving community based stroke rehabilitation services (Outpatient Service Trialists, 2002).

System Implications

- Organized and accessible stroke care available within communities
- Initial assessment performed by clinicians experienced in stroke and stroke rehabilitation.
- Timely access to specialized, interdisciplinary stroke rehabilitation services in the community.
- Timely access to appropriate type and intensity of rehabilitation for stroke survivors in the community.
- Optimization of strategies to prevent the recurrence of stroke.
- Stroke rehabilitation support provided to caregivers
- Long term rehabilitation services widely available in nursing and continuing care facilities, and in outpatient and community programs
- Definition, dissemination, and implementation of best practices for stroke rehabilitation across the continuum of care.
- Mechanisms for ongoing monitoring and evaluation, with a feedback loop for interpretation of findings and opportunities for quality improvement.

Performance Measures

   i.   **Percentage of stroke patients discharged to the community who receive a referral for ongoing rehabilitation prior to discharge from hospital (acute and/or inpatient rehabilitation).**

   ii.   **Median length of time between referral for outpatient rehabilitation to admission to a community rehabilitation program.**

   iii.   **Frequency and duration of services by rehabilitation professionals in the community.**

   iv.   **Change in functional status scores, using a standardized measurement tool, for stroke survivors engaged in community rehabilitation programs.**

   v.   Length of time between referral for ongoing rehabilitation to commencement of therapy.

   vi.   Percentage of persons with a diagnosis of stroke who receive outpatient therapy after an admission to hospital for a stroke event.

   vii.   Percentage increase in Telehealth/telestroke coverage to remote communities to support organized stroke care across the continuum and provide rehabilitation assessments and ongoing rehabilitation monitoring and management for stroke survivors in the community.

   viii.   Number of stroke patients assessed by: physiotherapy, occupational therapy, speech language pathologists, and social workers in the community.

Measurement Notes:

   a.   Many performance measures require targeted data collection through audits of rehabilitation records and community program records. Documentation quality by rehabilitation staff may create data availability and data quality concerns.

   b.   Information regarding frequency and duration of services by rehabilitation professionals would require a chart review or consistent use of reliable workload measurement tools that are implemented locally/regionally.

   c.   Data availability regarding community programs varies considerably across programs, regions and provinces. Efforts should be made to introduce standard audit tools for collection of this data.

Summary of the Evidence

"The efficacy of early supported discharge for acute stroke patients, evaluated by the Early Supported Discharge (ESD) Trialists, was first published in 2001 and was updated in 2004. The purpose of this

DRAFT   . .   08/11/2006

Figure 8-2A5. Example of CPG on stroke rehabilitation.

Canadian Stroke Strategy Recommendations

review was to determine whether ESD, with appropriate community support, could be as effective as conventional inpatient rehabilitation. ESD interventions were designed to accelerate the transition from hospital to home. Six of the trials provided coordinated interdisciplinary team care that was provided in the patients' home. One trial (Ronning & Guldvog 1998) provided a wide range of services, which were not centrally coordinated. A variety of outcomes were assessed comparing early supported discharge with conventional care at the end of scheduled follow up, which ranged from 3-12 months. While ESD programs were associated with shorter periods of initial hospitalization, their impact on the well being of caregivers remains unknown. The authors concluded that the "relative risks and benefits of this type of intervention remain unclear" and await the results of ongoing trials. Costing data were available for only two of the trials, both of which reported cost savings associated with ESD programs. However, the authors suggested that further data is required before recommendations can be made regarding potential cost savings" (Teasell et al, page 7, 2005).

Langhorne et al (2005) reported additional patient-level analysis from their original Cochrane review, which examined the effects of patient characteristics and differing levels of service provision (more coordinated versus less organized) on the outcome of death and dependency. The results from an unpublished study were included in this analysis. The levels of service included: 1. ESD team with coordination and delivery: an interdisciplinary team, which coordinated discharge from hospital and post discharge, care and provided rehabilitation therapies in the home 2. ESD team coordination: discharge and immediate post discharge plans were coordinated by a interdisciplinary care team, but rehabilitation therapies were provided by community-based agencies, and 3. No ESD team coordination-therapies were provided by uncoordinated community services or by health-care volunteers. As hypothesized by the authors, the increasing coordination of services was associated with an improved outcome. (Teasell et al, page 7-8, 2005)

"In a review of factors affecting functional outcomes following stroke, Cifu and Stewart (1999) reported the results of three "moderate quality" RCT's examining the differences in functional outcomes between groups of patients who had received either home based therapy or day hospital treatment (Gladman and Lincoln 1994, Tangemen et al. 1990, Young and Foster 1992)." (Teasell et al, pages 16-17, 2005). Teasell et al, 2005 concluded "Overall, the available literature demonstrates that participation in outpatient, home health, and day rehabilitation programs is strongly associated with improved functional outcomes after stroke".

In a systematic review of randomized controlled trials of stroke patients, the effects of therapy-based rehabilitation services targeted towards patients residing in the community was analyzed. Researchers identified and analyzed 14 randomized controlled trials of stroke patients (including 1617 patients) residing in the community and receiving a therapy intervention and compared this to conventional or no care. Electronic databases were searched for the years 1967-November 2001 to ensure identification of all potentially relevant trials were included in the review. Therapy services were defined as those provided by physiotherapy, occupational therapy, or by interdisciplinary staff working with patients primarily to improve task-oriented behaviour and hence increase activity and participation. The results indicated that therapy-based rehabilitation services reduced the odds of a poor outcome (Peto odds ratio 0.72 (95% CI 0.57 to 0.92; P = 0.009) and increased personal activity of daily living scores (standardized mean difference 0.14 (95% CI 0.02 to 0.25; P = 0.02). For every 100 stroke patients resident in the community receiving therapy-based rehabilitation services, 7 (95% CI 2 to 11) patients would be spared a poor outcome, assuming 37.5% would have had a poor outcome with no treatment. The authors concluded that therapy-based rehabilitation services targeted towards stroke patients living at home appear to improve independence in personal activities of daily living (Outpatient Service Trialists, 2002).

Figure 8-2A6. Example of CPG on stroke rehabilitation.

Cervical Manipulation Systematic Reviews

As indicated above, cervical manipulation is a clear example of where a systematic review is needed and should be updated when new evidence is available, given the potential interest from clinical, public, and policy sectors. Furthermore, a CPG might be useful to insure safer and better practice. We searched neck or cervical AND manipulation AND systematic reviews and kept all papers that addressed effectiveness or complications of manipulation. These were found.

Brand, P. L., Engelbert, R. H., Helders, P. J., & Offringa, M. (2005). Systematic review of the effects of therapy in infants with the KISS-syndrome (kinetic imbalance due to suboccipital strain). *Ned Tijdschr Geneeskd, 149*(13), 703-707.

Bronfort, G., Haas, M., Evans, R. L., & Bouter, L. M. (2004). Efficacy of spinal manipulation and mobilization for low back pain and neck pain: A systematic review and best evidence synthesis. *Spine Journal, 4*(3), 335-356.

Conlin, A., Bhogal, S., Sequeira, K., & Teasell, R. (2005). Treatment of whiplash-associated disorders—Part I: Non-invasive interventions. *Pain Resarch & Management, 10*(1), 21-32.

Cook, C., Hegedus, E., Showalter, C., & Sizer, P. S., Jr. (2006). Coupling behavior of the cervical spine: A systematic review of the literature. *Journal of Manipulative and Physiological Therapeutics, 29*(7), 570-575.

Ernst, E. (2001) Prospective investigations into the safety of spinal manipulation. *Journal of Pain and Symptom Management, 21*(3), 238-242.

Ernst, E. (2002). Manipulation of the cervical spine: A systematic review of case reports of serious adverse events, 1995-2001. *Medical Journal of Australia, 176*(8), 376-380.

Ernst, E. (2003). Chiropractic spinal manipulation for neck pain: A systematic review. *Journal of Pain, 4*(8):417-421.

Ernst, E., & Canter, P. H. (2006). A systematic review of systematic reviews of spinal manipulation. *Journal of the Royal Society of Medicine, 99*(4), 192-196.

Gemmell, H., & Miller, P. (2006). Comparative effectiveness of manipulation, mobilisation and the activator instrument in treatment of non-specific neck pain: a systematic review. *Chiropractic & Osteopathy, 14*, 7.

Gross, A. R., Hoving, J. L., Haines, T. A., Goldsmith, C. H., Kay, T., Aker, P., et al. (2004). A Cochrane review of manipulation and mobilization for mechanical neck disorders. *Spine, 29*(14), 1541-1548.

Gross, A. R., Kay, T., Hondras, M., Goldsmith, C., Haines, T., Peloso, P., et al. (2002). Manual therapy for mechanical neck disorders: A systematic review. *Manual Therapy, 7*(3), 131-149.

Hurwitz, E. L., Aker, P. D., Adams, A. H., Meeker, W. C., & Shekelle, P. G. (1996). Manipulation and mobilization of the cervical spine: A systematic review of the literature. *Spine, 21*(15), 1746-1759.

Inamasu, J., & Guiot, B. H. (2006). Intracranial hypotension with spinal pathology. *Spine Journal, 6*(5), 591-599.

Kay, T. M., Gross, A., Goldsmith, C., Santaguida, P. L., Hoving, J., & Bronfort, G. (2005). Exercises for mechanical neck disorders. *Cochrane Database of Systematic Reviews, 3*, CD004250.

Mior, S. (2001). Manipulation and mobilization in the treatment of chronic pain. *Clinical Journal of Pain, 17*(Suppl. 4), S70-S76.

Shekelle, P. G., & Coulter, I. (1997). Cervical spine manipulation: summary report of a systematic review of the literature and a multidisciplinary expert panel. *Journal of Spine Disorders, 10*(3), 223-228.

Verhagen, A. P., Karels, C., Bierma-Zeinstra, S. M., Burdorf, L., Feleus, A., Dahaghin, S., et al. (2006). Ergonomic and physiotherapeutic interventions for treating work-related complaints of the arm, neck or shoulder in adults. *Cochrane Database of Systematic Reviews, 3*, CD003471.

Vernon, H. T., Humphreys, B. K., & Hagino, C. A. (2005). A systematic review of conservative treatments for acute neck pain not due to whiplash. *Journal of Manipulative and Physiological Therapeutics, 28*(6), 443-448.

Weiner, D. K., & Ernst, E. (2004). Complementary and alternative approaches to the treatment of persistent musculoskeletal pain. *Clinical Journal of Pain, 20*(4), 244-255.

With permission of the lead developer and the publisher (Canadian Physiotherapy Association), we reproduce the CPG for cervical manipulation (short format).

Cervical Manipulation Clinical Practice Guideline (Figure 8-2B)

EXAMPLE 3—A CLINICAL PATHWAY COMPARISON IN TOTAL KNEE ARTHROPLASTY

Total knee arthroplasty is an increasingly large sector in rehabilitation. Surprisingly, there are few systematic reviews that address rehabilitation in this population. The focus in the literature tends to be on the surgery—not optimal rehabilitation. Literature synthesizes are appearing in other sources, so Medline may have missed some important information.

Systematic Reviews on Total Knee Arthroplasty Rehabilitation

We searched (arthroplasty AND systematic review AND knee) to find articles that might assist with rehabilitation. Of the 9 retrieved reviews, most dealt with medical issues and we list those that might have relevance to rehabilitation. The most relevant were as follows:

Ackerman, I. N., & Bennell, K. L. (2004). Does pre-operative physiotherapy improve outcomes from lower limb joint replacement surgery? A systematic review. *Australian Journal of Physiotherapy, 50*(1), 25-30.

Ethgen, O., Bruyere, O., Richy, F., Dardennes, C., & Reginster, J. Y. (2004). Health-related quality of life in total hip and total knee arthroplasty: A qualitative and systematic review of the literature. *Journal of Bone and Joint Surgery American, 86*-A(5), 963-974.

Kelly, M. A., & Clarke, H. D. (2003). Stiffness and ankylosis in primary total knee arthroplasty. *Clinical Orthopaedics & Related Research, 416,* 68-73

Schoderbek, R. J., Jr., Brown, T. E., Mulhall, K. J., Mounasamy, V., Iorio, R., Krackow, K. A., et al. (2006). Extensor mechanism disruption after total knee arthroplasty. *Clinical Orthopaedics & Related Research, 446,* 176-185.

A Clinical Pathway for Total Knee Arthroplasty Rehabilitation

A clinical team at St. Joseph's Health Care in London developed the following CP using a committee process. It is accessible at www.sjhc.london.on.ca/sjh/profess/cp/cp_clin.htm along with other institutional CPs and is used with permission (Figures 8-3A and 8-3B).

LEARNING AND EXPLORATION ACTIVITIES

1. Select one systematic review from the lists above and see if it is accurately reflected in the other form of evidence.

2. Contrast and compare the forms of evidence.

3. Select a treatment or patient group from the examples above and assume you are going to implement treatment with a patient tomorrow. List the information you derived (can derive) from either a systematic review or the CP, CPG, or algorithm. What additional information do you need and what steps are required to implement this tomorrow. Can you do it?

Clinical Practice Guideline on the Use of Manipulation or Mobilization in the Treatment of Adults with Mechanical Neck Disorders

Introduction

A working group of clinicians and researchers was formed to conduct a systematic review, develop evidence-based recommendations and generate a Clinical Practice Guideline (CPG).

Neck disorders are common and disabling, they can affect physical and social function, and result in large levels of health care use. Large proportions of the attributed health care costs are due to visits to health care providers. The mean cost per case of disablement and absenteeism due to neck pain is not clear but appears substantive. The CPG is intended to assist clinicians who perform manipulation and mobilization to do so in a manner which minimises adverse side effects or events and maximises the benefits of the procedure.

The CPG is a summary of a report published by Gross A.R., Kay T.M., Hurley L, et al. 2001 Clinical Practice Guideline on the Use of Manipulation or Mobilization in the Treatment of Adults with Mechanical Neck Disorders. Manual Therapy (submitted). The summary recommendations are reprinted with the permission of the Manual Therapy. Some reprints are available (please contact the College at 1-800-583-5885 or email info.collegept.org).

These recommendations apply to adults with symptomatic acute and chronic mechanical neck disorders with or without headache of cervical origin. This may include patients with degenerative disc disease or whiplash associated disorders.

Recommendations are based on systematic reviews, randomized controlled, and quasi-randomized controlled trials. The harm recommendations also utilized survey level trials. Consensus was not used to make recommendations in the absence of evidence.

Figure 8-2B1. Example of cervical manipulation systematic review.

Recommendations

Benefit

1. When choosing to apply manipulation or mobilization, incorporate them within an overall multi-modal[1] management strategy. The overall multi-modal management strategy demonstrates clear benefit.

Rationale
Based on a large number of trials restricted to the use of manual therapy, using both heterogeneous treatment approaches and comparisons, a multi-modal management strategy is proven beneficial in alleviating pain and achieving patient satisfaction. The effects on function are variable.

2. The recommended multi-modal treatment strategy to use in combination with manipulation or mobilization is exercise.

Rationale
Of the beneficial multi-modal strategies, the common element is exercise plus mobilization or exercise plus manipulation. The effect of other combinations of multi-modal treatment is less clear. The weight of the evidence suggests that there is less likely to be a benefit when either manipulation alone, mobilization alone, or a combination of the two are used, than when these manual therapies are used in combination with exercise.

3. Use your best judgement concerning other common multi-modal treatment strategies.

Rationale
The benefit of other therapies (e.g., drugs, relaxation, massage) or modalities (e.g., thermal agents, electrotherapies, phototherapies, orthoses) used in conjunction with manual therapy are unclear.

---

[1] A multi-modal treatment strategy is an inclusive description of a broad approach to treatment for patients with cervical neck disorders. The inclusive description includes the use of pain relieving medication, rare collar use, thermal agents, exercise, massage, relaxation, education, electrotherapies, and either manipulation or mobilization. The common beneficial element in all multi-modal approaches studied in published reports is the use of exercise.

Figure 8-2B2. Example of cervical manipulation systematic review.

4. We do not recommend using a single session of manipulation to decrease pain. However, the recommended frequency of manipulation to achieve optimal benefit is not known.

Rationale
Based on strong evidence, there is no benefit in using manipulation alone in a single session to decrease pain.

Risk

1. Advise your patients of the risk of complications from the use of manipulation or mobilization.

Rationale
The true risks are unclear. Available estimates are as follows. The lowest reported estimate for risk of irreversible injury when applying manipulation is one in 20,000. Estimates for serious risks following the application of mobilization have rarely been reported. The adverse event rate could not be determined from existing information.

Implications

Clinicians surveyed reflected a model of practice similar to the recommendations of the guideline. It is unlikely that dissemination and implementation of this guideline will significantly alter present practice.

Educative bodies need to stress effective communication strategies for clinicians in order to relay the risk information in an effective, clear and objective manner. Clinicians surveyed also expressed the need to further validate screening tests to ensure that patients who may present a risk are recognized

Payers should be aware choosing manipulation as a treatment option is a choice the clinician makes depending on the presenting risk factors, assessment findings, clinician's judgement, and patient preference. Attempting to enforce the use of a guideline through regulation would not be in the patient's best interest.

Patients should be informed of the relative risk of manipulation, screened for risk factors, informed of the benefits of manipulation in combination with other therapies, be informed of alternative choices of treatment, and provide informed consent before proceeding with manipulation.[2] Following manipulation, a reassessment should be performed to ensure no undue side effects have resulted.

---

[2] For further information on informed consent, please refer to *A Member's Reference Guide to the Health Care Consent Act,* College of Physiotherapists of Ontario, 1996.

Figure 8-2B3 . Example of cervical manipulation systematic review.

There were areas with insufficient evidence to make recommendations:

- Large randomized trials on single or multi-modal manual therapy care strategies are needed to better estimate their benefit. Due to a paucity of trials per category, it is unclear if certain variables such as methodological quality of the study, duration of symptoms and type of neck disorder influence the magnitude of the reported treatment effect.
- Optimal doses of response (frequency, intensity, duration) and technique selection are unclear.
- Existing studies on single manipulations and mobilization are mostly analytical in nature, and do not reflect the usual clinical approach, which would be to prescribe manipulation over some number of sessions in order to achieve an optimal therapeutic goal.
- No information about cost or patient preference was available.

Outcome measures

Ideal outcome measures should reflect long-term consequences, such as the effects of the manual therapy technique on morbidity or the incidence of certain complications (e.g., vertebral artery tear). However, due to the low complication rate, a large sample size would be needed to assess long-term consequences. For these reasons, the majority of studies employed measures of function, pain and patient satisfaction. These measures can not be considered surrogate measures for long-term outcomes.

All studies did not report on all outcomes that were measured. This was taken into account in the careful formulation of the recommendations.

This CPG is not designed to substitute clinical judgement in specific clinical circumstances.

Figure 8-2B4. Example of cervical manipulation systematic review.

CLINICAL PATHWAY - TOTAL KNEE

PATIENT'S NAME: _____

November, 1998

Date: _____
Date: _____

St. JOSEPH's	Preadmission	Preop/Same Day Admission Day 1 _____ 200__ Pre	Post	Day 2 Post Op Day 1 _____ 200__	Day 3 Post Op Day 2 _____ 200__	Day 4 Post Op Day 3 _____ 200__	Day 5 Post Op Day 4 _____ 200__	Day 6/Day 7 Post Op Day 5/6 _____ 200__
Consults/Referrals	Mandatory: • Nursing • Physio • Pharmacy • Orthopaedic Resident; Optional: • OT (G); • Medical consult (may have been pre-arranged) (G) • Anaesthesia consult (G) • Pastoral Care (G) • Social Work (G) • Dietician (G) • CCAC (G) • Rehabilitation (G)	• Pastoral Care	• Physio referral	• Chest physio if needed; • Pastoral Care if required	Ongoing Physio for ambulation & ROM >	> ; • OT Assessment * if needed for ADLs; • Assess need for Outpatient. Physio or CCAC Physio or Rehab	> ; • CCAC. if required • Pharmacist (if anticoagulant required upon discharge); > ; > >	• Review S/S infection/DVT • Stress importance of exercises. mobility and appropriate rest > ; • Review proper positioning • review discharge sheet - have patient sign and take copy
Patient/Family Teaching	• Give Total Knee Booklet (G) • PCA sheet (G) • Pharmacy anticoag teaching (G) • Nursing preop teaching (counselling): - SDA - DB&C • Physio (G) • Give Pastoral Care flyer (G)	• PCA Sheet (G) • Physio Sheet (G) • OR Record (G); • DB/C • Reinforce PCA-teaching (G)	> ; >	• Isometric exercises > ; • ↑ leg on pillow avoiding knee flexion and heel pressure	• Don't sit for longer than 1 h at a time • Review s/s infection and DVT • WBAT; • Sit in chair with feet on floor to encourage knee flexion (may use stool if necessary)	• Physio reviews mobility equipment needs > ; • OT for ADLs *	• If patient requires anticoagulant at home. arrange pharmacist to see patient (only if previous or current DVT. PE) > ; • Arrange for GP to monitor INRs > ; • Assess knowledge and understanding of knee exercises/positioning • Make sure patient has necessary equipment for home	
Tests	• CBC • S S ± • U/A • CXR ± • EKG ± • Knee x-ray ±	• CBC. SS (if not done Preadmission) • U/A • CXR ± • EKG ± • Knee x-ray ±	• knee x-ray in OR post OP	• CBC • SS • INR • Oxygen saturation (if on oxygen)	• INR	• CBC. SS. INR	• INR	

Figure 8-3A1. Example of clinical pathway for total knee arthroplasty.

	Preadmission	Preop/Same Day Admission Day 1 — Pre	Preop/Same Day Admission Day 1 — Post	Day 2 Post Op Day 1 ,200	Day 3 Post Op Day 2 ,200	Day 4 Post Op Day 3 ,200	Day 5 Post Op Day 4 ,200	Day 6/Day 7 Post Op Day 5/6 ,200
Treatments	•Explain Hibitane scrub and give sponge to take home	•Hib scrub if not done at home •DB/C •Start IV	•Oxygen as ordered •Skin care q4h •CSM q1h x4 then q4h •HMV - monitor and empty and record q12h (if no HMV - monitor dressing and reinforce as needed) •Maintain IV at rate ordered •I and O - q shift or more often as needed •VS q 1/2h on return from PACU x2 then q4h x 48hrs •may have femoral block which may effect CSM	•D/C HMV •monitor dressings q shift and PRN •CSM Q4h •VS q4h •I and O q shift •D/C oxygen if sat >92 •IV as ordered •Turn Q4h with skin care •Assess for abdominal and bladder distention q4h •Change to light dressing •Document drainage •Physio to initiate ROM exercises 2 times per day unless patient's pain uncontrolled	•Turn q4h with skin care •D/C IV/PCA if oral intake adequate and good pain control •CSM q4h •VS q4h •Assess for Homan's sign and edema	•Monitor wound/dressing; change PRN and document appearance of wound / drainage •VS q shift •CSM q shift •Turn Q4h with skin care while in bed	•Monitor wound/dressing - change PRN and document appearance of wound / drainage •VS daily •CSM q shift •Turn Q4h with skin care while in bed (teach how to turn independently) •Encourage independent turning while in bed every four hours	•Change dressing to light and assess wound before discharge •Give staple remover with instructions for G.P. to remove 2 weeks post op •VS before discharge
Medication	•Pharmacist to provide anticoagulant teachings and give Coumadin, for night before OR •List patient's meds •Advise patient which of own meds to take with sips in a.m. of OR according to Dr's orders	•Give pre-op meds as ordered •Antibiotic IV on call if ordered •Coumadin @ HS if ordered	•Antibiotic IV x 24h •PCA - monitor pain relief (if no PCA offer analgesia q4h) •Continue home meds as ordered •Post-op Coumadin (7.5 mgms) at HS	•Coumadin at HS	•Begin oral analgesia once PCA D/C'd (offer 1/2 hour before physio to see) •Continue home meds as ordered •Offer laxative as ordered per bowel routine			•Scripts for analgesic and/or any new medication started in hospital and to continue at home •D/C Coumadin
Diet	N/A	•NPO at 2400 day before OR	•Diet as tolerated (start with clear fluids)	•DAT - advance as tolerated •Encourage fluids	•DAT •Push fluids	•DAT	•DAT	•DAT
Activity	N/A		•Bed rest •Commode privileges	•Physio to see - up in chair as tolerated x2 •Encourage foot and ankle exercises and quad setting •Wear proper foot wear •Physio to see regarding ambulation WBAT and begin knee ROM •Document progress on physio sheet at bedside 2x day		•Ambulation/endurance in hall x2 •Teach independent transfers •Knee ROM with physio x2	•Continue to increase length of ambulation with supervision only •Attempt stairs •Continue knee ROM •Assess need for continuing physio at home	•OT D/C if needed •Independent with walking aid and with stairs •Physio/D/C •Referral for Outpatient physio or home care physio if needed •Independent with home exercise program

St JOSEPHs

Figure 8-3A2. Example of clinical pathway for total knee arthroplasty.

	Preadmission	Preop/Same Day Admission Day 1 ___ 200__ Pre	Post	Day 2 Post Op Day 1 ___ 200__	Day 3 Post Op Day 2 ___ 200__	Day 4 Post Op Day 3 ___ 200__	Day 5 Post Op Day 4 ___ 200__	Day 6/Day 7 Post Op Day 5/6 ___ 200__
Discharge Plan	• Community supports available (Booklet for seniors if needed) • Home resources • Make patient aware of expected length of stay • Convalescent care to be explored if required (Social Work) • Patient to get commitment from family members for assistance at discharge for ADLs/IADLs • Prepare and freeze meals ahead of time • Stress Home Care is generally not indicated but is available based on specific needs • Staple remover (check with GP's office if one available)				• Clarify home supports and discharge plans (ensure follow-up)	• Make appropriate referrals to Rehab/Social Work if required • Contact family if necessary regarding home supports • Instruct patient in TKA Home Exercise Program	• Reinforce discharge planning • Plan specific D/C day based on patient's progress to date • Assess need for continuing physio and arrange Outpatient or CCAC physio	• Discharge by 1000 • Follow-up appointment with surgeon for six weeks • Outpatient physio referral if required • Discharge sheet of exercises from physio
Other	• Nursing assessment/data collection (esp. previous mobility status) anaesthetic questionnaire: consent signed • HT/WT							
Expected Outcomes	• Patient and family verbalize understanding of pre-op teaching	• Chest clear • VS stable (within normal limits) • Able to dorsi flex (unless had spinal / block anaesthesia) • Patient verbalizes reasonable pain control		• Patient learns how to transfer bed/chair with assistance • Patient understands importance of turning q4h to maintain skin integrity ⌐⌐⌐⌐⌐⌐>	• Patient able to transfer bed/chair with one assistant • in chair for all three meals if able • begin to ambulate short distance in room with walker/crutches • Performs isometric exercises and ROM of knee (dorsi flexion and quads setting with physio 2x day and independently 3x day	• Bed/Chair transfers with minimal assistance • Ambulate to BR in room with one assistant and walking aid ⌐⌐⌐⌐⌐⌐> • Performs isometric exercises independently and continues to improve knee ROM independently • Identifies need for mobility aids	• Bed/Chair transfers with minimal assistance / independent • Ambulate in hall with supervision and walking aid • Walk to bathroom / supervision • Attempt stairs • Patient verbalizes readiness for discharge • D/C plans in place • Home support in place • Discharge plans made with community if required ⌐⌐⌐⌐⌐⌐>	• Manages stairs, transfers and ambulation independently • Patient and/or family independent with ADL's • Patient has all needed mobility equipment • Home has been modified for safety • Achieves ROM as outlined by physician ⌐⌐⌐⌐⌐⌐>
Signatures								

* Weight-Bearing Status   Discharge Location: _____

F:\wpfiles\maps\U z\tot\kne\iknee3-s.wpd

Figure 8-3A3. Example of clinical pathway for total knee arthroplasty.

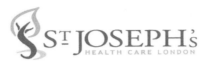

VARIANCE TRACKING SHEET

Date of Admission: **Clinical Pathway Name:**

Date of Discharge:

		VARIANCE	SOURCE			
Date	Actual Care Path Day	SPECIFY VARIANCE	Category (Select A to D)	Reason (Select 1-16)	Specify Reason for Variance	Sig./Status

CATEGORY	REASON	CATEGORY	REASON
A. Patient/Family	01-Patient condition 02-Pt/family decision 03-Pt/family availability 04-Pt/family other	C. Hospital	09-Bed/appt time availability 10-Information/date availability 11-Supplies/equipment availability 12-Dept. overbooked/closed
B. Care Giver/Clinician	05-Physician order 06-Caregiver(s) decision 07-Caregiver(s) response time 08-Caregiver other	D. Community	13-Hospital other 14-Placement/Home Care availability 15-Transportation availability 16-Community other

f:\wpfiles\maps\l-z\variance.wpd

Figure 8-3B. Example of variance tracking sheet.

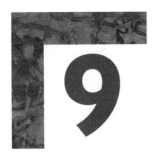

9

Evaluating the Evidence
Economic Evaluations

*Diane Watson, PhD, MBA, BScOT; Emma Housser, BSc;
and Maria Mathews, PhD, MHSA, BA, BSc*

LEARNING OBJECTIVES

After reading this chapter, the student/practitioner will be able to:
- Recognize the importance of assessing the value of intervention to ensure that it offers the most efficient treatment.
- Identify the different types of economic evaluations and when they are appropriate for use.
- Initiate research on a question related to economic analysis, including the development of a question and the use of various electronic databases.
- Critically appraise and communicate this research to his or her clients.

Over the past few years, evidence has increased regarding the effectiveness of certain types of occupational therapy and physical therapy services in enabling clients to attain specific, desirable outcomes. It would appear that clinical practitioners appropriately employ these interventions (Office of Inspector General, 1999) and are striving to shape their practice to become more evidence based. The next challenge is clear—rehabilitation professionals must assess the value of effective interventions to ensure that they offer the most efficient means of attaining these outcomes. Only then will clients and consumers be able to evaluate the costs and outcomes associated with the choices they face when determining whether to participate in or offer rehabilitation services (Watson, 2000).

Clients participate in health programs and receive these services to attain desirable outcomes at minimal cost and risk. We often assume that health services are beneficial, but some interventions can be harmful to one's physical and financial health. For example, it has been estimated that approximately 20% of patients receive contraindicated chronic care and 30% receive contraindicated acute care (Schuster, McGlynn, & Brook, 1998). In addition, between 45,000 to 195,000 individuals die each year as a result of medical errors (Kohn, Corrigan, & Donaldson, 1999; Leape 2004), and medical bills accounted for up to 50% of bankruptcies in the United

States in 2003 (Doty, Edwards, & Holmgren, 2005). These recent statistics draw attention toward the importance of balancing our understanding of potential benefits with insights regarding costs and risks.

Research evidence demonstrating the inappropriateness of some health services is mounting, and these findings are not unique to medicine. A recent review found that most Medicare patients in skilled nursing facilities who received occupational and physical therapy were appropriate candidates and benefited from intervention, but 10% of billed therapy was for services that were "not medically necessary" (Office of the Inspector General, 1999, p. 13). It was determined that patients who had similar diagnoses, goals, plans, and outcomes varied in the frequency and duration of the therapy services they received from different facilities. Evaluations such as this draw attention toward the importance of understanding the cost-effectiveness of rehabilitation services and excessive intervention.

The purpose of this chapter is to provide students, practitioners, administrators, and researchers with a basic understanding of, and appreciation for, research methods that have been used to appraise the costs and outcomes of health services. More extensive information regarding application of these methods to assess the value of rehabilitation services is published elsewhere (Watson, 2000). It is expected that this knowledge will enable these individuals to critically appraise and communicate evidence derived from the literature and stimulate enthusiasm among those who wish to conduct this type of evaluation. Other sections in this book highlight the process of seeking evidence regarding the effectiveness of specific services and incorporating this evidence into practice. By comparison, this chapter summarizes how research is conducted in order to evaluate the value of health services and describes how practitioners can obtain and appraise this evidence.

Assessing the Value of Rehabilitation Services to Clients: Economic Evaluation

Research methods have been developed to appraise, describe, and compare the relative value of health services. These methods have been called cost-effectiveness analyses (Russell, Gold, Siegel, Daniels, & Weinstein, 1996) and/or economic evaluations (Drummond, O'Brien, Stoddart, & Torrance, 1997). They are distinct from clinical evaluations in that they focus on costs and outcomes rather than the efficacy or effectiveness of a specific intervention. The effectiveness and appropriateness of a clinical intervention, however, should be established before being combined with an assessment of costs, as it would be wasteful to calculate the cost of providing ineffective services (Drummond, O'Brien, et al., 1997).

While effective research focuses on the impact of interventions on health, economic evaluations focus on the relative value of health services. Value refers to "a fair return or equivalent in goods, services, or money for something exchanged" (Merriam-Webster, 1984, p. 1303). Within the health care context, the term *value* refers to the relative worth, utility, or importance of a service in meeting the health needs of a defined clientele. For a service to be "valuable," clients should receive a fair return (i.e., service and outcome) for something exchanged (i.e., finances and time invested). In order to inform consumers and clients about the relative value of specific health and rehabilitation services for defined clientele, we must (a) conduct evaluations to determine whether specific interventions are effective at attaining desirable outcomes, (b) evaluate effective interventions to ensure that they offer the most efficient means of attaining specific outcomes, and (c) effectively communicate these results. Unfortunately, the number of evaluations that have been conducted to assess the relative value of rehabilitation services is small in comparison to the number of effectiveness studies (Watson & Mathews, 1998).

The intent and purpose of economic evaluations are to provide clients and consumers with information regarding value in order to inform their decisions. Therefore, these evaluations require that two or more services must be compared to assess "relative value." One of the comparisons, however, could be the "no service" alternative, which is equivalent to a control group in experimental research. In this context, a comparison would be made between the cost and benefit of receiving versus not receiving a rehabilitation service. For example, Meyer and colleagues (2005) conducted an economic evaluation in which they compared the cost and outcomes of providing versus not providing education and hip protectors for nurses to reduce the number of hip fractures for nursing home patients.

Types of Economic Evaluations

There are five different types of economic evaluation that have been defined in the literature: cost-consequence, cost-minimization, cost-effectiveness, cost-utility, and cost-benefit analyses (Canadian Coordinating Office for Health Technology Assessment, 1997; Drummond, O'Brien, et al., 1997). Table 9-1 illustrates how these different research methods might be applied to evaluate the relative worth of a rehabilitation service. Table 9-2 provides examples of economic evaluations that have been published in the literature and highlights the fact that investigators may conduct different types of economic evaluations when assessing the relative value of a health or rehabilitation service.

A cost-consequence analysis can be used to describe a health service or compare two or more health interventions. This type of analysis requires that investigators provide a descriptive profile of the costs (e.g., hospital costs, out-of-pocket expenses) and outcomes (e.g., impact on health and economic circumstances) of one or more interventions. For example, Patel, Knapp, Evans, Perez, and Kalra (2004) described the costs and outcomes of providing care giver training during rehabilitation of stroke patients.

A cost-minimization analysis is conducted to identify the least costly alternative when two or more services produce equivalent outcomes. Evidence that each service produces comparable outcomes must be demonstrated using evidence from the literature or tested as part of the analysis. When researchers determined that there was no significant difference in outcomes for patients who received hospital at home versus hospital inpatient care, a cost-minimization analysis was conducted to identify the least costly alternative (Jones et al., 1999).

A cost-effectiveness analysis is conducted when an investigator is interested in describing and comparing the relative costs and outcomes of two or more services. These evaluations require that the services being compared produce the same type of outcome. For example, Cochrane et al. (2005) compared the costs and outcomes of individuals who have lower limb osteoarthritis and receive water-based exercise or regular care. A cost-effectiveness analysis was used to study the value of each service option because the goal of each service was to achieve the same type of outcome (i.e., reduce upper extremity impairment and improve health status).

In contrast, cost-utility and cost-benefit analyses are conducted to compare the relative costs and outcomes of two or more services that produce different types of outcomes. Cost-utility analyses consider both health status and the value of that status to the client when evaluating outcomes, while cost-benefit analyses require that investigators measure the monetary value of outcomes. Consider the challenge of trying to determine which clients should receive occupational therapy given that demand for your services exceeds your ability to offer care. Should you offer occupational therapy services to individuals who have had a physical injury or to those who have a psychiatric condition? Consider making this decision on the basis of which alternative would maximize outcomes for the amount of cost (e.g., monetary and time) invested. One way to compare outcomes for services that produce different types of outcomes is to measure change in health status (i.e., cost-utility analysis). In other words, measure whether changes in the health

---

Table 9-1

APPLYING ECONOMIC EVALUATION METHODS
TO REHABILITATION SERVICES

Consider the Following Clinical Scenario and the Contribution of Economic Evaluation Methods to the Decision-Making Process:

Assume that people who have had a stroke in the last 10 to 15 days are given the choice to receive rehabilitation services using a number of different care approaches. Suppose that you have been given the responsibility to be a decision maker regarding the health care services received by this population. You have decided that his decision will primarily be based on the relative value (i.e., the relative costs and outcomes) of each alternative.

You have determined that the hospital offers poststroke rehabilitation services on a general unit or a specialized unit and that home-based rehabilitation services are available. Therefore, the following options are available: (1) hospital-based services on a general unit, (2) hospital-based services on a specialized unit, (3) early discharge from the hospital and home-based rehabilitation, or (4) early discharge and no rehabilitation services.

You have reviewed the literature to determine the relative value of institution-based versus home-based poststroke rehabilitation versus no intervention. A cost-consequences analysis would provide a descriptive profile of the costs and outcomes of each alternative and any evidence regarding significant differences between these alternatives. Assuming that the goals and objectives of the inpatient poststroke rehabilitation services were identical and, therefore, the types of outcomes expected of participants were similar, a cost-effectiveness analysis would provide insight regarding the relative value of the alternatives. Relative value would be measured by determining the cost per unit of health effect (e.g., cost per unit of change in functional status) derived from participation in each service delivery model in comparison to the no-service alternative.

Assume that the goals and objectives of the hospital-based programs were to increase independence in activities of daily living (ADL), while the goals of the home-based programs were to enhance participation of individuals who have experienced a stroke in community-based activities and support programs. In this context, it would be appropriate to conduct a cost-utility and/or cost-benefit analysis to compare the relative value of service alternatives that are directed toward different outcomes (i.e., independence in ADL versus enhanced community participation). Both outcomes, however, impact health-related quality of life (HRQL). Therefore, a cost-utility analysis would require a comparison of the costs and HRQL of these two service alternatives. Alternatively, a cost-benefit analysis could be conducted to compare the costs, monetary outcomes, and net financial impact of participating in either of these two service alternatives.

status of patients with physical injuries are more, less, or the same as those with psychiatric conditions. Another way to compare outcomes is to measure outcomes in financial terms (i.e., cost-benefit analysis). See Tables 9-1 and 9-2 for more examples of economic evaluations.

Table 9-2

EXAMPLES OF ECONOMIC EVALUATIONS IN THE REHABILITATION LITERATURE

Type of Evaluation	Health Service Area	Example Evaluation
Cost-consequence	Community-based geriatric case management program for frail elderly	Duke, 2005
	Training versus no training for care givers of stroke patients	Patel, Knapp, Evans, et al., 2004
Cost-minimization	Stroke rehabilitation: home or hospital	Anderson et al., 2000; Jones et al., 1999
	Use of hip protectors in the prevention of hip fractures in frail institutionalized elderly	van Schoor et al., 2004
Cost-effectiveness	Water-based exercise therapy versus usual care for lower limb osteoarthritis	Cochrane, Davey, & Edwards, 2005
	Use of hip protectors in nursing homes	Meyer et al., 2005
	Home exercise program or no intervention for knee pain	Thomas et al., 2005
	High-intensity exercise program or conventional physical therapy for individuals with rheumatoid arthritis	van den Hout et al., 2005
Cost-utility	Hospital-based rehabilitation or conventional care after an acute coronary event	Briffa et al., 2005
	Home or group-based rehabilitation programs for women with breast cancer	Gordon et al., 2005
	Early discharge of elderly persons	Miller et al., 2005
	Stroke unit, stroke team, or domiciliary stroke care	Patel, Knapp, Perez, Evans, and Kalra, 2004
	Cardiac rehabilitation prevention program versus conventional therapy	Yu et al., 2004
Cost-benefit	Individual placement and support versus regular employment placement service for mental health patients	Chalamat, Minalopoulos, Carter & Vos, 2005
	Needle exchange program to prevent HIV transmission	Gold, Gafni, Nelligan, & Millson, 1997
	Providing versus not offering a fall prevention program	Rizzo, Baker, McAvay, & Tinetti, 1996
	Home versus institutional-based psychiatric services	Margolis & Petti, 1994

Conducting Economic Evaluations

Economic evaluations are conducted using a multistep process (Mathews & Watson, 2000). A research question is initially posed to define the purpose and scope of the assessment. The question should describe a service or identify interventions being described or compared, outline the perspective and time horizon of the analysis, specify the scope of the intervention, and detail the costs and outcomes considered. Economic evaluations can be descriptive, comparative, or both. Descriptive evaluations simply describe the goals and objectives of the service, the population for whom the program was provided, the type of intervention offered, the costs of providing and/or consuming the intervention service, and the outcomes or effects of the service. Comparative assessments require that two or more services be compared with appropriate alternative interventions or no intervention. The perspective of the analysis is important to consider and identify prospectively, as evaluations that are conducted from the same viewpoint as the "user" of the assessment tend to be more relevant and useful (Stoddart, 1982). Evaluations can be conducted from the perspective of society, payers, providers, and/or consumers. The important and relevant costs and outcomes should be specified and included in an evaluation. These elements can be identified through a process that considers the goals, objectives, and activities of the health service; the needs of the target population and service recipients; and the preference of the audience for whom the evaluation report is intended. The most relevant and important costs and outcomes to include are those that are valued by all stakeholders. The majority of economic evaluations published in the literature appear to be authored by a team of investigators who have diverse backgrounds. It appears, therefore, that the successful generation of evidence regarding the cost and outcomes of medical and rehabilitative services may require a team of individuals who have clinical, research, methodological, and health economic backgrounds.

A literature review is important to conduct during the initial planning stages of an evaluation to enhance the understanding of the particular issue and to capitalize on what others have previously done. Evidence regarding the costs and/or the effectiveness of the services being described and/or compared is compiled and evaluated. The process by which evidence can be located in the literature and critically appraised is profiled in Chapters 5 and 6. Economic evaluations should employ rigorous methodologies to determine the efficacy and effectiveness of an intervention and estimate as realistically as possible the true costs of intervention.

Good evaluations should include an assessment regarding the robustness of the findings. These assessments—termed *sensitivity analyses*—are required, as investigators must make a number of judgments or assumptions throughout the course of the analysis. A sensitivity analysis presents the range of possible values resulting from variations of a critical judgment (Drummond, O'Brien, et al., 1997). Evaluators should also make judgments regarding the internal and external validity of their assessments. Sources of bias, contamination, and noncompliance should be described and documented. All studies are hampered by limitations, but a final report that includes a description of these shortcomings will ultimately help decision makers to weigh the merits of the evaluation and, thereby, make judgments based on evidence and reason.

Critically Reviewing Economic Evaluations

The characteristics that describe rigorous economic evaluation projects are those that can be used to critically appraise those articles summarizing the findings of one of these evaluative efforts. Table 9-3 provides a listing of questions that can be used when evaluating evidence in the literature regarding the relative value of health service interventions. This list was developed after reviewing formats that have been used by others to appraise the quality of economic evaluation evidence (Drummond, O'Brien, et al., 1997; Drummond, Richardson, O'Brien, Levine, & Heyland, 1997).

> **Table 9-3**
>
> ## CRITICALLY APPRAISING THE INTERNAL AND EXTERNAL VALIDITY OF ECONOMIC EVALUATIONS
>
> *Internal Validity*
>
> - Did the research question clearly and accurately define the options compared?
> - Was the perspective of the analysis defined?
> - Were the important and relevant costs and outcomes identified?
> - Were the costs and outcomes properly measured and valued?
> - How rigorous was the methodology that was used to establish costs?
> - How rigorous was the methodology that was used to establish the effectiveness of the service alternatives?
> - Were the differences in costs and outcomes between the options analyzed and compared?
> - Was appropriate allowance made for uncertainties in the evaluation by including a sensitivity analysis incorporating clinically sensitive variations in important variables?
>
> *External Validity*
>
> - Are the outcomes worth the costs?
> - Could my patients expect similar health outcomes?
> - Could I expect similar costs?

The National Health Service Research and Development Centre for Evidence-Based Medicine (CEBM) in Oxford, England was established in 1995 to promote the teaching and practice of evidence-based health care. The CEBM has published guidelines for ranking the level of evidence of effectiveness studies and economic evaluations, and this document is available on the World Wide Web at www.cebm.net/index.aspx?o=1025.

Locating Economic Evaluations in the Literature

Economic evaluations that have been published in the literature can be found using traditional databases. The National Library of Medicine provides free Internet access to enable people to search online databases such as MEDLINE and HealthSTAR. The World Wide Web address for these resources is www.nlm.nih.gov. MEDLINE is considered to be a premier bibliographic database that contains references and abstracts for journal articles in life sciences with a concentration on biomedicine and the clinical sciences. HealthSTAR is the bibliographic database that provides access to the published literature of health services technology, administration, and research. The National Information Centre on Health Services Research and Health Care Technology provides free Internet access to enable people to search their on-line databases. The World Wide Web address for this resource is http://text.nlm.nih.gov/hsrsearch/hsr.html.

There are two databases that provide abstracts and critical appraisals of economic evaluations. The National Health Service Centre for Reviews and Dissemination at the University of York in the United Kingdom offers free Internet access to their Economic Evaluation Database (NHS EED). The World Wide Web address for this valuable resource is www.york.ac.uk/inst/crd/. This database contains structured abstracts and critical appraisals of economic evaluations from 1994 onward. The Office of Health Economics and the International Federation of Pharmaceutical

Manufacturers Association offers access to their Health Economic Evaluations Database (HEED) on a subscription basis. This database contains abstracts and structured reviews of economic evaluations, cost analyses and cost of illness studies from 1967 onward. HEED is available in CD format or via the Internet and can be accessed at most university libraries.

CONCLUSION

The number of evaluations that have been conducted to evaluate the effectiveness of rehabilitation interventions and programs has grown rapidly in the last few years. By comparison, the number of evaluations that have been conducted to assess the relative value of these services is small. This is not unexpected, as it is important to establish clinical effectiveness before calculating costs. It would be wasteful to determine the relative cost of providing ineffective services.

Research methods have been established to appraise the costs and outcomes of health services to provide clients and consumers with information regarding relative value. It is hoped that these insights will inform their decisions. There are five types of economic evaluations, but these methodological approaches simply differ in how they measure and/or quantify outcomes. A number of good evaluations have been published in the literature, and Table 9-2 provides examples of studies that may be of interest to rehabilitation professionals. Information has been provided to enable the reader to locate and appraise this literature in hopes that this exercise will inform clinical practice and stimulate enthusiasm among those who wish to conduct this type of research. The next challenge for the rehabilitation profession is clear. We must assess the value of effective interventions to ensure that they offer the most efficient means of attaining specific outcomes and effectively communicate these findings to our clients.

TAKE-HOME MESSAGES

✔ Rehabilitation professionals must assess the value of effective interventions so that clients and consumers can evaluate costs and outcomes when deciding to participate and so that they can offer the most efficient types of interventions.

✔ We cannot always assume that the potential benefits from receiving a service outweigh the costs and risks.

✔ When making a decision about which service to offer or which intervention to receive, clinicians and clients must consider the costs, risks, and outcomes of each alternative.

Economic Evaluation

- Focus on appraising, describing, and comparing the relative value of specific interventions in order to inform decision making.

- Value is the relative worth, utility, or importance of a service in meeting the health needs of a defined clientele.

- There are three aspects to an economic evaluation:

  1. Evaluate whether specific interventions are effective at attaining outcomes.

  2. Evaluate effective interventions to ensure they offer the most efficient means.

  3. Effectively communicate these results.

Types of Economic Evaluations

- Cost-consequence—Descriptive profile of the costs and outcomes of one or more interventions.
- Cost-minimization—Identifies the least costly alternative for services that result in equivalent outcomes.
- Cost-effectiveness—Describes and compares the relative costs and outcomes of two or more interventions that result in the same type of outcome.
- Cost-utility—Describes and compares the relative costs and outcomes of two or more interventions in which the outcomes of interest include health status and the value of the status to the individual.
- Cost-benefit—Describes and compares the relative costs and outcomes of two or more interventions in which both the costs and outcome can be measured in monetary values.

Conducting Economic Evaluations

- Research question defines the purpose and scope of assessment.
- Descriptive analysis or comparative assessment.
- Important to consider the perspective of the analysis (i.e., from society, payers, providers, and/or consumers).
- Evaluators of economic analyses should make judgments regarding the internal and external validity of their assessments, including source of bias, contamination, and noncompliance.
- When critically analyzing economic analyses, it is important to look at both internal and external factors.

Locating Economic Evaluations in the Literature

- Research can be found with traditional databases like MEDLINE and HealthSTAR.
- National Health Service Centre for Reviews and Dissemination (University of York, UK) contains structured abstracts and critical appraisals of economic evaluations from 1994 onward (Web-based).
- Health Economic Evaluations Database contains abstracts and structured reviews from 1967 onward (subscription).

LEARNING AND EXPLORATION ACTIVITIES

The purpose of this chapter is to provide a basic understanding and appreciation of the research methods that have been used to appraise the costs and outcomes of health services. Upon completion of this chapter, students should be aware of the role that economic evaluations play in evidence-based practice.

1. You are the manager for a program providing home-based rehabilitation services for older adults discharged home after total hip replacement surgery. It is important to conduct economic evaluations of this program. For each type of economic analysis, describe the purpose of the evaluation and what specific information would be collected to complete such an evaluative study:

    a. Cost-consequences

    b. Cost-minimization

    c. Cost-effectiveness

    d. Cost-utility

    e. Cost-benefit analyses

2. Select one of the economic evaluation studies listed in Table 9-2. Using the questions in Table 9-3, complete a critical appraisal of this article. What are the implications of the findings for rehabilitation practice?

3. This activity is very similar to the one above, with a different spin.

Snoezelen rooms, originating from the Dutch words "to sniff" and "to doze" (Chung & Lai. 2005), have been created as multisensory environments that provide participants with visual, auditory, olfactory, and tactile stimuli (Baker, Dowling, Wareing, Dawson, & Assey, 1997). Adults with dementia have become the newest population to use Snoezelen rooms as therapy (Chung & Lai, 2005). Snoezelen rooms may be effective for increasing positive behaviors (i.e., interaction), and decreasing negative behaviors (i.e., aggression and depressed mood) in the short-term when used as a form of therapy (Baillon et al., 2004; Baker et al., 2003; Chung & Lai, 2005). However, there is often a hefty price tag that comes with this very technological equipment, and the effects may not generalize, nor extend to the longer term (Baker et al., 2004; Chung & Lai, 2005). A clinician is left wondering if the positive effects of Snoezelen rooms warrant the expenses associated with them?

How can this clinical question be answered using the five different types of economical evaluation? What research question would address each type of economic evaluation regarding the use of Snoezelen rooms with adults with dementia?

REFERENCES

Anderson, C., Mhurchu, C. N., Rubenach, S., Clark, M., Spencer, C., & Winsor, A. (2000). Home or hospital for stroke rehabilitation? Results of a randomized controlled trial. II: Cost minimization analysis at 6 months. *Stroke, 31*, 1032.

Baillon, S., Van Diepen, E., Prettyman, R., Redman, J., Rooke, N., & Campbell, R. (2004). A comparison of the effects of Snoezelen and reminiscence therapy on the agitated behaviour of patients with dementia. *International Journal of Geriatric Psychiatry, 19*(11), 1047-1052

Baker, R., Dowling, Z., Wareing, L., Dawson, J., & Assey, J. (1997). Snoezelen: Its long term and short term effects on older people with dementia. *British Journal of Occupational Therapy, 60*(5), 213-218.

Baker, R., Holloway, J., Holtkamp, C., Larsson, A., Hartman, L., Pearce, R., et al. (2003). Effects of multi-sensory stimulation for people with dementia. *Issues and Innovations in Nursing Practice, 43*(5), 465-477.

Briffa, T. G., Eckerman, S. D., Griffiths, A. D., Harris, P. J., Heath, M. R., Freedman, S. B., et al. (2005). Cost-effectiveness of rehabilitation after an acute coronary event: A randomized controlled trial. *Medical Journal of Australia, 183*, 450-455.

Canadian Coordinating Office for Health Technology Assessment. (1997). *Guidelines for economic evaluation of pharmaceuticals: Canada* (2nd ed.). Ottawa, ON: Author.

Chalamat, M., Mihalopoulos, C., Carter, R., & Vos, T. (2005). Assessing cost-effectiveness in mental health: Vocational rehabilitation for schizophrenia and related conditions. *Australian and New Zealand Journal of Psychiatry, 39*, 693-700.

Chung, J. C., & Lai, C. K. (2005). Snoezelen for dementia. *Cochrane Database of Systematic Reviews, 3.*

Cochrane, T., Davey, R. C., & Edwards, S. M. M. (2005). Randomised controlled trial of the cost-effectiveness of water-based therapy for lower limb osteoarthritis. *Health Technology Assessment, 9*(31), 1-114.

Doty, M. M., Edwards, J. N., & Holmgren, A. L. (2005). Seeing red: Americans driven into debt by medical bills. *Issue Brief (Commonw Fund), 837,* 1-12

Drummond, M. F., O'Brien, B. J., Stoddart, G. L., & Torrance, G. (1997). *Methods for the economic evaluation of health care programmes* (2nd ed.). Oxford, UK: Oxford University Press.

Drummond, M. F., Richardson, W. S., O'Brien, B. J., Levine, M., & Heyland, D. (1997). Users' guide to the medical literature. How to use an article on economic analysis of clinical practice: Are the results of the study valid? *Journal of the American Medical Association, 277,* 1552-1557.

Duke, C. (2005). The Frail Elderly Community-Based Case Management Project. *Geriatric Nursing, 26,* 122-127.

Gold, M., Gafni, A., Nelligan, P., & Millson, P. (1997). Needle exchange programs: An economic evaluation of a local experience. *Canadian Medical Association Journal, 157,* 255-262.

Gordon, L. G., Scuffham, P., Battistutta, D., Graves, N., Tweeddale, M., & Newman, B. (2005). A cost-effectiveness analysis of two rehabilitation support services for women with breast cancer. *Breast Cancer Research and Treatment, 94,* 123-133.

Jones, J., Wilson, A., Parker, H., Wynn, A., Jagger, C., Spiers, N., et al. (1999). Economic evaluation of hospital at home versus hospital care: Cost minimization analysis of data from randomized controlled trial. *British Medical Journal, 319,* 1547-1550.

Kohn, L., Corrigan, J., & Donaldson, M. (1999). *To err is human: Building a safer health system.* Washington, DC: National Academy Press.

Leape, L. (2004). 195,000 Annual deaths linked to in-hospital errors, study says. *Quality Letters for Healthcare Leaders, 16*(9), 10-11.

Margolis, L. H., & Petti, R. D. (1994). An analysis of the costs and benefits of two strategies to decrease length in children's psychiatric hospitals. *Health Services Research, 29,* 155-167.

Mathews, M., & Watson, D. (2000). Designing and managing an evaluation. In D. E. Watson (Ed.), *Evaluating costs and outcomes: Demonstrating the value of rehabilitation services* (pp. 25-42). Bethesda, MD: American Occupational Therapy Association.

Merriam-Webster. (1984). *Merriam-Webster's ninth new collegiate dictionary.* Springfield, MA: Author.

Meyer, G., Wegscheider, K., Kersten, J. F., Icks, A., & Mühlhauser, I. (2005). Increased use of hip protectors in nursing homes: Economic analysis of a cluster randomized, controlled trial. *Journal of the American Geriatric Society, 53,* 2153-2158.

Miller, P., Gladman, J. R. F., Cunliffe, A. L., Husbands, S. L., Dewey, M. E., & Harwood, R. H. (2005). Economic analysis of an early discharge rehabilitation service for older people. *Age and Ageing, 34,* 274-280.

Office of Inspector General. (1999). *Physical and occupational therapy in nursing homes: Medical necessity and quality of care.* Washington, DC: Department of Health and Human Services.

Patel, A., Knapp, M., Evans, A., Perez, I., & Kalra, L. (2004). Training care givers of stroke patients: Economic evaluation. *British Medical Journal, 328,* 1102-1107.

Patel, A., Knapp, A., Perez, I., Evans, A., & Kalra, L. (2004). Alternative strategies for stroke care. Cost-effectiveness and cost-utility analyses from a prospective randomized controlled trial. *Stroke, 35,* 196-203.

Rizzo, J. A., Baker, D. I., McAvay, G., & Tinetti, M. E. (1996). The cost-effectiveness of a multifactorial targeted prevention program for falls among community elderly persons. *Medical Care, 34,* 954-969.

Russell, L. B., Gold, M., Siegel, J. E., Daniels, N., & Weinstein, M. C. (1996). The role of cost-effectiveness analysis in health and medicine. *Journal of the American Medical Association, 276,* 1172-1177.

Schuster, M., McGlynn, E., & Brook, R. (1998). How good is the quality of health care in the United States? *Milbank Quarterly, 76,* 517-563.

Stoddart, G. L. (1982). Economic evaluation methods and health policy. *Evaluation and the Health Professions, 5*, 393-414.

Thomas, K. S., Miller, P., Doherty, M., Muir, K. R., Jones, A. C., & O'Reilly, S. C. (2005). Cost effectiveness of a two-year home exercise program for the treatment of knee pain. *Arthritis and Rheumatism, 53*, 388-394.

Watson, D. E. (2000). *Evaluating costs and outcomes: Demonstrating the value of rehabilitation services.* Bethesda, MD: American Occupational Therapy Association.

Watson, D. E., & Mathews, M. (1998). Economic evaluation of occupational therapy: Where are we at? *Canadian Journal of Occupational Therapy, 65*, 160-167.

van den Hout, W. B., de Jong, Z., Munneke, M., Hazes, J. M. W., Breedveld, F. C., & Vliet Vlieland, T. P. M. (2005). Cost-utility and cost-effectiveness analyses of a long-term, high-intensity exercise program compared with conventional physical therapy in patients with rheumatoid arthritis. *Arthritis and Rheumatism, 53*, 39-47.

van Schoor, N. M., de Bruyne, M. C., van der Roer, N., Lommerse, E., van Tulder, M. W., Bouter, L. M., et al. (2004). Cost-effectiveness of hip protectors in frail institutionalized elderly. *Osteoporosis International, 15*, 964-969.

Yu, C., Lau, C., Chau, J., McGhee, S., Kong, S., Cheung, B. M., et al. (2004). A short course of cardiac rehabilitation program is highly cost effective in improving long-term quality of life in patients with recent myocardial infarction or percutaneous coronary intervention. *Archives of Physical Medicine and Rehabilitation, 85*, 1915-22.

SECTION IV:
USING THE EVIDENCE

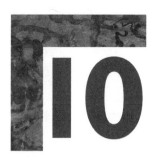

Strategies to Build Evidence in Practice

Mary Law, PhD, OTReg(Ont), FCAOT; Joy MacDermid, PT, PhD;
and Jessica Telford, BA

LEARNING OBJECTIVES

After reading this chapter, the student/practitioner will be able to:

- Develop an understanding of building evidence for practice/of how to incorporate evidence into clinical practice.

- Apply strategies to limit the influence of potential barriers to the implementation of evidence for practice.

- Understand the different tools available to enhance EBP such as CATs, critically appraised papers (CAPs), and EBP resource sites and other technologies (e.g., literature searching services).

- Identify the essential components and different types of CATs.

- Understand and explain the use of CATs in EBP.

Using EBP as an occupational therapist or a physical therapist means processing and organizing a lot of information from the research literature. This task can seem quite challenging in a busy practice setting (e.g., Law, Pollock, & Stewart, 2004). Each time you use your evidence evaluation skills (i.e., identifying new clinical questions, searching for relevant studies in the literature, and integrating your findings into practice), you will be exposed to vast amounts of information. So much information can seem overwhelming. Instead of inundating yourself with evidence about the many interventions that could be used, it is vital that you implement strategies to quickly locate the evidence you require. Remember that evidence for practice is not only about using research evidence, but using it in partnership with excellent clinical reasoning and paying close attention to the client's stated goals, needs, and values.

IMPLEMENTATION MODELS

Researchers have proposed models or strategies to help therapists implement evidence for practice more efficiently and effectively. We outline some of these models below.

In describing EBM, the originators described a five-step process (Sackett,1997; Sackett, Straus, Richardson, Rosenberg, & Haynes, 2000):

1. Convert your information needs into answerable questions.

2. Track down, with maximum efficiency, the best evidence with which to answer them.

3. Critically appraise that evidence for its validity and usefulness.

4. Integrate this appraisal with your clinical expertise and apply it in practice.

5. Evaluate your performance.

A similar step-by-step model for therapists to follow has been suggested by several researchers (Corcoran, 2006; Law, Pollock, & Stewart, 2004; Tickle-Degnen, 2000). Once a clinical problem or issue is identified, the therapist can carry out the following steps:

- Write a clinical question/formulate a relevant practice question.

- Search for evidence related to the question.

- Evaluate/critically appraise evidence to determine the evidence that best informs the clinical question.

- Speak with the client and their family and decide in partnership with them whether to act upon the evidence.

- Evaluate the outcomes of these actions.

- Save the evidence-based information you have acquired for future reference for you and your colleagues; post this information on a Web site (e.g., www.otevidence.info).

When formulating the practice question (step one), it is helpful to break it down into components (Bennett & Bennett, 2000). For example, think about the primary client, the occupational performance or health issues, the outcome you want, and whether the focus of the practice encounter is assessment, intervention, or both (Law et al., 2004). The various components can help you formulate different search words to use in the literature search (Bennett & Bennett, 2000).

When searching for evidence (step two), it may be necessary to search multiple databases, redesign your search for each database, and use thesaurus terms and text searches. When determining whether to act upon the evidence (step four), clinicians should determine whether the evidence "fits" with the features of the client's context (personal skills, living environment, and daily activities). Factors such as the environment in which the client lives and his or her cultural beliefs, priorities, and values ultimately determine the usefulness of research evidence for informing clinical practice. Consideration is also given to the practice setting, clinical expertise, and resources available to the therapist.

Corcoran (2006) includes a step-by-step model *within* her concept about what busy practitioners need to do to incorporate evidence into practice. She says that "making positive changes requires attitude, knowledge and skills" (p. 127). In terms of attitude, Corcoran urges clinicians to consider the importance of staying current with and implementing literature to provide clients with the best possible treatments. Such practices also encompass a professional and ethical obligation toward continuous learning. In terms of knowledge, practitioners can learn about evidence and how to apply it. This is where the step-by-step model fits best. Finally, she states that "you will need to develop skills that make using evidence a vital part of everyday clinical reasoning" (p. 128). To do this one should do the following:

- Familiarize yourself with the evidence for practice resources that are available via the Internet.

- Bookmark the sites that will help you quickly obtain the best information.

- Learn how to use keywords.

- Look for services that find information for you (these will be discussed later in this chapter).

Gillespie and Gillespie (2003) have outlined a similar approach regarding where and how to find useful information. They suggest that clinicians can perfect the art of searching by moving through three stages of questioning:

1. Patient-focused questioning to ascertain specific functional problems.

2. Primary research questioning.

3. Secondary research questioning.

They then suggest that clinicians become familiar with search terms, exploding/focusing terms, and combining terms and that they should learn to use search databases such as PEDro and the Cochrane Libraries. See Chapter 5 of this book for information on searching for evidence.

Bennett and Bennett's (2000) model is based on the notion that evidence for practice is a process that involves clinical expertise, relevant research, colleague support, and family and client choice. To integrate evidence for practice into practice, clinicians must do the following:

- Ask a clinical question classified into diagnosis, treatment prevention, or prognosis.

- Formulate the question into P. I. C. O. (patient/disease, intervention, comparative intervention, outcome), and search the literature using that information. Hierarchies of evidence relevant to each question are presented. They caution users to focus on peer-related journals.

- Critically appraise the evidence that you find by deciding if the information is valid and clinically significant (see Chapter 6 as well). This can be accomplished by asking four questions:

  1. Do the results apply to my client?

  2. Does the treatment fit into my client's values and preferences?

  3. Do I have the resources to implement this treatment?

  4. Do I have the training or skill necessary to implement these interventions?

McCluskey and Cusick (2002) believe that managers are extremely important to the implementation of evidence for practice and may need to lead and support the change within an organization. Managers can facilitate the use of evidence in practice by championing its use and ensuring that evidence for practice is a core value for their service. Manager support promotes positive attitudes toward evidence for practice and confirms that the use of evidence is valued by the organization. Managers can also work closely with therapists to identify real and potential barriers to implementation. Through strategic planning and the use of SWOT analysis (strengths, weaknesses, opportunities and threats), managers and therapists together can plan opportunities and strategies most suitable to the organization in order to facilitate evidence for practice.

Remember, change takes time. According to Drake, Torrey, and McHugo (2003), there are three stages to implementing evidence for practice:

1. Motivational or educational interventions to prepare for change

2. Enabling or skill building interventions to enact a new practice

3. Reinforcing structural or financing interventions to sustain change

As Drake et al. (2003) state:

> *Multifaceted changes that involve all stakeholders, rearrange daily workflow to sup-port new practices and are reinforced by financing and regulatory strategies are more likely to succeed than those focusing exclusively on changing practitioners' behaviour... Program implementation is most likely to be successful when it matches the values, needs and concerns of practitioners.*

Specific information about what all stakeholders can do help implement evidence for practice will take place later in this chapter.

EVIDENCE-BASED PRACTICE: BARRIERS AND SOLUTIONS

Bennett et al. (2003) studied the attitudes of EBP in a group of occupational therapists and found that while most participants felt that evidence for practice was important and helpful in improving client care, they most frequently made decisions based on their clinical experience. Therefore, it is important to look at many of the common barriers to practicing evidence for practice that people describe as well as effective solutions that have been put in place. Several research studies have found that the barriers and solutions that clinicians note to implementing evidence for practice include the following:

Barriers

- Difficulty finding the time to search for evidence and then appraise and implement it (Bennett et al., 2003; Law, Pollock, & Stewart, 2004).
- Limited quantity of evidence in specific practice areas (Bennett et al., 2003).
- Lack of resources such as staff shortages (Curtin & Jaramazovic, 2001).
- Insufficient quality of evidence (Hebert, Sherrington, Maher, & Mosseley, 2001).
- Lack of access to computers and journal articles that are needed to carry out evidence for practice (Bennett et al, 2003; Curtin & Jaramazovic, 2001).
- Lack of training about evidence for practice and how to carry it out (Curtin & Jaramazovic, 2001).
- The influence of personal factors (those who are self-motivated, have a personal interest in evidence for practice, and are willing to work evidence for practice into their work and personal time are more likely to actively use evidence for practice) (Curtin & Jaramazovic, 2001).
- Research does not provide certainty since findings cannot be applied to individual patients (Hebert et al., 2001).
- Clinical research does not tell of client's experiences (Hebert et al., 2001).

Solutions

- Support from managers (Curtin & Jaramazovic, 2001).
- Access to and effective distribution of relevant resources (Curtin & Jaramazovic, 2001).
- Personal factors (self-motivated, personal interest) (Curtin & Jaramazovic, 2001).
- Postgraduate education was linked to greater use of current research literature (Bennett et al., 2003).

- Use of alerting services, technology services.

- The role of clinical trials is to provide information about the size of treatment effects, not to tell if something will or will not definitely work in every situation; clinical trials cannot tell how an individual client will react to a therapy, however, they do give an idea of a likely result based on certain criteria.

In order to deal with these problems, clinicians need the support of mangers and to be given access to necessary resources such as computers, journals, and ongoing training (Curtin & Jaramazovic, 2001). Haynes (1998) suggests that managers and organizations do the following:

- Produce guidelines for how to develop evidence-based clinical guidelines.

- Use information systems that integrate evidence and guidelines with patient care.

- Develop facilities and incentives to encourage effective care and better disease management systems.

- Improve effectiveness of educational and quality.

- Improvement programs for practitioners.

Therapists in turn need to make EBP a priority for themselves. They need to be self-motivated and willing to spend some personal time learning to use evidence for practice (Curtin & Jaramazovic, 2001) because the more time spent searching, appraising, and applying evidence, the easier and, therefore, less time consuming it will become (Hebert et al., 2001).

Specific instructions on how to overcome evidence for practice barriers were given by Bennett and Bennett (2000, p. 178):

- Seek out continuing education opportunities.

- Make use of evidence for practice resources such as Web sites and journal clubs.

- Participate in research evaluating interventions within your discipline.

- Participate in or establish a journal club.

- Seek out or contribute to evidence based clinical practice guidelines.

- Negotiate work time to search and appraise research.

ISSUES RELATED TO SKILL LEVEL

A major problem reported by clinicians was a lack of skill level in finding, appraising, and applying research evidence. Clinicians do not always know how to determine the quality of the evidence or how it should be applied to their own practice. Bennett et al. (2003) found that most occupational therapists were confident in finding literature (60.8%) and determining clinical significance of results (49.6%). They were less sure of how to determine study design (37%) and validity (37%) and using Cochrane databases (15%) (p. 19).

In addition to utilizing the implementation strategies discussed at the beginning of this chapter and looking for continuing education opportunities as discussed above, therapists should familiarize themselves with the numerous evidence for practice resources that are available to them. For example, the Internet contains evidence for practice directories that provide access to articles and instructions on how to carry out evidence for practice, free sites that give access to electronic databases, and systematic reviews. There are also methods that help you organize your searches and that search, summarize, evaluate, and even rank methodology and study implications for you (Bennett et al., 2003; Corcoran, 2006; Hebert et al., 2001). These and other methods for enhancing EBP will be discussed in detail later in this chapter.

Issues Related to the Quantity and Quality of Research Evidence

There are areas within the research literature in which there is so much evidence that it can be overwhelming for clinicians both because of the amount of research and also the complexity of the research (Haynes, 1998). The amount of evidence available to therapists is growing daily. Therefore, it is very difficult for therapists to keep up with the research literature in their area of practice. There are also topic areas in which it is difficult to find any relevant research literature (Bennett & Bennett, 2000; Hebert et al., 2001). Finally, it has been found that clinicians feel that the quality of evidence is not always good enough (Hebert et al., 2001).

Again, in cases where there is too much information, complicated information, or when you are unsure of the quality of the study methodology, make use of resources such as those that abstract, synthesize, and evaluate the information for you (Haynes, 1998). Practice your evidence for practice skills and continue to look for educational opportunities about research methods. Also, it may be helpful to know that search databases such as PEDro have increased RCTs scores (from 3 to 5) in an attempt to weed out the more inferior RCTs for you (Hebert et al., 2001).

Using Technology to Support Evidence-Based Practice

Recent innovations in technology and the use of push-out services are changing this situation. New evidence-based services (such as electronic databases, systematic reviews, and journals that summarize evidence) are now being developed and will make accessing current best evidence feasible and easy in clinical settings.

PEDrO (www.pedro.fhs.usyd.edu.au/index.html) and OTSeeker (www.occupational thera-pistseeker.com) are Web sites that contain abstracts and appraised information about systematic reviews and RCTs relevant to physical therapy and occupational therapy. By searching these sites, therapists can access information easily and be assured that it has been rated using a stan-dard quality rating system. Therapists can use the information on these two databases to judge whether a particular intervention is appropriate for specific clients. Both of these databases are growing rapidly. For example, as of April 2006, OTSeeker listed 912 reviews relevant to occupational therapy.

An example of an innovative use of push-out technology is McMaster PLUS (McMaster Premium LiteratUre Service). MacPLUS was originally developed for physicians with funding from the Ontario Ministry of Health and Long-Term Care in Canada and provides an innovative solution to these problems by "pushing-out" valuable current evidence. Specifically, MacPLUS 1) identifies the clinical interest of individual practitioners; 2) rates the scientific merit, clinical relevance, and newsworthiness of new evidence; 3) alerts practitioners about new high-quality research findings in their area; and 4) provides a cumulative database so that practitioners can look up information when needed. The service does not duplicate library services but enhances their functionality." Currently, there is a rehabilitation version of MacPLUS in development (see http://hiru.mcmaster.ca/PLUS for more information).

Therapists can also access information to support EBP from Web resource sights on the Internet. Web portal sites, with links to many evidence for practice resources, are also beginning to be developed. An example recently completed for occupational therapy is at www.otevidence.info. The American Physical Therapy Association (APTA) has "Hooked on Evidence" that allows members to access and contribute to a database of article extractions, Web sites, and resources that support EBP and tutorials on using the Guide to Physical Therapist Practice (located at www.hookedonevidence.com). Other sites are listed at the end of this chapter. Therapists can also sign up for email alert services. For example, the Gerontological Society of America (GSA) will alert users to publication of articles that match key words or authors previously identified by the user as does PubMed.

What to Do When There Is Little Evidence

There are likely to be clinical areas where there is little research evidence. In clinical areas where there appears to be little or no research evidence available, the problem may be that the clinicians are unaware of the research that is available or can be useful. Bennett et al. (2003, p. 12) suggest that a useful strategy is to ensure that evidence from other disciplines is searched and used.

> *Our search strategies may be limiting our access to available and relevant evidence. For example, using the phrase "occupational therapy" when searching bibliographic databases may restrict the ability to find all research that can inform occupational therapy practice. Using the phrase 'occupational therapy' to search the Database of Systematic Reviews within the Cochrane Library yields about 35 systematic reviews. A thorough hand search of this database however, indicated that there are approximately 90 systematic reviews relevant to occupational therapy.*

Some forms of evidence may never have "level 1 evidence." While many trials suggest patient education is important in rehabilitation, the specific information patients need or should follow, to set goals is not usually explicit nor can its best format be easily evaluated by the RCT design. It is unlikely to this topic and others will be studied in this way. Therefore, the specific in formation that is necessary to implement best practice may not be readily available. Using alternative forms of evidence including expert panels, Delphi consensus processes, and qualitative studies may enrich our understanding of these issues.

BARRIERS AND SOLUTIONS
REQUIRING HELP FROM ALL STAKEHOLDERS

Some of the barriers associated with evidence for practice are difficult for rehabilitation practitioners to deal with on their own. These barriers include current health policies, organizational barriers, and biases within the research evidence (Maher, Sherrington, Elkins, Hebert, & Moseley, 2004). Maher et al. (2004) suggest that clinicians and researchers need to work together and do the following:

- Publish all RCTs, regardless of outcome.
- Petition MEDLINE and CINAHL for complete coverage of (rehabilitation) journals.
- Expand free access to databases.
- Expand access to free text.
- Include translations of non-English research.
- Use relevant research to predict the treatment effect and adjust that prediction based on clinical experience.

Other suggestions on how to narrow the gap between research and practice are for research professionals to demand or "emphasise the timely transfer of research and theoretical knowledge into practice" (Law et al., 2004) and to create linkages and partnerships between researchers and practice participants (Forsyth, Summerfield-Mann, & Kielhofner, 2005; Hayes, 2000). A model proposed and tested by Forsyth et al. (2005) drew the following conclusions:

- In order to create an evidence-based practice, there must be a research alliance with all key stakeholders (i.e., researchers, students, administration, and clinicians).
- These stakeholders can join to form a community of practice or community of "practice scholars."
- In order to successfully close the gap between theory and practice, three factors should be considered:
  1. Those who use knowledge should be involved in helping to generate and refine it.
  2. Development of a scholarship of practice to create new educational and research opportunities.
  3. Models developed should show clear links between theoretical concepts and the everyday work of therapists.
- A centralized agency should oversee the transfer of knowledge between all practice scholars.

Burns (2003) suggested that research studies should be carried out in the field to involve practitioners to begin with and ensure that studies are relevant to current practice. Burns proposed a Clinic/Community Intervention Development Model as follows (p. 164):

- Develop research question in the setting where it is to be treated
- Initial efficacy trial under controlled conditions to determine potential benefit
- Single case applications in clinical setting
- Initial effectiveness trial in clinic
- Full test of effectiveness under everyday practice conditions
- Effectiveness of treatment variations
- Assessment of goodness of fit with host organization, practice setting or community
- Dissemination of information to other organizations (p. 964)

Illot (2003) describes "a systemic approach" to evidence for practice. This approach is based on the notion that a supportive system is needed in order for clinicians to provide high-quality services. The parts of the system that work together are as follows:

- Research (required for evidence for practice)
- Service standards, clinical guidelines, care pathways, and patient information (ways that evidence for practice is implemented)
- Audits and benchmarks (are standards being met?)
- Outcome measures (to evaluate clinical change, patient experience, organizational issues)

How to Enhance Evidence-Based Practice

There are specific strategies that therapists can use to enhance their use of evidence in practice. The CAT is one method for organizing your thoughts and keeping your evidence straight.

Critically Appraised Topics

CATs are the preferred categorization format for quick studies in EBP. The CAT was originally developed at McMaster University (Sauve et al., 1995), but several CAT formats have evolved since then. Simply put, a CAT is a one- or two-page "summary of a search and critical appraisal of the literature related to a focused clinical question, which should be kept in an easily accessible place so that it can be used to help make clinical decisions" (Center for Evidence-Based Emergency Medicine, n.d.a). The most essential characteristics of CATs are that they be simultaneously brief, informative, and useful.

Figure 10-1. Table used for diagnostic calculations. (Reprinted with permission from Centre for Evidence-Based Medicine.)

	Disease Positive	Disease Negative
Test Positive	a	b
Test Negative	c	d

To give a more general understanding of the basis for CATs, it is important to be able to place them in the complete evidence for practice process. The University of Oxford's Centre for Evidence-Based Medicine (n.d.) breaks up the evidence-based information search process into five parts. They suggest that once you have realized that you have an information need, you should do the following:

1. Translate these needs into answerable questions.

2. Track down the best evidence to answer them.

3. Appraise that evidence for its validity and applicability.

4. Integrate that evidence with clinical expertise and apply it in practice.

5. Evaluate the performance of the intervention.

This definition meshes with that of the Centre for Evidence-Based Emergency Medicine's (n.d.b) definition of a CAT, which states, "A CAT is a one- or two-page summary of all of the preceding steps involved in your evidence-based approach to the literature. It provides immediate access to your method and results."

CATs have a hand in all of the steps of the evidence-based process. They require that one have a focused question, categorize the evidence found, allow for the evaluation of that evidence, and produce a clinical bottom line that will be developed into practice. Finally, CATs can be reviewed on a regular basis and their successes passed on for further analysis and use.

Different Types of Critically Appraised Topics

There are five major types of CATs:

1. Diagnosis/screening

2. Prognosis

3. Evaluating risk and harm in a case-control study

4. Evaluating risk and harm in a cohort study

5. Treatment, prevention, and screening

Diagnosis/Screening

CATs for diagnosis are one of the easiest to understand. This type of CAT involves finding relevant studies that identify disease symptoms and assessing the diagnostic accuracy of those symptoms. If the symptom in question is present, how likely is it that the patient has the disease or condition? Diagnostic CATs compare new diagnoses with the "gold standard," or the most highly accurate diagnostic test that currently exists. The CAT for diagnosis has a two-by-two table for entering the evidence numbers (Figure 10-1) and a formula for calculating the likelihood ratios (LRs) for the new diagnosis, or how likely it is that a person has the disease if he or she shows the symptom.

A LR is a simple calculation of the probability that a client has a certain condition given the results of a test. There are two equal and opposite types of results to consider when examining the results of clinical tests—sensitivity and specificity. These two factors interplay with each other to produce results. The sensitivity of a diagnostic test is the proportion of people who actually have the disease or problem in question who come up with a positive test. The specificity of a test is the equal and opposite result—the proportion of people who do not have the disease who come up (rightfully) with a negative test. From the above graphic:

- Sensitivity = a
  (a + c)

- Specificity = d
  (b + d)

Thus, the LR is the sensitivity of the test (the chance that it will rightly include clients with the condition) divided by the opposite of the specificity (1 - specificity, or the chance that it will wrongly exclude clients with the condition). A LR (LR) is thus:

- LR = sensitivity
  (1 - specificity)

- LR = a
  (a + c)

  b
  (b + d)

If this is still unclear, we suggest that you consult a medical statistics textbook or online resource such as the Centre for Evidence-Based Medicine's Glossary, which is located at www.cebm.net/index.aspx?o=1116. LRs are most often used by physicians for medical diagnostic questions, but they are also used in rehabilitation for screening issues (e.g., the identification of a developmental delay).

Prognosis

A CAT for prognosis will assess the ability of a symptom to forecast probable outcomes. The difference between a diagnosis CAT and a prognosis CAT is that diagnosis CATs attempt to establish whether or not persons have a condition, while prognosis CATs try to predict the future of a condition for one person. An example in rehabilitation is the predictive validity of screening tests, such as the Motor Assessment of Infants.

Risk and Harm in Case-Controlled Studies

Risk is very simply defined as the probability that an event will occur, and the next two types of CATs discussed attempt to find the risk for patients with a certain condition in two different ways. A case-controlled study is "a study that starts with identification of people with the disease or outcome of interest (cases) and a suitable control group without the disease or outcome" (Cochrane Reviewer's Handbook Glossary version 4.1.6, 2003).

The case-controlled CAT, therefore, analyzes information on the presence of risk factors using a statistical technique called an odds ratio (OR). An OR is simply the odds of a patient in the experimental group suffering an adverse event relative to the odds of a patient in the control group suffering the same event. There are two numbers to consider when calculating an OR: the experimental event odds (EEO) and the control event odds (CEO). The OR is:

- OR = EEO
  1 − EEO

- CEO
  1 – CEO

Once again, if this is not clear, consult a text or the CEBM (NHS Research and Development, n.d.a).

Risk and Harm in Cohort Studies

Cohort studies differ from case-controlled studies in that the two types of studies approach populations differently. Cohort studies are studies in which subsets of a defined population are identified. These groups may or may not be exposed to factors hypothesized to influence the probability of the occurrence of a particular outcome. The cohorts are then followed forward in time to determine differential outcomes based on exposure or no exposure.

In cohort studies, it is necessary to calculate the relative risk of the experimental and control groups.

A relative risk is simply the number of people exposed to a risk factor who developed the unwanted outcome taken as a percentage of the whole. The relative risk will differ for groups that are categorized differently, as the population considered is different. An easy analogy that illustrates this concept is the example of taxation. Each year, a percentage of citizens in a country who file tax returns are randomly chosen and are subjected to an in-depth audit. The number of citizens audited taken as a percentage of the total number of citizens who file tax returns is the relative risk of an audit. For those who are not legally required to file tax returns (e.g., children), the relative risk of an audit is different; for those who decide to illegally refrain from filing a tax return, the relative risk of an audit is different again. It is crucial to understand that while each subgroup has its own relative risk, the complete sample (the entire population of the country) has its own relative risk as well (which would be a weighted average of the relative risks of its subgroups).

Intervention Studies (Treatment, Prevention, and Screening)

CATs in this category deal with the strongest type of available evidence—RCTs. This type of CAT distills information from an article on a treatment into a final conclusion on the number needed to treat (NNT).

The NNT, as defined by the NHS Research and Development Centre (n.d.b), is as follows:

The Number Needed to Treat (NNT) is the number of persons you need to treat to prevent one additional bad outcome (stroke, poor function, etc.) ...An NNT of 5... means you have to treat 5 people with the intervention to prevent one additional bad outcome.

Elements Present in Reliable Critically Appraised Topics

No matter what type of CAT you use, whether you use a general form or tailor it specifically to each individual situation, there are elements of the CAT that will always be present. Those elements and a discussion of their purpose in the CAT are provided below.

The Date of Completion

Although this seems straightforward, all CATs that require a date of completion be prominently displayed. As will be discussed, CATs are inherently transitory creations, with a "shelf life" hovering between a few months and a few years (depending on the advance of knowledge in the field). When you are reviewing your CATs, or if others are examining them for use with their clients, it is imperative that they know when you completed your evidence-based analysis of the literature and whether or not they should do their own search to find out if any advances in knowledge have been made in the interim.

The Question

At the heart of the CAT is your clinical question. Care should be taken in preparing and wording this question as its structure will dictate the course of your research. It has been suggested (Richardson, Wilson, Nishikawa, & Hayward, 1995) that a question's "anatomy" should consist of the following four parts:

1. The person or problem being addressed (P)
2. The intervention or exposure being considered (I)
3. The comparison intervention or exposure, when relevant (C)
4. The outcomes of interest (O)

If a question encompasses all four aspects (P.I.C.O.), it will be usable in a literature search and will likely yield results that will be helpful. A sample question could be phrased as follows: For persons with condition A, will treatment X be more effective than treatment Y in leading to outcome P, or increasing function in outcome P? If a question cannot be made to fit these criteria, more work needs to be done in defining it.

The Clinical Bottom Line

The clinical bottom line is where you summarize your findings for yourself and others to have readily available. After your examination of the evidence (discussed next), your final evaluation and the actions you will take based on that evidence are briefly summarized here. The clinical bottom line is more than the results of the article you read. Rather, you should report your critical evaluation of the evidence you have reviewed and your clinical judgment on how those results could be generalized to apply to your client.

The Evidence

As this is EBP, there is room on the CAT to list the evidence you have found that pertains to the question. It is a good idea to summarize the evidence you are using to make your case. The CAT is your clinical lifeline; it is the backup you have for your decision on a person's treatment. If required, you can refer back to the CATs and explain them as the basis for your clinical judgment. It is important to cite the article's source on the CAT and, if your institution uses paper CATs, advisable to attach the article and proof you found to the final document. The information (or critical review) written up in the CATs also includes the numerical and statistical bases of the evidence.

The Gold Standard

On CATs that specifically have to do with diagnosis or screening (e.g., asking if test A can accurately diagnose condition B), there is room to describe the current "gold standard" test. The gold standard will be a known, valid diagnostic or screening tool. Your diagnostic tool (based on the evidence you have found) should be offered up for comparison to the gold standard in its LRs. You can also input information gleaned from journal articles to calculate LRs (discussed previously). Other types of CATs, such as those for evaluating risk and harm, do not have a "gold standard" treatment with which to be compared, but they should be measured against other existing treatments for the specific condition in question.

Notes

This section, sometimes titled "comments" or "additional information," is where information goes that does not fit into any of the other categories but which you feel should be added to the CAT. It is a good idea to note any important issues that came up in the critical appraisal or any other costs or consequences of a proposed "clinical bottom line" that were not mentioned before. This section could also be used to record your personal reflections on the evidence you have found and its application. This section will be especially helpful if your CAT is used by others in the field, as it provides a human dimension to the making of the CAT.

Sample Critically Appraised Topic Format

The sample CAT format (Table 10-1) was developed by the Centre for Evidence-Based Emergency Medicine. A template developed by Annie McCluskey for the OTCATs Web site is available from www.otcats.com/template/index.html. We have included a sample completed CAT as Appendix J to this chapter. Students should look at the following sample CATs:

- www.otcats.com
  - This Web site is a resource for CATs and CAPs. Many of the CATs and critically appraised papers (CAPs) on the site have been completed by practitioners.
  - The CATs on this site are reviewed by an academic faculty member prior to posting them on the site.
- www.rehab.queensu.ca/cats
  - This Web site contains CATs completed by graduate students in rehabilitation at Queen's University, Canada.

Finally, the Centre for Evidence-Based Medicine has developed a software program called the CATmaker, which assists in the creation of computerized CATs. A demonstration version of the software is available for download at http://www.cebm.net/index.aspx?o=1216.

Using Critically Appraised Topics

As was stated at the beginning of this chapter, CATs are used to summarize and organize evidence for specific clinical situations in practice. However, they are even more useful if they are available to a network of health care professionals. Some health care centers have set up collections of CATs called CATbanks that contain all of the CATs their staff have put together. This way, each practitioner's evidence-based work is made available to the entire unit. Several good examples of CATbanks include the following:

- The University of Washington EBM page: www.mebi.washington.edu/ebm-uwsom/index-body.html
- University of North Carolina CATs: www.med.unc.edu/medicine/edursrc/!catlist.htm
- University of Michigan CATs: www.med.umich.edu/pediatrics/ebm/cat.htm
- University of Western Sydney: www.otcats.com

Drawbacks of Critically Appraised Topics

Despite their usefulness as a tool in EBP, CATs have their drawbacks. Each CAT is the product of either one individual or a small group of individuals and, as such, is subject to error, bias, and other limitations that are inherent to non–peer-reviewed material. CATs are designed to be dated as well and are only used as short-term or interim guides until more conclusive evidence in the form of RCTs or systematic reviews can provide more conclusive evidence on the topic in question. Sauve et al. (1995) suggest that "when others research and reappraise the same clinical

---

Table 10-1

SAMPLE CAT

Title

This is the same as the clinical question. Identify the type of question that has been asked (therapy, diagnosis, prognosis, harm).

Reviewer

Name of CAT author.

Search

The resource selected (MEDLINE, EMA, etc.) and the specific search strategy used are summarized, including MeSH terms, specification of publication type(s), and years searched. The number of citations found and the number selected are given.

Date

Date of the search and the proposed date for re-evaluation of the topic. Base the latter upon your estimate of how fast knowledge in this area is changing.

Citation(s)

Use a standardized format such as MEDLINE or *Annals of Emergency Medicine,* and use standard abbreviations for journal identification.

Summary of Study

Summarize the study using the following format:
- **Population**—What patients were included and excluded.
- **Interventions**—Therapeutic interventions, diagnostic interventions, exposures, time.
- **Outcomes**—What was measured and/or counted.
- **What happened**—Track flow through study, how many patients presented, were excluded, dropped out, completed protocol, etc.

Appraisal

- **Validity check list**—A one- or two-line summary of the results of the validity tests for your question type.
- **Results**—Summarize results of appraisal. Calculate important parameters such as NNT, LR, include confidence intervals or P values whenever possible.
- **Applicability**—Review clinical significance, applicability to your patient population and potential tradeoffs between harm and benefit.

Conclusion

Two- or three-line summary and conclusions. Do not make recommendations stronger than justified by the literature. Make value judgments explicit (e.g., "This is not a good test for X *because* of this clinical reason.").

Reprinted with permission from Center for Evidence-Based Emergency Medicine. (n.d.b). Formulating a critically appraised topic. Retrieved January 11, 2002, from http://www.ebem.org/cats/forumlate.html

problem the next time a client presents it, the old CAT may be used as the starting point rather than the last word."

Summary of Critically Appraised Topics

CATs are quick, easy, and intuitive organizational tools for using EBP. They can be created around a variety of topics and methods of looking at evidence. Despite some differences in format, they consist of several basic categories that must be completed. CATs are useful in that they can be collected and can serve as a pool of the EBP knowledge created by a specific unit; however, CATs can be flawed because of the inherent speed of their creation. CATs represent an advance in the organization and dissemination of research-transfer knowledge and should be integrated into the repertoire of the evidence-based practitioner.

CRITICALLY APPRAISED PAPERS

The CAP is very useful in helping practitioners quickly figure out the quality of a newly published research study and how to apply it. CAPs are similar to CATs but specific to individual papers. Their characteristics include the following:

- They are "succinct appraisal of a single research study… comprised of a declarative title, a structured abstract and a commentary" (Canadian Association of Occupational Therapists, n.d.).
- They are written by a clinician or methodologist who describes the strengths and weaknesses of a study, "places the study in the context of other research, and discusses implications for practice, education and future research" (Canadian Association of Occupational Therapists, n.d.).

The *Australian Journal of Occupational Therapy* regularly publishes CAPs that are peer reviewed. The Canadian Association of Occupational Therapists (www.caot.ca/default. asp?pageid=1295) has developed a web resource for CAPs that is free to members or can be purchased by emailing publications@caot.ca. The CAPS on this site are peer reviewed. Queen's University, Canada has a Web site for CATs in rehabilitation science that have been completed by students in their programs (see www.rehab.queensu.ca/cats).

CAPs are useful because they cover many different types of evidence, including RCTs, qualitative studies, systematic reviews, and meta-syntheses of qualitative research. They are easy to share amongst colleagues or at meetings (www.otcats.com).

CAPs also have limitations. Many CAPs have more of a medical than a rehabilitation focus. Not all CAPs have been peer reviewed so it is important to take note of this. CAPs are meant to provide a guide since they are based on someone else's interpretation of the methods, results, and statistics of a paper. These interpretations may not always be accurate and the suggestions on implications for practice might not apply to your own situation, setting, or specific client.

Sample Critically Appraised Papers and How to Use Them

Information on how to use CAPs and sample CAPs can be accessed at the following Web sites:

- www.otcats.com (see description in CATs section above)
- The Canadian Association of Occupational Therapists: www.caot.ca/default.asp?pageid =1295
    - The CAPs on this site are free to members or can be purchased by emailing publications@caot.ca.

- Online discussion forums also exist on this site so that therapists can speak with each other about how to apply findings.
  - The CAPS on this site are peer reviewed.
- Many other CAP samples are available on the Internet and can be found by typing "critically appraised paper" into your Web browser. Examples:
  - NSW (New South Wales, Australia) Speech Pathology Evidence-Based Practice Interest Group: Sample CAP: www.ciap.health.nsw.gov.au/specialties/ebp_sp_path/pdf/Sellars%20et%20all%201998%20pulse%20oximetry.pdf
  - Critical Care Research Newsletter published a sample CAP: www.criticalcareresearch.net/newsletter/Fall01.PDF#search=%22critically%20appraised%20paper%20(CAP)%22

WEB-BASED RESOURCE SITES

Numerous sites exist to teach therapists about EBP and how to search, appraise, evaluate, and apply evidence. These sites often contain links to other sites on the topic. One of the most comprehensive of these sites is the new Evidence-Based Occupational Therapy Web Portal. This site is a one-stop destination containing most of the information that therapists need for finding and using evidence. The Web site includes up-to-date articles on evidence for practice as well as lists of search databases and systematic reviews. The site is located at: www.otevidence.info

Searchable databases are very useful in supporting evidence for practice. Therapy specific sites include:

- OTSeeker
  - Contains abstracts of systematic reviews and RCTs "that have been critically appraised and rated to assist you to evaluate their validity and interpretability. These ratings will help you to judge the quality and usefulness of trials for informing clinical interventions" (OTSeeker, n.d.).
  - As of April 2006, OTSeeker (www.otseeker.com) listed 912 reviews relevant to occupational therapy (Bennett et al., 2003).
- RehabTrials.org: www.rehabtrials.org
- PEDro: www.pedro.fhs.usyd.edu.au/index.html

Additional Web resources useful for EBP include the following:

- Clinical Guidelines: www.guidelines.gov
- Primary care practice guidelines: www.medicine.ucsf.edu/resources/guidelines
- Exeter medical library: www.ex.ac.uk/library/eml/guidelin.html
- The Ottawa Hospital library service: www.ottawahospital.on.ca/library/internetresources/index-e.asp
- Orthopaedic Web links: www.orthopaedicweblinks.com
- SUM search: http://sumsearch.uthscsa.edu
- TRIP database: www.tripdatabase.com
- EBM guidelines (by subscription): www.ebm-guidelines.com

Sources of systematic reviews and trials include the following:

- The Cochrane Library: www.update-software.com/cochrane

- National Health Service Center for Reviews and Dissemination: www.york.ac.uk/inst/crd/
- PEDro: www.pedro.fhs.usyd.edu.au
- Clinical evidence: www.clinicalevidence.com
- Orthopaedic Web links: www.orthopaedicweblinks.com
- SUM search: http://sumsearch.uthscsa.edu
- TRIP database: www.tripdatabase.com
- Getting hooked on evidence: www.apta.org

TAKE-HOME MESSAGES

✔ Evidence for practice is not only about using research evidence, but using it in partnership with excellent clinical reasoning and paying close attention to the client's stated goals, needs, and values.

✔ Use of a step-by-step model to gather and use evidence will improve the process of building evidence for your practice.

Critically Appraised Topics

- A CAT is a one- or two-page summary of a search and critical appraisal of the literature related to a focused clinical question.
- CATs are brief, informative, and useful.
- Five types of CATs: diagnosis/screening; prognosis; evaluating risk/harm in a case controlled study; evaluating risk/harm in a cohort study; treatment, prevention, and screening.
- Necessary elements of CATs: date of completion, question, clinical bottom line, evidence, gold standard, notes.
- CATs are a quick, easy and intuitive tool, but are also subject to error or bias.
- Should be seen as a starting point in a decision-making process rather than a final word.

LEARNING AND EXPLORATION ACTIVITIES

The purpose of this chapter is to introduce the definition and uses of CATs. The following exercises allow you to practice developing and using CATs so that they become an effective tool of EBP.

1. Compare the different CAT templates suggested in this chapter. Which one makes the most sense to you? Which information do you think is the most crucial in a CAT? Which the least important? Why? Using the CAT templates given as examples, create your own CAT template and incorporate the information you feel is essential.

2. Choose a topic in rehabilitation and make a CAT about it. This can be something you have been studying in class or a topic of personal interest. Do this exercise along with a number of your classmates, and when you have finished, exchange CATs and discuss their strengths and weaknesses. If you are really energetic, the class may want to create a paper or electronic CATbank of your collected CATs, which can be expanded as you collectively continue your studies in evidence for practice.

REFERENCES

Bennett, S., & Bennett, J. (2000). The process of evidence based practice in occupational therapy: Informing clinical decisions. *Australian Journal of Occupational Therapy, 47*, 171-180.

Bennett, S., Tooth, L., McKenna, K., Rodger, S., Strong, J., Ziviani, J., et al. (2003). Perceptions of evidence based practice: A survey of Australian occupational therapists. *Australian Occupational Therapy Journal, 50*, 13-22.

Burns, B. (2003). Children and evidence based practice. *Psychiatric Clinics of North America, 26*, 955-970.

Canadian Association of Occupational Therapists. (n.d.). Critically appraised papers: An introduction for readers. Retrieved October 11, 2006, from: http://www.caot.ca/default.asp?pageid=1295

Center for Evidence-Based Emergency Medicine. (n.d.a). Critically appraised topics bank. Retrieved January 11, 2002, from http://www.ebem.org/cats/catbank.html

Center for Evidence-Based Emergency Medicine. (n.d.b). Formulating a critically appraised topic. Retrieved January 11, 2002, from http://www.ebem.org/cats/forumulate.html

Cochrane Reviewer's Handbook Glossary version 4.1.6. (2003). Retrieved October 11, 2006, from http://www.york.ac.uk/inst/crd/GLOSSARY1.doc

Corcoran, M. (2006). A busy practitioner's approach to evidence-based practice. *American Journal of Occupational Therapy, 60*, 127-128.

Curtin, M., & Jaramazovic, E. (2001). Occupational therapists views and perceptions of evidence based practice. *British Journal of Occupational Therapy, 64*, 214-221.

Drake, R. E., Torrey, W. C., & McHugo, G. J. (2003). Strategies for implementing evidence-based practices in routine mental health settings. *Evidence-Based Mental Health, 6*, 6-7.

Forsyth, K., Summerfield-Mann, L., & Kielhofner, G. (2005). Scholarship of practice: Making occupation-focused, theory-driven evidence-based practice a reality. *British Journal of Occupational Therapy, 68*(6), 260-268

Gillespie, L., & Gillespie, W. (2003). Finding current evidence: Search strategies and common databases. *Clinical Orthopaedics and Related Research, 413*, 133-145.

Hayes, RL. (2000). Viewpoint: Evidence-based occupational therapy needs strategically-targeted quality research now. *Australian Occupational Therapy Journal, 47*(4), 186-190.

Haynes, B. (1998). Barriers and bridges to evidence based clinical practice. *British Medical Journal, 317*, 273-276.

Hebert, R., Sherrtington, C., Maher, C., & Moseley, A. (2001). Evidence-based practice: Imperfect but necessary. *Physiotherapy Theory and Practice, 17*, 201-211.

Illot, I. (2003). Challenging the rhetoric and reality: Only an individual and systemic approach with work for evidence-based occupational therapy. *American Journal of Occupational Therapy, 57*(3), 351-354.

Law, M., Pollock, N., & Stewart, D. (2004). Evidence-based occupational therapy: Concepts and strategies. *New Zealand Journal of Occupational Therapy, 51*, 14-22.

Maher, C., Sherrington, C., Elkins, M., Hebert, R., & Moseley, A. (2004). Challenges for evidence-based physical therapy: Accessing and interpreting high quality evidence on therapy. *Physical Therapy, 84*(7), 644-654.

McCluskey, A., & Cusick, A. (2002). Strategies for introducing evidence-based practice and changing clinician behaviour: A managers toolbox. *Australian Occupational Therapy Journal, 49*(2), 63-70.

NHS Research and Development Centre for Evidence-Based Medicine. (n.d.a). Odds ratios. Retrieved January 14, 2002, from http://cebm.jr2.ox.ac.uk/docs/oddsrats.html

NHS Research and Development Centre for Evidence-Based Medicine. (n.d.b). NNT. Retrieved January 14, 2002, from http://cebm.jr2.ox.ac.uk/docs/nnt.html

OTSeeker. (n.d.). Welcome to OTSeeker. Retrieved August 30, 2007. From http://www.otseeker.com/default.htm

Richardson, W., Wilson, M., Nishikawa, J., & Hayward, R. (1995). The well-built clinical question: A key to evidence-based decisions. *ACP Journal Club, 123*, A12-13.

Sackett, D. L. (1997). Evidence-based medicine. *Seminars in Perinatology, 21*, 3-5.

Sackett, D. L., Straus, S. E., Richardson, W. S., Rosenberg, W., & Haynes, R. B. (2000). *Evidence-based medicine: How to practice and teach EBM* (2nd ed.). Toronto, ON: Churchill Livingstone.

Sauve, S., Lee, H. N., Meade, M. O., Lang, J. B., Faroukh, M., Cook, D. J., et al. (1995). The critically appraised topic: A practical approach to learning critical appraisal. *Annals of the Royal College of Physicians and Surgeons of Canada, 28*(7), 396-8.

Tickle-Degnen, L. (2000). Evidence-based practice forum: Communicating with clients, family members, and colleagues about research evidence. *American Journal of Occupational Therapy, 54*, 341-343.

University of Oxford Centre for Evidence-Based Medicine. (n.d.). What is a CAT? Retrieved January 11, 2002, from http://www.jr2.ox.ac.uk/ceb/docs/cats/catabout.html

Other Resources

CATs

- Centre for Evidence-Based Medicine—Oxford University: www.cebm.net/cats.asp
- University of Rochester: www.med.unc.edu/medicine/edursrc/!catlist.htm
- OTCATS: www.otcats.com

Using CATs

- The Center for Evidence-Based Medicine CATbank: www.cebm.net/cats.asp
- The University of Washington Pediatric EBM page: http://dev.hsl.washington.edu/content-Browser.jsp?ctype=17
- The University of Rochester: www.cebm.net/cats.asp
- University of North Carolina CATs: www.med.unc.edu/medicine/edursrc/!catlist.htm
- University of Michigan CATs: www.med.umich.edu/pediatrics/ebm/Cat.htm
- CATwalk—RocketCAT: The CAT Evaluation Sheet: /www.library.ualberta.ca/subject/healthsciences/catwalk
- School of Rehabilitation Therapy at Queen's University, Canada prepared the critically appraised topics (CATs): www.rehab.queensu.ca/cats/

  CATs—UBC and McMaster University: www.mrsc.ubc.ca/site_page.asp?pageid=98

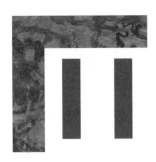

Practice Guidelines, Algorithms, and Clinical Pathways

Joy MacDermid, PT, PhD

LEARNING OBJECTIVES

After reading this chapter, the student/practitioner will be able to:
- Identify the key characteristics of CPGs, algorithms, and clinical pathways (CPs).
- Identify the steps required to formulate EBP guidelines.
- Be aware of CPG resources pertaining to rehabilitation.
- Be able to critically evaluate CPG using a structured critical appraisal instrument.
- Use the appropriate terminology associated with CPs.
- Recognize barriers to implementing practice guidelines and CPs and suggest potential solutions.
- Recognize and understand administrative, technological, and legal factors involved in implementation.

BACKGROUND

CPGs, algorithms, and CPs have only recently emerged in the health care field. With increasing amounts of research information and a philosophical belief that evidence should be used as a basis for clinical decision making, comprehensive documents that guide clinical practice are now seen as a fundamental step to ensuring that the latest evidence is used to promote best practices. Nationally funded health care systems (Burgers, Cluzeau, Hanna, Hunt, & Grol, 2003; Cluzeau & Littlejohns, 1999; Graham, Beardall, Carter, Tetroe, & Davies, 2003) and professional associations (Burgers, Grol, Klazinga, van der, Makela, & Zaat, 2003) have often been the first to take on leadership roles in developing such documents. The methodology to develop, critically appraise, and implement these formalized documents and processes has only recently emerged as a scientific methodology in its own right. The process is not without controversy but has been shown to provide reduced variations in health care delivery and in some cases, improved outcomes (Bahtsevani, Uden, & Willman, 2004; Grimshaw & Hutchinson, 1995). Historically, in some areas of health care, including rehabilitation practice, "protocols" were developed based on expert opinion alone. Such documents have little role in evidence-based practice. CPGs have also been referred to as practice parameters, practice policies, appropriateness criteria, or consensus statements, although these terms are more generic and do not necessarily imply the same specific components. Ideally, CPGs should be based on strong evidence that would provide clear and comprehensive recommendations regarding all the relevant issues on a particular clinical topic or intervention, would provide a framework for evaluating the outcome of implementing the CPG into clinical practice, and would incorporate a regular review and updating process. In addition, useful CPGs would incorporate tools, customized for the different end-users, to assist with the implementation of best practices. This ideal situation can be difficult to attain, particularly in rehabilitation practice where it is well known that barriers exist to conducting high-quality clinical trials and where multiple interventions may be required at a single point in time and then modified over time. For this and other reasons, rehabilitation has lagged behind other fields in the development of evidence-based CPGs and processes. Only recently have studies started to appear in rehabilitation literature regarding the quality of available rehabilitation CPGs (Brooks et al., 2005; Brosseau et al., 2004; MacDermid, 2004).

This chapter will focus on strategies designed to provide "front-end" support to EBR: CPGs, algorithms, and CPs. A CPG is a protocol or practice statement that is developed by synthesizing research and other evidence using a consensus process to formulate specific recommendations regarding the management of a specific problem/diagnosis or the application of a specific treatment technique. An algorithm is a structured process that guides clinicians through a set of sequential steps using decision trees, computations, and/or tables to improve and standardize clinical decision making. A CP is a cause-and-effect framework that incorporates clinical standards that are measured against a timeline. The CP may or may not be based on an existing CPG.

CLINICAL PRACTICE GUIDELINES

The Institute of Medicine defines CPGs as "systematically developed statements that assist practitioner and patient decisions about appropriate health care for specific clinical circumstances" (Canadian Medical Association, 1994; Field & Lohr, 1992). In 1994, the Canadian Medical Association adopted this definition (Canadian Medical Association, 1995). The medical profession has invested heavily in guideline development and the majority of guidelines listed on the National Guideline Clearinghouse (www.guideline.gov) relate to medical practice. Rehabilitation professions have recognized the potential benefits of CPG and have recently become more engaged in this process. Occupational and physical therapy associations are increasingly focusing on the role of evidence-based CPG. For example, the American Society of Hand Therapists is currently in the process of replacing expertise opinion-based CPG with EBP guidelines. APTA has similar initiatives linking CPG development with previous initiatives such as the *Guide to Practice* and more recent knowledge from ICF and high-quality evidence.

Practice guidelines are sometimes produced by professional associations, interest groups, or rehabilitation departments. The rigor of development varies widely. The rigor of development is fundamental to the confidence in recommendations contained within a CPG. Any CPG that is not based on a systematic review of the evidence is prone to bias and does not fit the current definition of CPG or EBP.

CPGs are increasingly appearing in rehabilitation literature where they have been subject to peer review (Duncan et al., 2005; Gross et al., 2002; Johnston, Wood, Stason, & Beatty, 2000; Rodin, Saliba, & Brummel-Smith, 2006; Scholten-Peeters et al., 2002). Brooks and co-authors

(2005) published a paper summarizing the quality of 50 CPGs used in physical therapy, demonstrating wide variability in quality (rigor of development was 53 +/- 29%). When comparing mean quality scores of CPGs developed prior to 2000 with those developed in 2000 or later, the newer CPGs scored higher for stakeholder involvement, rigor of development, and editorial independence, suggesting that increased awareness of proper methodology for developing and evaluating CPGs has resulted in improved quality.

The Development Process

Sufficient experience on the process of developing CPG now exists so that a number of key elements to the process are recognized (Table 11-1). CPGs are developed by teams with sufficient breath of professional, content, and methodological skill to proceed through the detailed, systematic process required to ensure that relevant high-quality information is synthesized. It is recommended that patients and/or their representatives be included on this team to provide a consumer perspective. In rehabilitation practice, substantial barriers to the development of CPG have included the following:

- The lack of sufficient high-quality evidence
- Substantial gaps between the interventions used in practice and those investigated in the clinical literature
- The complex nature of rehabilitation practice
- The multidimensional nature of rehabilitation outcomes

The focus of the CPG is defined by the development team and can be written as a specific clinical question. The population and condition to be addressed, the range of interventions to be considered, and the extent and nature of the multidisciplinary team define this clinical question. CPG developers must develop a strategy to search/retrieve high-quality evidence, to include lower quality evidence where necessary, and to develop meaningful recommendations in areas of practice where published evidence is absent. Practice pattern reviews or surveys are a useful strategy to identify the scope of interventions used, the perceived efficacy of such interventions, and the gaps between clinical practice and research evidence. These have been used effectively by some developers to support guideline development processes (Bitzer, Klosterhuis, Dorning, & Rose, 2003; Gulich, Engel, Rose, Klosterhuis, & Jackel, 2003). Strategies for identifying and evaluating evidence are key elements of guideline development and have been addressed in earlier chapters.

One of the key features of a properly designed guideline is that it provides clear recommendations associated with statements about the level of evidence supporting those recommendations. For example, a CPG on the management of lymphedema following breast cancer surgery listed some recommendations that were based on high-quality evidence, while others were clearly identified as not derived from scientific research but based solely on recommendations from clinicians and patients (Harris, Hugi, Olivotto, & Levine, 2001) (Table 11-2). In dealing with both types of evidence, they were able to provide more comprehensive recommendations to clinicians (examples are provided in Table 11-2). Development teams must also decide on a process for arriving at consensus on clinical recommendations and how those recommendations will be formatted in various publications arising from CPG development process. A formal consensus process can promote efficiency and circumvent group members dominating the process or decisions (Pagliari & Grimshaw, 2002; van der Sanden, Mettes, Plasschaert, Grol, & Verdonschot, 2004).

It is common for well-developed guidelines to be associated with scientific publications as well as other nontraditional publications like executive summaries, exhaustive and detailed literature synopsis, and implementation tools. Broad dissemination and lay publication can be important elements in ensuring guidelines are implemented. Guideline development committees may wish

Table 11-1

PROCESS FOR DEVELOPING A CLINICAL PRACTICE GUIDELINE FOR CLINICAL PATHWAY IN REHABILITATION

1. Assemble a development team. The team should contain:

- Multidisciplinary representation
- A range of content expertise required
- A range of methodological expertise required
- Prior experience in development of guidelines
- Patients/consumers and/or their representatives

2. Define the clinical question:

- The clinical population(s)
- The range of interventions to be addressed
- The outcomes of interest
- The disciplines involved

3. Define current clinical practice (to define scope of practice in areas that should be addressed within the guidelines; in some cases it will be necessary to draw on clinical practice patterns where evidence is lacking):

- Clinical populations treated, important clinical subgroups
- Range of interventions used
- Clinical and/or patient surveys on efficacy or treatment mediators

4. Devise and document a strategy to locate the best quality evidence on the clinical question, as defined:

- Retrieve all relevant systematic reviews
- Determine search terms and databases to locate primary studies
- Identify what quality cutoffs will be used in areas where there is a substantial number of primary studies
- Identify what quality cutoffs will be used where there are few primary studies
- Identify a strategy to deal with areas where there is no evidence (expert consensus may be useful in this case)
- Identify a strategy to integrate patient opinions and their preferences with evidence

5. Identify a strategy for evaluating quality of the available evidence:

- Identify an appropriate rating system for labeling the levels of evidence (suggest www.cebm.net/levels_of_evidence.asp)
- Identify an appropriate rating process, including a method for resolving disagreements on ratings (establish a defined consensus process)
- Use steps 4 and 5 to produce an updated literature synthesis

6. Identify a process for documenting specific conclusions or recommendations and the associated level of evidence:

- Identify and document process/forms for retrieving specific conclusions from primary studies
- Identify and use a consistent process within the CPG for presenting clinical recommendations and identifying the level of evidence supporting it

continued

Table 11-1, continued

PROCESS FOR DEVELOPING A CLINICAL PRACTICE GUIDELINE FOR CLINICAL PATHWAY IN REHABILITATION

7. Establish outcome measures that could be used to monitor the impact of the CPG/pathway implementation:
- Standardized, reliable, and valid measures that fit within a rehabilitation framework
- Consider process and outcomes
- Consider qualitative and quantitative elements

8. Consider whether the CPG or a series of guidelines can be used to establish a clinical pathway or algorithm:
- Consider treatment or outcome mediators
- Consider contraindications
- Consider the rate of progression and how patients move from one element/stage of the rehabilitation program to the next level
- Consider where guidelines can be linked to form clinical pathways

9. Identify forms of documentation to be used for dissemination and implementation:
- Identify the needs of stakeholders in terms of receiving and implementing the guideline

10. Consider the use of clinical tools, executive summaries, primary and secondary publications, research and training presentations, different vehicles for information exchange:
- Establish the process timeline for developing each component

11. Establish a process for external review of the completed guidelines:
- Include all disciplines involved
- Include a range of expertise
- Implement a pilot testing where possible

12. Revise based on feedback.

13. Devise a schedule and process for updating the guideline (every 3 years suggested):
- Updating the literature review and recommendations
- Re-evaluating and revising tools and communications
- Fixing problems identified

14. Disseminate and participate in ongoing knowledge exchange and transfer regarding CPG.

These steps were developed by Joy MacDermid (2006).

Table 11-2

INTERVENTIONS RECOMMENDED
FOR MANAGEMENT OF LYMPHEDEMA

Recommend Patients Based on High-Quality Evidence (level 1 or 2)	*Recommendations Based on Lower-Quality Evidence (>2)*	*Recommendations Based on Clinician or Patient Feedback*
One randomized trial has demonstrated a trend in favor of pneumatic compression pumps compared with no treatment. Further randomized trials are required to determine whether pneumatic compression provides additional benefit over compression garments alone.	Practitioners may want to encourage long-term and consistent use of compression garments by women with lymphedema.	Clinical experience supports encouraging patients to consider some practical advice regarding skin care, exercise, and body weight.
	Complex physical therapy, also called complex decongestive physiotherapy, requires further evaluation in randomized trials. In one randomized trial no difference in outcomes was detected between compression garments plus manual lymph drainage versus compression garments alone.	

Adapted from Harris, S. R., Hugi, M. R., Olivotto, I. A., & Levine, M. (2001). Clinical practice guidelines for the care and treatment of breast cancer: 11. Lymphedema. *CMAJ, 164,* 191-199.

to include experts in knowledge exchange and transfer (see Chapter 13) to assist with these processes. The developed CPG should provide comprehensive, high-quality, specific recommendations on the management of the clinical question as defined. This initial draft document must then be reviewed by novice and expert clinicians across the different disciplines involved, as well as methodology experts. Based on this feedback and pilot testing, if possible, a final document is drafted. Supplemental publications are then prepared and disseminated.

CPGs are intended to be updated on a regular basis to ensure that errors are fixed and evidence is current. Three years has been suggested as the optimal time frame for this reevaluation. It can be problematic to find groups who have an ongoing commitment to update CPGs, particularly when one considers that it may take 3 years to develop a single evidence-based CPG. For this reason, it is beneficial to have the involvement of professional associations who may support an ongoing commitment.

Standard Recommendation Language

Recommendations for common language and grouping of clinical recommendations within a CPG are listed. These are adapted by Joy MacDermid from basic principles of EBP and the standard language recommendation used by the United States Public Service at http://www.ahrq.gov/clinic/ajpmsuppl/harris3/htm#translating

Recommendation: A

Language: The guideline committee recommends that clinicians routinely provide the following services [list service] to eligible patients. There is found good evidence that these interventions provide clinically important health outcomes and that benefits substantially outweigh harms.

Recommendation: B

Language: The guideline committee recommends that clinicians routinely provide the following services [list services] to eligible patients. There is at least fair evidence that these interventions provide positive health outcomes and that benefits outweigh harms.

Recommendation: C

Language: The guideline committee makes no recommendation for or against routine provision of these services [list service]. There is at least fair evidence that these interventions can improve health outcomes, but the overall impact or balance of the benefits and harms is too close or uncertain to justify a general recommendation. Clinicians making specific decisions will have to provide a case-by-case rationale.

Recommendation: X

Language: The guideline committee recommends against routinely providing these interventions to patients. There is at least fair evidence that these interventions are either ineffective or that harms outweigh benefits.

Recommendation: I

Language: The guideline committee concludes that the evidence is insufficient to recommend for or against routinely providing these interventions [list]. Evidence to support or refute these interventions is lacking, of poor quality, or conflicting and the balance of benefits and harms cannot be determined.

Recommendation: S

Language: The guideline committee concludes that there is insufficient scientific evidence to support or refute the following practices. However, patient representatives and/or survey data obtained from patients or other stakeholders suggest that these practices or considerations are considered meaningful or beneficial to patients AND is it unlikely that they would have harm. The stakeholder groups who have supported these recommendations are identified in brackets (e.g. patients, general public, administrators, clinicians, payors, employers, families, injured worker).

Clinical Practice Guideline Resources

Currently, there are thousands of CPGs available, most on medical issues. Definitions, examples, explanations, and a list of these can be obtained from the Canadian Medical Association (CMA) Web site (www.cma.ca/cpgs/index.htm) or the National Guidelines Clearinghouse Web site (www.guideline.gov). This Web site provides open access to some guidelines, whereas others must be obtained from national associations or developers. National Guidelines Clearinghouse offers a sign-up service so that subscribers can receive regular e-mail updates about newly developed guidelines. A description and quality rating of some of the CPGs that pertain to rehabilitation practice have been described in publications that address published CPGs (Brooks et al., 2005; MacDermid, 2004), as well as those available on the Internet (Brosseau et al., 2004). Table 11-3 lists examples of some of the CPGs with high rigor of development.

The Agency for Health Care Policy & Research (AHCPR) initially developed CPGs but now restricts its activity to dissemination (as opposed to development and approval) of guidelines that are available in formats suitable for health care practitioners, the scientific community, educators, and consumers. Rehabilitation and professional groups are becoming increasingly involved in the development and dissemination of CPGs, and a number of professional associations not only support guidelines development but also maintain web sites that link their members to other guideline resources (see Web site links provided).

Barriers to Implementation and Uptake of Clinical Practice Guidelines

Although the benefits of implementing CPGs appear obvious (evidence-based practice, standardized approach/reduced variation, increased practitioner and patient knowledge, enhanced quality, efficiency, accountability, and effectiveness), practitioners continue to be reluctant to embrace them for many reasons. Some of the controversies around CPGs have dealt with clinicians being uncomfortable with prescriptive statements, or a concern that CPGs fail to address important elements of practice that are generally accepted within a clinical specialty (Farquhar, Kofa, & Slutsky, 2002; Garfield & Garfield, 2000). Clinicians may feel that their expertise is insufficiently recognized when CPGs are implemented (Garfield & Garfield, 2000). More specifically, it is sometimes perceived that their ability to be client-centered or use their clinical experience to optimize treatment will be impeded by a CPG (Farquhar et al., 2002). Some suspect that cost reduction, not quality, is the primary motivation for their implementation (Browman, 2000). Some practitioners might also be concerned that CPGs might pose a liability issue (Farquhar et al., 2002), as not all clinics/practitioners may be able to provide interventions for which there is supporting evidence. A realistic concern is that low-quality CPGs may adversely affect practice (Savoie, Kazanjian, & Bassett, 2000). This concern is reinforced when clinicians observe different CPGs that make different recommendations or contradict each other. Fortunately, CPGs developed more recently tend to have higher quality (Brooks et al., 2005).

Practical barriers to the implementation of guidelines also exist. These include:

- Development of guidelines is a time consuming and labour intensive effort.

- Current information and reporting systems are inadequate.

- To succeed in implementing, there must be intense, multimodal dissemination efforts, including clinical tools to assist with implementation and a variety of methods of communication. Strategies that involve direct contact with clinicians are effective, but time consuming.

- Many of the guidelines developed are not executable at the point of care (too complicated, time consuming, or inconvenient). Few guidelines contain sufficient information on how to perform recommended interventions.

- There is often no system for monitoring the impact of the guideline on current practice, no feedback mechanism, and no process for iterative refinement.

Table 11-3

TEN HIGH-QUALITY CPGs IN REHABILITATION

Title of Clinical Practice Guideline	*Source*	*Quality Rating on AGREE Instrument**
Guidelines for the Management of Soft Tissue (Musculoskeletal) Injury With Protection, Rest, Ice, Compression, and Evaluation (PRICE) During the First 72 Hours	The Chartered Society of Physiotherapy, 1998	97
A Clinical Practice Guideline on Peri-operative Cardiorespiratory Physical Therapy	Brooks, Crowe, et al., 2001	94
Management of Early Rheumatoid Arthritis	Scottish Intercollegiate Guidelines Network, 2002	92
Smoking Cessation Guidelines for Health Professionals: A Guide to Effective Smoking Cessation Interventions for the Health Care System	Raw, McNeill, & West, 1998	91
Post-Stroke Rehabilitation	US Department of Health and Human Services (Public Health Service, 1995)	90
Clinical Practice Guideline on the Use of Manipulation in the Treatment of Adults with Mechanical Neck Disorders	College of Physiotherapists of Ontario, 2002	90
The Recognition and Assessment of Acute Pain in Children	Royal College of Nursing, 1999	90
Clinical Practice Guideline for Suctioning the Airway of the Intubated and Nonintubated Patient	Brooks, Anderson, et al., 2001	89

continued

Table 11-3, continued		
TEN HIGH-QUALITY CPGs IN REHABILITATION		
Title of Clinical Practice Guideline	*Source*	*Quality Rating on AGREE Instrument**
Pressure Ulcer Prevention and Treatment Following Spinal Cord Injury: A Clinical Practice Guideline for Health Care Professionals	Consortium for Spinal Cord Medicine Clinical Practice Guidelines, 2001	88
Urinary Incontinence in Adults: Acute and Chronic Management	US Department of Health and Human Services (Public Health Service, 1996)	87

This information was adapted from a published review of the quality of CPG in physical therapy (Brooks et al., 2005).

Factors for Ensuring Successful Implementation of Clinical Practice Guidelines

A systematic review that addressed guideline implementation (Davis & Taylor-Vaisey, 1997) suggested that it is problematic. Variables that are known to affect the adoption of guidelines include qualities of the guidelines, characteristics of the health care professional, characteristics of the practice setting, incentives, regulation, and patient factors. Specific implementation strategies were grouped into two categories: primary strategies involving mailing or publication of the actual guidelines, and secondary interventional strategies to reinforce the guidelines. The traditional interventions were shown to be weakly effective (didactic, traditional, continuing medical education, and mailings). More user-centered interventions were moderately effective (audit and feedback, especially when targeted to specific providers and delivered by peers or opinion leaders). Relatively strong interventions included reminder systems, academic detailing, and multiple interventions. Effective CPG implementation strategies will require that this information be incorporated into a clear plan and an ongoing commitment to these more time consuming and resource intensive interventions (Moulding, Silagy, & Weller, 1999). A review conducted with respect to physicians provided "a differential diagnosis for why physicians do not follow practice guidelines, as well as a rational approach toward improving guideline adherence and a framework for future research" (Cabana et al., 1999).

Critical Appraisal of Clinical Practice Guidelines

Figure 11-1 presents an algorithm for defining and evaluating an appropriate CPG. One key difference between searching for primary studies and CPGs is the source location is less clear for CPGs. It is advisable to develop separate search strategies for databases like PubMed and CINAHL and those required to identify CPGs through the Internet (e.g., Google). A number of associations or guideline developers have now published the full text of their guidelines (which are often quite large) on the Internet, whereas scientific publications contain a concise

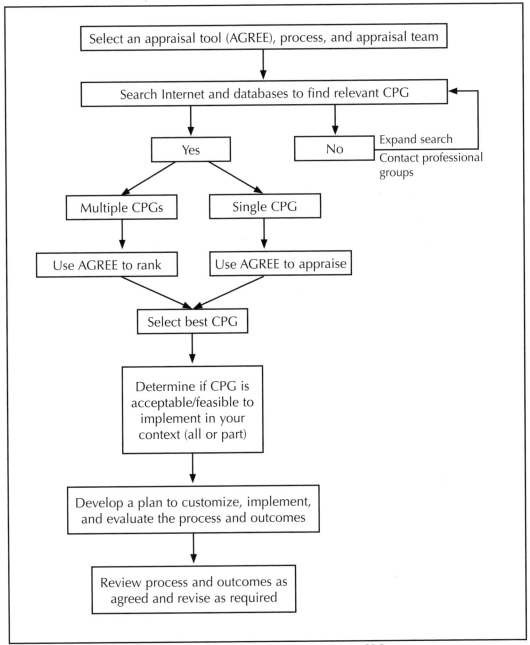

Figure 11-1. Algorithm for defining and evaluating an appropriate CPG.

version. Some CPGs are only available by contacting developers or professional associations. Some CPGs may only be located through National Guideline Clearinghouse (www.guideline. gov) or by searching for "CPG" using an Internet search engine.

The other key element in identifying CPGs most useful to one's practice is to perform a critical appraisal. A variety of instruments have been developed to evaluate CPGs. Graham, Calder, Hebert, Carter, & Tetroe (2000) reviewed 12 guideline appraisal instruments according to their context, developer information, methods, recommendations, dissemination, implementation, and evaluation.

Although numerous guideline appraisal instruments exist, the most commonly used instrument in current literature is the AGREE (Appraisal of Guidelines Research and Evaluation), located at www.agreetrust.org. This instrument itself has undergone an evolution. The original instrument was based on a yes/no scale, whereas the more recent version uses a four-point Likert scale (Cluzeau & Littlejohns, 1999; Cluzeau, Littlejohns, Grimshaw, Feder, & Moran, 1999; The AGREE Collaboration, 2003a).

One of the benefits of using the AGREE is that it has the most rigorous validation and ongoing support. The original validation study (The AGREE Collaboration, 2003b) demonstrated a strong foundation for the AGREE and this was further substantiated by a similar study that reproduced these findings when physical therapists used the AGREE to evaluate CPGs developed for a spectrum of rehabilitation issues (MacDermid et al., 2005). A list of items contained in the AGREE is listed in Table 11-4 and full documentation of the AGREE and how it is applied and scored are obtained at the AGREE Web site (www.agreecollaboration.org).

Using the Evidence: Why Implement Clinical Practice Guidelines (or Care Pathways)?

Given the controversy and potential resistance to implementation of CPGs (or CPs), it is especially imperative that evidence establishes that the substantial effort and cost to develop these processes are warranted. Anticipated effects include less variation in services delivered, better outcomes, and potentially lower costs (Grimshaw & Hutchinson, 1995). As yet, the evidence is inconclusive on those issues. Fritz, Delitto, & Erhard (2003) examined the effectiveness of a classification-based physical therapy intervention with that of therapy based on CPG for patients with acute, work-related low back pain. They found that after adjusting for baseline factors, subjects receiving classification-based therapy showed greater change on the Oswestry and the SF-36 physical component at 4 weeks. Patient satisfaction and work status were also better in the classification-based group. After 1 year, the direction (not size) of this difference remained. Median total medical costs for 1 year after injury were $1003.68 for the guideline-based group and $774.00 for the classification-based group. Thus, a clinically based classification system was shown to be superior to a guideline for this problem.

Even when the search is extended beyond rehabilitation, evidence on the role for CPGs remains weak (Bahtsevani et al., 2004). A review of this topic located only eight relevant studies, concluding that the scientific foundation was poor. The review did find some support that evidence-based CPG, when put to use, improve outcomes for some patients, but given the paucity and variability of the evidence-based CPG, were unable to make meaningful generalizations.

The evidence around CPs is equally sparse. Clinical pathway implementation is perhaps most common in lower extremity arthroplasty, where it has been shown to result in significant reduction in the length of stay (reducing costs) without compromising outcome (Pennington, Jones, & McIntyre, 2003). Another study compared the use of CP in above- or below-knee amputation, managed using either no clinical pathway, a consultation to rehabilitation services in the postoperative stay, or a rehabilitation-focused clinical pathway. The results of the study indicated more patients were able to return home from acute care and rehabilitation with a CP (Schaldach, 1997). Implementation of a clinical pathway was also reported to reduce health care cost without impairing quality of care in the treatment of decubitus ulcer patients (Dzwierzynski, Spitz, Hartz, Guse, & Larson, 1998). CPs have been used so extensively in stroke rehabilitation that a recent systematic review was published on this topic. The authors concluded,

Table 11-4

THE 23 ITEMS EVALUATED BY THE AGREE

No.	Domain	Item
1	Scope and purpose	The overall objective(s) of the guideline is (are) specifically described.
2	Scope and purpose	The clinical question(s) covered by the guideline is (are) specifically described.
3	Scope and purpose	The patients to whom the guideline is meant to apply are specifically described.
4	Stakeholder involvement	The guideline development group includes individuals from all the relevant professional groups.
5	Stakeholder involvement	The patient's views and preferences have been sought.
6	Stakeholder involvement	The target users of the guideline are clearly defined.
7	Stakeholder involvement	The guideline has been piloted among target users.
8	Rigor of Development	Systematic methods were used to search for evidence.
9	Rigor of development	The criteria for selecting the evidence are clearly described.
10	Rigor of development	The methods used for formulating the recommendations are clearly described.
11	Rigor of development	The health benefits, side effects, and risks have been considered in formulating the recommendations.
12	Rigor of development	There is an explicit link between the recommendations and the supporting evidence.
13	Rigor of development	The guideline has been externally reviewed by experts prior to its publication.
14	Rigor of development	A procedure for updating the guideline is provided.
15	Clarity and presentation	The recommendations are specific and unambiguous.
16	Clarity and presentation	The different options for management of the condition are clearly presented.

continued

Table 11-4, continued

THE 23 ITEMS EVALUATED BY THE AGREE

No.	Domain	Item
17	Clarity and presentation	Key recommendations are easily identifiable.
18	Clarity and presentation	The guideline is supported with tools for application.
19	Applicability	The potential organizational barriers in applying the recommendations have been discussed.
20	Applicability	The potential cost implications of applying the recommendations have been considered.
21	Applicability	The guideline presents key review criteria for monitoring and/or audit purposes.
22	Editorial independence	The guideline is editorially independent from the funding body.
23	Editorial independence	Conflicts of interest of guideline development members have been recorded.

Care pathways should, intuitively, improve the quality of stroke care; however, surprisingly, evidence does not support this conclusion. It is not clear why this occurs. Care pathways may simply reinforce rather than change practice. This suggests that imposing a blueprint of care, rather than individualizing treatment, does not improve outcomes. Therefore, although organized interdisciplinary stroke rehabilitation units have been shown to improve outcomes, care pathways do not appear to be contributing to this success. (StrokEngine, 2007)

A caveat should be considered before CPGs and CP processes are cast in too negative a light. Firstly, the methodologies are new and evolving. The pressures for enhanced quality are forcing positive improvements in quality and implementation so newer CPGs and CPs may be more useful. The related field of knowledge exchange and transfer is itself in its infancy, so the potential benefits may be underestimated because of a failure in implementation. In fact, evidence supports that results are better when implementation is better. The guideline or pathway process is expected to contribute to the following potentially valuable consequences:

- Reduce uncertainty and inappropriate variations in clinical management within specific conditions

- More effective processes to influence clinical behaviour than traditional journal articles

- Mechanisms to help clinicians assimilate large amounts of rapidly evolving scientific evidence

- Provide a vehicle for public/patient participation into medical decision-making

- A respectable process to respond to the demands of third-party funding and quality monitoring agents for guidance on and succinct recommendations about appropriate rehabilitation practice

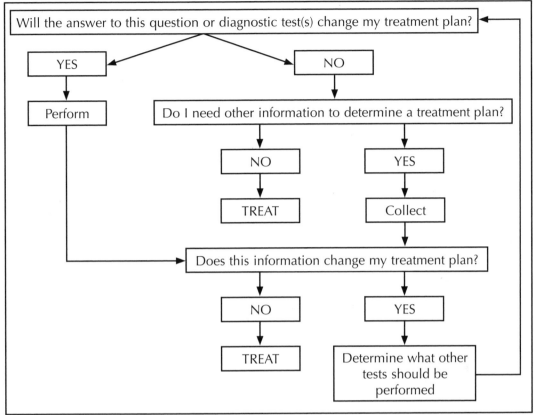

Figure 11-2. Example of a simple decision tree.

ALGORITHMS

To facilitate the move to EBP and the development of CPGs and CPs, practitioners who are unfamiliar with these strategies may find it useful to begin the process by developing algorithms or decision trees. Algorithms are "written guidelines to stepwise evaluation and management strategies that require observations to be made, decisions to be considered, and actions to be taken" (Hadorn, McCormick, & Diokno, 1992). They can be formulated by taking information from CPGs and arranging it in a decision-tree format. Other algorithms synthesize information from diagnostic test studies and support a diagnostic process. Rehabilitation practitioners may be familiar with the algorithm concept found in the well-known outcome measure, the Functional Independence Measure. Developers of CPGs have found that algorithms facilitate decision making for practitioners, making it easier to list essential clinical steps to be used during the development of a guideline and a subsequent CP. For example, in overall management of persons with stroke, the results of the history and physical examination could lead to the use of a guideline for management of poststroke. The recommendations concerning routine tests and other diagnostic procedures could be incorporated into the "tests/diagnostics" section of a CP (see section on CPs for more detailed information regarding pathways). The development of an algorithm can be a straightforward way to introduce the process of development for CPGs and pathways to practitioners who may not be familiar with these concepts. Algorithms help clarify the key decision points requiring action. A generic simple algorithm is illustrated in Figure 11-2, which might be used to teach students how to proceed when constructing an examination plan. A more complex (realistic) algorithm on the management of low back pain developed by the Alberta Workers Compensation Board is provided in Chapter 8.

CLINICAL PATHWAYS

It has been recognized that the way in which CP developed in the United Kingdom differs from that of the United States (Currie & Harvey, 1998; McKenna et al., 2006). In the United States the concept of clinical pathway was used as a framework for balancing costs and quality whereas in the United Kingdom and Canada, CPs are more viewed as a way of achieving a continuum of care across care settings. A recent systematic review tried to deal with the definition more precisely and found 82 out of 263 eligible papers provided a definition. A total of 84 definitions were found. They suggested the definition below.

Definition

One definition of a clinical pathway is "a cause and effect grid or framework, which identifies expected measurable patient/client outcomes (or behaviours) against a timeline for a specific case-type or group" (Zander & Hill, 1995). A more precise definition is given by De Bleser et al. (2006):

> *A clinical pathway is a method for the patient-care management of a well-defined group of patients during a well-defined time period. A clinical pathway explicitly states the goals and key elements of care based on evidence-based medicine guidelines, best practice and patient expectations by facilitating communication, coordinating roles and sequencing the activities of the multidisciplinary care team, patients and their relatives; by documenting, monitoring and evaluating variances; and by providing the necessary resources and outcomes. The aim of a clinical pathway is to improve the quality of care, reduce risks, increase patient satisfaction and increase efficiency in the use of resources.*

The clinical pathway is a tool that sets locally agreed clinical standards, based on the best available evidence, for managing specific groups of clients. It can form part or all of the clinical record and enables the care given by members of the multidisciplinary team, together with the progress and outcome, to be documented. Variations from the pathway are recorded, and analysis allows a continuous evaluation of the effectiveness of clinical practice. Information obtained is used to revise the pathway to improve the quality of client care (Kitchiner & Bundred, 1996, 1999).

History of Care Pathways

CPs have been developed in an attempt to improve quality of care and patient satisfaction and to reduce variations in practice, complications, errors, resource utilization, and costs. They identify anticipated outcomes, health care provider interventions, and anticipated intervention times. Pathways have been utilized in the American health care system since the late 1980s when Karen Zander of the Center for Case Management developed a patented model named CareMap. The model applied the engineering project management principles of those effective critical paths utilized since the late 1950s and early 1960s in the automotive industry and manufacturing, first gaining international recognition in the American Aerospace Industry at the National Aeronautics and Space Administration. The concept, which began as a nursing and case management initiative in Boston's New England Medical Center in 1985, was quickly adopted by the hospital sector both in the United States and larger centers in Canada, as well as internationally. Soon after this, we began to see the trend to focus care planning in American health care organizations for clusters of patient/clients with similar conditions called case mixed groups (CMGs) or diagnostic-related groups (DRGs). Subsequent to this, the American health care system moved to capping service by dictating maximum costs based on the projected episode of care in a model known as managed care.

We are now experiencing an explosion of coordinated care models both in the United States and Canada similar to Zander's original CareMap model. These models use names synonymous with the original, but unique to each particular setting and application, both for the purpose of avoiding copyright issues and to achieve user participation by ensuring provider involvement during development and commitment to the use of the pathway. See Chapter 8 for an example of a CP.

Framework for Care Pathways

Developers have coined a multitude of names for their particular coordinated care models—case path, care path/plan/pathway/compass/track/guide, multidisciplinary action plan, target track, critical path, anticipated recovery path, clinical pathway, care management/case management, collaborative care path, care process—but the framework and components of all are similar and recognizable as having roots in the CareMap concept. We have also seen the emergence of other copyrighted systems, sold for profit, and providing education and support for development and implementation within a unique setting. The obvious advantages of using a purchased system include time and cost savings by avoiding the prolonged and expensive development process. They facilitate the comparability of results across other settings and institutions using the same tool and provide expert support for implementation and evaluation. In some cases, the tool is based on solid research evidence.

Home-Built or Manufactured Pathways?

Drawbacks to commercial systems include lack of buy-in from staff who may refuse to support what is perceived as cookie-cutter health care, possible poor fit of a generic model with a unique service, and little opportunity for consumers to be involved in development of the care plan. Furthermore, they may fail to address the process, health care model, and environmental issues of the setting. Although home-built pathways are generally viewed by staff with less suspicion than purchased systems, some concerns may still be expressed by staff who are newly introduced to the concept. Pathways may be seen as cookbook health care or cost-cutting mechanisms for administrators. Difficulty may be experienced when attempting to address co-morbidity since most pathways address just one diagnosis or condition. Implementing one pathway that addresses multiple conditions or using more than one pathway concurrently with an individual receiving care may result in unmanageable complexities (e.g., a person with diabetes and congestive heart failure who has suffered a CVA). Conversely, pathways may be perceived as too simplistic, inflexible, and just one more piece of paper to complete. There may also be the fear that information collected will be used to penalize performance.

Structure

Clinical pathway models have a matrix listing interventions along one axis and a timeframe along another. Interventions typically include consultations and referral, assessments and observations, tests, treatments, measurements and diagnostics, nutrition, medication, activity and mobility, safety, patient/client and family education/teaching, and discharge planning. Within the timeline, factors identified may include typical problems, desired clinical outcomes, intermediate goals or key indicators, as well as physician orders. Some "next generation" pathways now incorporate not only variance tracking records but also admission and discharge indicators/status, as well as key indicator and outcome records (clinical and client/patient).

Pathway Development

Choosing Case Types

Experts with experience in developing pathways recommend a systematic review be undertaken of the particular population served such as cost of care, volume, level of risk, etc. When choosing a particular area for development of a pathway, the greatest impact will be achieved if the initial focus is directed toward groups with the following factors identified:

- High volume
- High cost
- High risk
- High practice variability
- Potential for improvement
- Potential to cross multiple settings and disciplines in continuum
- Predictable course
- Provider interest
- Physician interest, initiative, and acceptance

Using the Evidence: Pathway Development Strategies

Many of the first pathways developed were based on current practice because of the paucity of available research in rehabilitation and lack of support from organizations for the time and effort in literature searching. Currently, most developers recognize the importance of basing their pathways on best practice supported by solid research evidence. Developers begin building pathways by reviewing background information, including critically reviewing similar pathways in use within other sites. This should be complemented by an extensive literature review focused on similar pathways, as well as the effectiveness of interventions for the pathway being developed. Many developers begin the process by bringing together key partners involved in care for the case type to be addressed and provide key research articles, samples of pathways, and a description of the development task. The development committee then researches information on their specific practice for the specific client group. If multiple agencies are involved in development, each agency reviews and provides current data regarding practice for comparative purposes. In this way, if evidence in the literature is lacking in a particular area, preimplementation data provide a foundation for further investigation and evaluation following implementation of the pathway. Since all members of the development team must have a thorough understanding of the concept and philosophy of the clinical pathway model, it is necessary to provide staff with education and teaching materials regarding pathway models prior to embarking on the development task.

Evolution of Pathway Models

First-generation pathways were usually diagnosis-based (as in the management of stroke, diabetes, acute myocardial infarction), or symptom-based (as for the investigation and treatment of clients presenting with chest pain). They also focused on a specific procedure (total joint replacement, coronary artery bypass graft, transurethral resection of prostate) or encouraged the use of therapeutic guidelines such as postoperative analgesia. Second-generation pathways are now emerging that highlight activity or function (continence, enteral feeding, memory loss, self-injection, fine motor/handwriting) with a resulting focus on education, teaching, and client outcomes rather than specific medical interventions.

Continuum Pathways

The first pathways to emerge usually reflected only the activity within a single institution or service, but developers are now realizing the importance of linking pathways along the continuum of care (e.g., hospital to home; home to long-term care). This enables the person receiving care to have knowledge of the entire episode of care, while providers ensure that gaps between settings and services are minimized. Chronic conditions such as asthma, obstructive pulmonary disease, diabetes, and palliative care have been managed through the development of pathways that coordinate care across the primary-secondary care interface (Dowsey, Kilgour, Santamaria, & Choong, 1999).

Benefits

The effort involved in developing such transorganizational, multidisciplinary pathways is enormous but the benefits do outweigh the risks. Studies are now emerging that show better client outcomes are achieved when pathways are introduced (Ellershaw, Foster, Murphy, Shea, & Overill, 1997). Results indicate that pathways contribute to client-focused care, as they constantly monitor quality and any deviation from the pathway identifies complications early. The plan of care is clearly defined and shared with the client and in some instances, clients are involved in the actual development of the plan. Discharge or transition planning is facilitated since the median length of stay is defined and length of stay can often be reduced without an increase in complications or unscheduled readmissions.

When developing such continuum pathways, it is important for developers to do the following:

- Work together to choose the target group for which the pathway will be developed
- Concentrate on the interface between the pathways and clearly define the transition status (functional level or point at which the client/patient moves from one setting to another)
- Reach consensus regarding common definitions, (e.g., develop a multi-site terminology guide)
- Use international diagnostic codes
- If computerized, use a common electronic interface

Often, the resulting side benefits of developing and implementing continuum pathways for the care providers are the emergence of new partnerships and increased collaboration between agencies, decreased duplication of effort, increased knowledge of available services, and recognition for expertise.

Pathway Development Teams

It is important that the development team selects the specific client group for the pathway to ensure interest and enthusiasm for the task at the front line rather than solely at an administrative level. Many excellent pathways have failed simply because those affected by the tool were not involved with its formulation and implementation. As a result, they were disinterested and did not see the importance of the work. Interested participants who are involved in the actual care delivery must be identified and selected to form working groups. In situations in which providers have never had the opportunity of debating practice or reviewing literature, it may be necessary to form single discipline working groups prior to moving to multidisciplinary groups. In this way, scope of practice for each discipline can be determined and agreed upon prior to determining the scope of the pathway (beginning and end). If the literature search identifies any related CPGs that direct practice for the client group for which a pathway is being developed, the CPG can become the foundation for the pathway with the addition of a timeline, plus admission and discharge indicators or criteria.

Documentation System

CPs and their documentation systems have often been implemented without follow-up such as chart audits and milestone tracking. In the past, there has been a lack of congruence between clinical pathway tools and nonpathway tools such as flow charts and outcome measures. When they were first developed, CPs were tools used only as a guide, often housed in policy and procedure manuals. With some pathways, staff were asked to "sign-off" at the end of a shift. Others were used in conjunction with flow sheets to facilitate compiling information over an episode of care.

The introduction of CPs is an entirely new approach of recording and charting, requiring the development of a documentation system to complement the model and ensure that organizational, legal, and professional standards are met. If documentation is not integrated, there is the danger that staff may see the clinical pathway as an "add-on" or "one more form to sign."

Advantages

CPs facilitate the move to a charting-by-exception model, resulting in many immediate advantages. Any trends in a client's or a group of clients' status can be seen immediately. Abnormal data recorded on a client's record are quickly highlighted and easily retrieved. Transcription and duplication of charting are eliminated, resulting in significant decreases in documentation time. Information that has already been recorded is not repeated. Clients are evaluated against well-defined goals since assessments are standardized so providers evaluate and document findings consistently. All providers use the same approach for each case type and begin to compare outcomes without being dependent on formalized research. This occurs because an accurate representation of the course of treatment, changes in condition, and care rendered for the particular case type are readily available—an ideal format for conducting applied research.

CLINICAL PATHWAY EVALUATION

Preimplementation Appraisal Instrument of Care Pathways

In deciding to implement a clinical pathway developed by others, a process of critically evaluating the clinical pathway should be undertaken. Unlike CPGs, few validated tools have been designed for this purpose. A recent paper evaluated tools developed for CPGs as a potential way to fulfill this role (Vlayen, Aertgeerts, Hannes, Sermeus, & Ramaekers, 2005). The study concluded that the AGREE with most suitable, but would require modification to customize it to this new application (Vlayen et al., 2005). Another systematic review addressed clinical pathway audit tools, providing a detailed analysis of seven potential instruments (Vanhaecht, De Witte, Depreitere, & Sermeus, 2006). One instrument was found to be the only tool to be validated by a study published in the peer-reviewed literature, although its use was yet to be cited in a peer-reviewed publication, illustrating the recent emergence of scientific rigor in this area. The

The Integrated Care Pathway Appraisal Tool (ICPAT) (Whittle, McDonald, & Dunn, 2004). Example questions include the following:

- Does the CP have an identified start point?
- Are there clear instructions on how to use the documentation?
- Is there a record of the decisions made and discussion concerning the content of the pathway?
- Has an ongoing training program for the staff users been established?
- Is someone nominated to maintain the CP?

Postimplementation Review of Process and Experience

Evaluation following initial implementation of a clinical pathway should collect data from multiple sources, including surveys or focus groups for users (staff surveys), consumers, families, and physicians. Chart audits should be carried out to validate information collected from surveys and provide important information regarding documentation practices. It is helpful to develop a data collection template with details that have been chosen for review such as length of stay and visit frequencies, client's discharge status, clinical (functional status) and client outcomes (negotiated goals achieved), as well as any positive or negative variances along the pathway.

Identifying Outcomes: Variances

By tracking information on CPs, it is possible to identify critical success factors for case types that will define optimal steps in clinical processes, reduce unnecessary variation in these processes, and provide data for continuous improvement. When making a decision regarding the process by which to define patient/client progress and outcome, it is necessary to carefully consider the plan for analysis and the available supports (clerical, technical, systems, etc.). Many large institutions embarking on the clinical pathway model have made the error of implementing complex tracking systems for determining outcomes only to be quickly overwhelmed by data without having the ability to make changes based on the reports generated.

Definition

A variance is defined as the difference between what is expected and what actually happens. Variances can be the result of client, practitioner, or system issues and can be either positive or negative. Factors usually resulting in a variance include the following:

- The client's condition such as an unexpected complication or unanticipated rapid progress
- An issue of the support network such as availability of informal supports or burden of care
- A provider or agency issue such as presence of a wait list or availability of test results
- Provision of equipment and supplies (e.g., delivery, availability)
- Environmental issues (e.g., unsanitary conditions, lack of water, heat, electricity, food, telephone)

If the recording and reporting system is computerized, it may be possible to track variances concurrently (at the same time the variance is identified) and address the variance immediately. However, since most agencies lack this degree of technical support, variances are usually tracked retrospectively (after the client has been discharged from the pathway). Variances that focus on the program level rather than client level include factors such as length of stay, number and frequency of visits, readmission rates, infection rates, and length of time waiting for service. The example in the Chapter 8 includes a variance tracking record used for total knee arthroplasty.

Identifying Outcomes: Key Indicators

The concept of refining variance data leads to the identification of key performance indicators. More recently, this has resulted in a move away from variance tracking towards identification of performance capability that indicates the client's recovery status—a type of health report card. These key indicators or outcomes form milestones that coincide with a change in level of care or resource utilization, such as weight-bearing status for an orthopaedic intervention, ability to self-inject insulin for diabetes care, or first day of ambulation following stroke. With this move has also come a new focus away from "micromanaging" an episode of care (e.g., extubation, catheter removal, tolerance of fluids) to a broader focus on the continuum of care, identifying key admission and discharge indicators to facilitate a smooth transition throughout levels of care. Key indicators such as length of stay, readmission rates, or incidence of complications have statistical value that can provide a direction over time of a specific process (see Exercise 3). Standard tools used for quality improvement such as control charts are useful methods for interpreting and presenting the data collected. Standardized outcome measures may also be identified within the pathway (assessments/tests/measurements), providing the foundation for the measurement of the key indicators and outcomes chosen. In this manner, specific benchmarks can be identified at several points along the timeline of the pathway and progress towards a goal within the specific timeframe can be clearly identified. The exercises at the end of this chapter contain templates for developing key indicator records and are included for student practice in identifying decision points within a plan of care.

PATHWAY COMPUTERIZATION AND IMPACT OF TECHNOLOGY

A systematic review on the effects of computer-based clinical decision support systems on physician performance and patient outcomes revealed the trends for physicians answering questions regarding their practice. The study showed that 76% asked colleagues, 14% used CPGs, and 10% accessed MEDLINE (Hunt, Haynes, Hanna, & Smith, 1998). The implementation of an electronic system that includes links to supporting evidence has been shown to facilitate access for the users to the evidence supporting the guidelines and pathways at the point of care. This can result in more effective uptake of new protocols.

Point of care tools that allow timely data access/capture, plus order entry/result reporting help to facilitate concurrent interdisciplinary documentation. They allow multiple user access to information and have the potential for comparison of data on many levels (provider, agency, provincial, national, international). As well as the benefit of reduced documentation time and the potential for concurrent variance analysis (impossible with a paper-based system), information can be integrated across the continuum of care so that data can be easily shared and are only entered once. This allows all providers to retrieve complete and current information from a common health database. It is then possible to build in decision support and education tools (staff and client/patient) consistent with the protocol.

Internet-Based Design

Several emerging Internet-based novel design concepts called "clinical or disease guidance systems" enhance the management of clients/patients through the use of "just-in-time, evidence-based medical literature and practice guidelines" (Penn, Lau, & Wilson, 1996). Not only do these systems generate a set of client care activities or orders individualized to each person, but it is done in such a way that the individual activities are linked to available evidence, providing practitioners the ability to enroll clients into active research trials via the Internet. All components of the system, literature, and guidelines are maintained and distributed by a robust publishing system through an expanded Web technology which allows commercial control of copyright and royalties. Several international (United States, United Kingdom, Netherlands, Germany) evaluation studies are underway to determine the effectiveness of such clinical guidance systems. Other computer-based projects underway include the Alberta WellNet, an initiative that links pharmacy information, providing distance health services and development of a common financial system; StrokeNet, a collaborative effort researching best practice for stroke care; and CQIN, the Clinical Quality Improvement Network, linking randomized controlled trial evidence and its application in clinical practice.

LEGAL IMPLICATIONS OF CARE PATHWAYS AND CLINICAL PRACTICE GUIDELINES

Integration of CPs and CPGs into a documentation system that moves to charting by exception often raises legal questions from practitioners regarding the security of the electronic chart, rigor of the record in a court of law, and professional documentation responsibility (notion that if it isn't documented, it was not done). In response to such concerns, lawyers indicate that the use of practice standards does not create significant new risks and actually may reduce the risk and cost of litigation when the tool is approved as a permanent part of the care record (Stradiotto, 1997). Signatures must follow completion of interventions, outcomes must be entered, and variances identified and documented as lack of progress with identification of plans to deal with them. The opinion in the legal community is that exception charting is likely stronger documentation than the documentation consistently recorded in the previous system since casebooks are filled with examples showing poor record keeping and conflicting professional notes as sources of liability. CPs provide a complete plan of care, encourage clear communication, and enhance uniform record keeping (Burke & Murphy, 1995). Exception charting provides consistent documentation of standards of care and meets government as well as professional standards. It is a legally and financially defensible documentation system, if followed consistently by those who use it. If documentation policy is consistently applied and staff can testify to consistent application of policy, while understanding the importance of switching to detailed charting as soon as there is any reason to believe the client/patient has fallen outside the norm, defence should not be difficult (Hill, 1995).

CLINICAL PRACTICE GUIDELINES, ALGORITHMS, AND CARE PATHWAYS: REVIEW

Table 11-5 is provided to highlight the similarities and differences between CPGs and CPs. Although it is not essential to develop a CPG or algorithm before developing a pathway, they can be an excellent foundation upon which a clinical pathway may be built.

DEVELOPING CARE PATHWAYS

Material is provided in exercises 1 to 3 to assist the practitioner who is beginning to develop CP or to practice some of the conceptual issues addressed by CP. The sample CP in Chapter 8 and the Web sites that direct practitioners to CPs available online can be used to provide more exposure to the ways that CPs can be developed and formatted.

Table 11-5	

COMPARISON OF CLINICAL PRACTICE GUIDELINES AND CARE PATHWAYS

Clinical Practice Guidelines	Care Pathways
Focus on identifying best clinical option	Focus on operationalizing options
Useful across clinical settings; apply generally	Setting/institution specific; tailored to fit local conditions
May or may not be provider specific	Require multi/transdisciplinary approach
Based on evidence, may also include expert opinion or consensus	Based on evidence from research studies and practice settings (including process and outcomes)
Developed and supported by a group of experts	Produced by a multidisciplinary team
Guide practice in an explicit manner; focus on linking evidence to recommendations	Define optimum sequence and timing of interventions

DEFINITIONS

algorithm: Written guidelines to stepwise evaluation and management strategies that require observations to be made, decisions to be considered, and actions to be taken.

case mixed group: A grouping of clients based on the different types (mix) of diagnoses (cases) for which they are being treated.

charting by exception: A method of documenting normal findings about a client (sometimes using symbols) and based on clearly defined guidelines for practice (i.e., plan of care, predicted outcomes).

clinical pathway: A multidisciplinary tool that makes explicit the usual client problem and activities that must occur to facilitate the achievement of expected client outcomes in a defined length of time (The Center for Case Management, n.d.).

concurrent variance analysis: The immediate review of current variance data for a particular population or individual client to identify the need to alter interventions.

CPGs: Clinical practice guidelines are systematically developed statements to assist practitioner and patient decisions about appropriate health care for specific clinical circumstances (Field & Lohr, 1990).

diagnostic related group: A code of classifying illnesses according to principal diagnosis and treatment requirements.

key indicator: An event or intervention deemed to be critical for achieving the anticipated outcome. May also be called milestones or benchmarks.

negative variance: A deviation that occurs when the client progresses at a rate slower than anticipated, usually resulting in a longer length of stay or a greater number of visits per episode of care.

outcomes: Factors that identify the results of the interventions (e.g., functional health status, morbidity, mortality, quality of life, satisfaction, cost).

performance indicator: A measurement tool, screen, or flag that is used as a guide to monitor, assess, and improve the quality of client care, support services, and organizational functions that affect outcomes.

positive variance: A deviation that occurs when the client progresses at a rate faster than anticipated, usually resulting in a shorter length of stay or fewer visits per episode of care.

protocol: A written statement or plan that defines the management of broad client problems or issues and may include decision trees, algorithms, flowcharts, and research plans.

retrospective variance analysis: The analysis of aggregated variance data for a particular population after discharge to identify patterns and trends.

standards of care: A level of performance or a set of conditions considered acceptable by some authority or by the individual(s) engaged in performing or maintaining the set of conditions in question.

standards of practice: Desired and achievable levels of performance against which actual performance can be compared (Canadian Council on Health Services Accreditation, n.d.).

variance analysis: The process of collecting, managing, reviewing, analyzing, and reporting variance occurrences.

variance: A deviation in the implementation or occurrence of a stated critical indicator (i.e., the difference between what is expected to happen and what actually happens).

TAKE-HOME MESSAGES

Recent Trends in Health Care
✔ It is important to adopt new models of service delivery that blend quality with responsiveness and focus on accountability, quality, efficient utilization of health-care services, and standardization of care.
✔ Care pathways are based on CPGs or protocols standardization which is accountable to funders and consumers.

Clinical Practice Guidelines
✔ Systematically developed statements that assist practitioner and client decisions about appropriate health care for specific clinical circumstances.
✔ Best approach to development is to combine evidence-based and expert consensus.
✔ Ensuring success of CPGs: Single, well-defined clinical problem; participation of practitioners; resulting documents which are simple and clear in language, reduction of administrative barriers, *strength of evidence.*

Algorithms
✔ CGPs in a decision-tree format.
✔ Facilitate decision-making for practitioners by clarifying key decision points while maintaining a simplistic approach.

Clinical Pathways
✔ Built upon foundation of evidence from CPGs.

✔ A cause-and-effect grid that identifies expected measurable client outcomes against a time-line for a specific group.

✔ Developed using a range of tools for *specific* needs of clients and clinicians who will use the tool.

✔ Evaluate through a preimplementation review for design and a postimplementation review of process and experience.

Implementation

✔ Move away from tracking variance toward identification of performance capability and broader focus on continuum of care.

✔ Increasing implementation of electronic systems for linking clinical pathways to supporting evidence.

✔ Evidence-based approach that achieves a balance between benefit, harm, and cost.

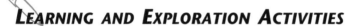

LEARNING AND EXPLORATION ACTIVITIES

Clinical Practice Guidelines

Obtain a CPG of clinical interest and critically apprise it using the AGREE. Compare your results to a colleague. Discuss how you might implement this CPG in your practice. What barriers would you need to overcome? What process changes would you make?

Care Pathways

The purpose of this chapter is to introduce the concept of CPs as a means through which to standardize practice and ensure its accountability. Through these exercises, the student can develop the necessary skills in actively developing pathways and outcome statements. The following templates should be used to assist the student in the exercise and to help provide practical experience.

1 *Developing a Specific Pathway:* Use the following template for developing a specific pathway. Begin by choosing a particular diagnostic group or condition and record the expected admission status, critical interventions, timeline, and discharge status.

2. *Developing Outcomes*: Complete the outcome statements for each of the conditions listed.

Exercise 1: Template for Development of Clinical Pathways

Case Type (Description): _____

Length of Stay: _____

Frequency of Visits: _____

Focus	Visit 1	Visit 2	Visit 3
Observations/ Assessments			
Tests/ Measurements			
Functional Level Safety			
Treatments			
Teaching/ Education			
Discharge Planning			
Consultation/ Referral			

Admissions Criteria:	Discharge Criteria:
1.	1.
2.	2.
3.	3.
4.	4.

Exercise 2: Developing Outcomes

Complete the Outcome Statements listed below for the following client conditions:

I. Cardiovascular Accident

II. Congestive Heart Failure

III. Major Joint Replacement

IV. Bipolar Disorder

V. Parkinson's Disease

VI. Early Onset Dementia

1   The client understands and demonstrates knowledge of _____

_____

_____

_____ by visit number: _____ .

2. The client's status is stabilized/is improving as evidenced by _____

_____

_____

_____ by visit number: _____ .

3. The client's (family, caregiver, workplace, etc.) understands and demonstrates knowledge of:_____

_____

_____

_____ by visit number: _____ .

4. The client can identify the following safety precautions or prevention factors: _____

_____

_____

5. The client can identify the following risks related to the health concern/treatment:

_____

_____

_____

Exercise 3: Blank Clinical Pathway

Complete this template for a patient group you deal with using the goals/processes from the previous 2 steps. Then think of some of the variances you have experienced in your own practice. Complete the CP, recording the actual variance in the comments column.

Clinical Pathway for _____			Diagnostic Code _____					
Client Name _____		**Date CP Initiated** _____			**D/C Date** _____			
Expected Number of Treatments _____			**Expected D/C date** _____					
Date	Visit #	Goals/ Expected Outcomes	Date Met	Not Met	Variance Code	Variance Date	Comments	
Team Members					**Variance Code** 1. Patient choice 2. Patient Co-morbidity/ Complication 3. Patient Non-medical issues 4. Health Care provider 5. Health care institution (internal) 6. Health Care system (external) 7. Other system-External factors			

WEB LINKS

- *Canadian Medical Association Info Base*
  www.cma.ca/cpgs or http://mdm.ca/cpgsnew/cpgs/index.asp
  Source of CPGs and other evidence.

- *National Guidelines Clearinghouse (NGC)*
  http://www.guideline.gov/
  A look-up and sign-up service that has extensive coverage and evaluation of CPGs. A standardized format presents information on development and access to guidelines. User may receive regular updates. Most are medically focused.

- *New Zealand Guidelines Group.*
  www.nzgg.org.nz/index.cfm

- *Centre for Evidence-Based Mental Health*
  www.cebmh.com.

- *Alberta Wellnet*
  www.health.gov.ab.ca or www.albertawellnet.org.

- *Veteran's Affairs Guidelines*
  www.oqp.med.va.gov/cpg/cpg.htm.

- *Evidence-Based Medicine Resource Center*
  www.ebmny.org/cpg.html
  List of CPGs.

- *eGuidelines*
  www.eguidelines.co.uk
  A Web site that provides comprehensive coverage of United Kingdom guidelines and information for patients.

- *Guidelines Advisory Committee*
  www.gacguidelines.ca/
  The Guidelines Advisory Committee (GAC) is an independent partnership of the Ontario Medical Association and the Ontario Ministry of Health and Long-Term Care and contains a listing of many guidelines; summaries in Word or for PDAs and full text is usually downloadable.

- *Primary Care Clinical Practice Guidelines*
  medicine.ucsf.edu/resources/guidelines/index.html

- *How to Use a Clinical Practice Guideline*
  www.cche.net/usersguides/guideline.asp
  Guide to using CPG.

- *Clinical Practice Guidelines and Protocols in British Columbia*
  www.healthservices.gov.bc.ca/msp/protoguides/index.html

- *The Ottawa Hospital*
  www.ottawahospital.on.ca/library/internetresources/cpg-e.asp
  A detailed list of CPG resources.

- *Respiratory Care*
  www.rcjournal.com/online_resources/cpgs/cpg_index.asp
  List of CPGs in respiratory care.

Clinical Pathways

- *The European Pathway Association*
  www.e-p-a.org/index2.html
  This association is an international network of clinical pathway/care pathway networks, user groups, academic institutions, supporting organizations and individuals who want to support the development, implementation, and evaluation of clinical/care pathways. If you want up-to-date information, you can join for free.

- *The European Pathway Association*
  www.the-npa.org.uk

- *Journal of Integrated Care Pathways*
  www.rsmpress.co.uk/jicp.htm

- *American Academy of Physical Medicine and Rehabilitation*
  www.aapmr.org/hpl/clinpath.htm
  List of CPs.

- *Center for Case Management, South Natick, MA*
  www.cfcm.com
  Lists CareMap pathways for purchase, educational resources, online copy of *The New Definition* newsletter.

- *Royal Children's Hospital Melbourne*
  www.rch.org.au/rch_clinpath/pathways.cfm?doc_id=4393
  List of CPs.

- *Australian Government Department of Veterans' Affairs*
  www.dva.gov.au/health/provider/community_nursing/pathways/pathindex.htm#cp
  List of CPs.

- *Children's Hospital Central California*
  www.childrenscentralcal.org/Portal2.asp?ID=606
  List of CPs.

- *St. Joseph's Health Care London, Ontario*
  www.sjhc.london.on.ca/sjh/profess/cp/cp_clin.htm
  List of a number of multidisciplinary CPs and a sample variance tracking sheet.

- *National Library for Health Protocols and Care Pathways Database*
  www.library.nhs.uk/pathways

REFERENCES

Bahtsevani, C., Uden, G., & Willman, A. (2004). Outcomes of evidence-based clinical practice guidelines: A systematic review. *International Journal of Technology Assessment in Health Care, 20*, 427-433.

Bitzer, E. M., Klosterhuis, H., Dorning, H., & Rose, S. (2003). Developing an evidence based clinical guideline on cardiac rehabilitation--Phase 2: comparative analysis of the present level of service provision in cardiac rehabilitation based on the KTL statistics. *Rehabilitation (Stuttgart), 42*, 83-93.

Brooks, D., Crowe, J., Kelsey, C. J., Lacy, J., Parsons, J., & Solway, S. (2001). A clinical practice guideline on peri-operative cardiorespiratory physical therapy. *Physiotherapy Canada, 53*(1), 9-25.

Brooks, D., Anderson, C. M., Carter, M. A., Downes, L. A., Keenan, S. P., Kelsey, C. J. et al. (2001). Clinical practice guidelines for suctioning the airway of the intubated and nonintubated patient. *Canadian Respiratory Journal, 8*, 163-181.

Brooks, D., Solway, S., MacDermid, J., Switzer-McIntyre, S., Brosseau, L., Graham, I. D. (2005). Quality of clinical practice guidelines in physical therapy. *Physiotherapy Cananad, 57*(2), 123-134.

Brosseau, L., Graham, I., Casimiro, L., MacLeay, L., Cleaver, S., Dumont, A., et al. (2004). What is the quality of clinical practice guidelines accessible on the World Wide Web for the treatment of musculoskeletal conditions in physiotherapy? *Physiotherapy Theory Practice, 20*(2), 91-105.

Browman, G. P. (2000). Improving clinical practice guidelines for the 21st century: Attitudinal barriers and not technology are the main challenges. *International Journal of Technology Assessment in Health Care, 16*, 959-968.

Burgers, J. S., Cluzeau, F. A., Hanna, S. E., Hunt, C., & Grol, R. (2003). Characteristics of high-quality guidelines: Evaluation of 86 clinical guidelines developed in ten European countries and Canada. *International Journal of Technology Assessment in Health Care, 19*, 148-157.

Burke, L., & Murphy, J. (1995). *Charting by exception applications: Making it work in clinical settings.* Albany, NY: Delmar Publishers.

Cabana, M. D., Rand, C. S., Powe, N. R., Wu, A. W., Wilson, M. H., Abboud, P. A., et al. (1999). Why don't physicians follow clinical practice guidelines? A framework for improvement. *Journal of the American Medical Association, 282*, 1458-1465.

Canadian Council on Health Services Accreditation. (n.d.). Retrieved October 22, 2007, from http://www.cchsa.ca

Canadian Medical Association (1994). *Guidelines for Canadian clinical practice guidelines.* Ottowa: Author.

Canadian Medical Association (1995). *Care maps and continuous quality improvement.* Ottowa: Author.

Cluzeau, F. A., & Littlejohns, P. (1999). Appraising clinical practice guidelines in England and Wales: The development of a methodologic framework and its application to policy. *Joint Commission Journal on Quality Improvement, 25,* 514-521.

Cluzeau, F. A., Littlejohns, P., Grimshaw, J. M., Feder, G., & Moran, S. E. (1999). Development and application of a generic methodology to assess the quality of clinical guidelines. *International Journal for Quality in Health Care, 11,* 21-28.

College of Physiotherapists of Ontario. (2002). Clinical practice guidelines (CPG) on the use of manipulation on the treatment of adults with mechanical neck disorders. [On-line].

Consortium for Spinal Cord Medicine Clinical Practice Guidelines. (2001). Pressure ulcer prevention and treatment following spinal cord injury: a clinical practice guideline for health care professionals. *Journal of Spinal Cord Medicine, 24*(Suppl. 1), S40-S101.

Currie, L., & Harvey, G. (1998). Care pathways development and implementation. *Nurs Stand, 12*(30), 35-38.

Davis, D. A., & Taylor-Vaisey, A. (1997). Translating guidelines into practice: A systematic review of theoretic concepts, practical experience and research evidence in the adoption of clinical practice guidelines. *Canadian Medical Association Journal, 157,* 408-416.

De Bleser, L., Depreitere, R., De Waele, K., Vanhaecht, K., Vlayen, J., Sermeus, W. (2006). Defining pathways. *Journal of Nursing Management, 14*(7), 553-563.

Dowsey, M. M., Kilgour, M. L., Santamaria, N. M., & Choong, P. F. (1999). Clinical pathways in hip and knee arthroplasty: a prospective randomised controlled study. *Medical Journal of Australia, 170,* 59-62.

Duncan, P. W., Zorowitz, R., Bates, B., Choi, J. Y., Glasberg, J. J., Graham, G. D., et al. (2005). Management of adult stroke rehabilitation care: A clinical practice guideline. *Stroke, 36,* e100-e143.

Dzwierzynski, W. W., Spitz, K., Hartz, A., Guse, C., & Larson, D. L. (1998). Improvement in resource utilization after development of a clinical pathway for patients with pressure ulcers. *Plastic and Reconstructive Surgery, 102,* 2006-2011.

Ellershaw, J., Foster, A., Murphy, D., Shea, T., & Overill, S. (1997). Developing an integrated care pathway for the dying patient. *European Journal of Palliative Care, 4,* 203-207.

Farquhar, C. M., Kofa, E. W., & Slutsky, J. R. (2002). Clinicians' attitudes to clinical practice guidelines: a systematic review. *Medical Journal of Australia, 177,* 502-506.

Field, M., & Lohr, K. N. (1990). *Clinical practice guidelines: Directions for a new program.* Washington, DC: National Academy Press.

Field, M., & Lohr, K. E. (1992). Guidelines for clinical practice: From development to use. Retrieved October 18, 2007, from http://www.nap.edu/openbook.php?record_id=1863&page=R1

Fritz, J. M., Delitto, A., & Erhard, R. E. (2003). Comparison of classification-based physical therapy with therapy based on clinical practice guidelines for patients with acute low back pain: A randomized clinical trial. *Spine, 28,* 1363-1371.

Garfield, F. B., & Garfield, J. M. (2000). Clinical judgment and clinical practice guidelines. *International Journal of Technology Assessment in Health Care, 16,* 1050-1060.

Graham, I. D., Beardall, S., Carter, A. O., Tetroe, J., & Davies, B. (2003). The state of the science and art of practice guidelines development, dissemination and evaluation in Canada. *Journal of Evaluation in Clinical Practice, 9,* 195-202.

Graham, I. D., Calder, L. A., Hebert, P. C., Carter, A. O., & Tetroe, J. M. (2000). A comparison of clinical practice guideline appraisal instruments. *International Journal of Technology Assessment in Health Care, 16,* 1024-1038.

Grimshaw, J. M., & Hutchinson, A. (1995). Clinical practice guidelines: Do they enhance value for money in health care? *British Medical Bulletin, 51,* 927-940.

Gross, A. R., Kay, T. M., Kennedy, C., Gasner, D., Hurley, L., Yardley, K. et al. (2002). Clinical practice guideline on the use of manipulation or mobilization in the treatment of adults with mechanical neck disorders. *Manual Therapy, 7,* 193-205.

Gulich, M., Engel, E. M., Rose, S., Klosterhuis, H., & Jackel, W. H. (2003). Development of a guideline for rehabilitation of patients with low back pain—phase 2: Analysis of data of the classification of therapeutic procedures. *Rehabilitation* (Stuttgart), *42*, 109-117.

Hadorn, D. C., McCormick, K., & Diokno, A. (1992). An annotated algorithm approach to clinical guideline development. *Journal of the American Medical Association, 267*, 3311-3314.

Harris, S. R., Hugi, M. R., Olivotto, I. A., & Levine, M. (2001). Clinical practice guidelines for the care and treatment of breast cancer: 11. Lymphedema. *Canadian Medical Association Journal., 164*, 191-199.

Hill, M. (1995). Integration of CareMap tools into the documentation system. In K. Zander (Ed.), *Managing outcomes through collaborative care: The application of core mapping and case management*. Chicago, IL: American Hospital Publishing.

Hunt, D. L., Haynes, R. B., Hanna, S. E., & Smith, K. (1998). Effects of computer-based clinical decision support systems on physician performance and patient outcomes: a systematic review. *Journal of the American Medical Association, 280*, 1339-1346.

Johnston, M. V., Wood, K., Stason, W. B., & Beatty, P. (2000). Rehabilitative placement of poststroke patients: reliability of the Clinical Practice Guideline of the Agency for Health Care Policy and Research. *Archives of Physical Medicine and Rehabilitation, 81*, 539-548.

Kitchiner, D. J., & Bundred, P. E. (1996). Integrated care pathways. *Archives of Disease in Childhood, 75*, 166-168.

Kitchiner, D. J., & Bundred, P. E. (1999). Clinical pathways. *Medical Journal of Australia, 170*, 54-55.

MacDermid, J. C. (2004). The quality of clinical practice guidelines in hand therapy. *Journal of Hand Therapy, 17*, 200-209.

MacDermid, J. C., Brooks, D., Solway, S., Switzer-McIntyre, S., Brosseau, L., & Graham, I. D. (2005). Reliability and validity of the AGREE Instrument used by physical therapists in assessment of clinical practice guidelines. *BMC Health Services Research, 5*, 18.

McKenna, H. P., Keeney, S., Currie, L., Harvey, G., West, E., Richey, R. H. (2006). Quality of care: A comparison of perceptions of health professionals in clinical areas in the United kingdom and the United States. *J Nurs Care Qua, 21*(4), 344-351.

Moulding, N. T., Silagy, C. A., & Weller, D. P. (1999). A framework for effective management of change in clinical practice: Dissemination and implementation of clinical practice guidelines. *Quality in Health Care, 8*, 177-183.

Pagliari, C., & Grimshaw, J. (2002). Impact of group structure and process on multidisciplinary evidence-based guideline development: An observational study. *Journal of Evaluation in Clinical Practice, 8*, 145-153.

Penn, A., Lau, F., & Wilson, D. (1996). An internet-based clinical guidance system for managing stroke. [On-line].

Pennington, J. M., Jones, D. P., & McIntyre, S. (2003). Clinical pathways in total knee arthroplasty: A New Zealand experience. *Journal of Orthopedic Surgery* (Hong Kong), *11*, 166-173.

Raw, M., McNeill, A., & West, R. (1998). Smoking cessation guidelines for health professionals. A guide to effective smoking cessation interventions for the health care system. Health Education Authority. *Thorax, 53*(Suppl. 5)Pt. 1, S1-19.

Rodin, M., Saliba, D., & Brummel-Smith, K. (2006). Guidelines abstracted from the Department of Veterans Affairs/Department of Defense clinical practice guideline for the management of stroke rehabilitation. *Journal of the American Geriatrics Society, 54*, 158-162.

Royal College of Nursing. (1999). Clinical guidelines for the recognition and assessment of acute pain in children. Recommendations and technical report. Retrieved October 18, 2007, from http://www.rcn.org.uk/development/practice/clinicalguidelines/pain

Savoie, I., Kazanjian, A., & Bassett, K. (2000). Do clinical practice guidelines reflect research evidence? *Journal of Health Services Research & Policy, 5*, 76-82.

Schaldach, D. E. (1997). Measuring quality and cost of care: evaluation of an amputation clinical pathway. *Journal of Vascular Nursing, 15*, 13-20.

Scholten-Peeters, G. G., Bekkering, G. E., Verhagen, A. P., Der Windt, D. A., Lanser, K., Hendriks, E. J., et al. (2002). Clinical practice guideline for the physiotherapy of patients with whiplash-associated disorders. *Spine, 27*, 412-422.

Scottish Intercollegiate Guidelines Network (2002). Managementt of early rheumatoid arthritis. A national clinical guideline. Retrieved October 22, 2007, from http://www.sign.ac.uk/pdf/sign48.pdf

Stradiotto, R. (1997). Clinical pathways in the continuum of care: Are they a defence to medical malpractice claims? Presentation to Clinical Pathways, Toronto, ON.

StrokEngine. (2007). Retrieved 4 September 2007, from www.medicine.mcgill.ca/Strokengine/index-en.html.

The AGREE Collaboration. (2001). Appraisal of guidelines for research and evaluation (AGREE) instrument. www agreecollaboration org. Retrieved October 18, 2007, from www.agreecollaboration.org.

The AGREE Collaboration (2003a). Appraisal of Guidelines for Research and Evaluation. http://www agreecollaboration org/pdf/aitraining pdf. Retrieved October 18, 2007, from http://www.agreecollaboration.org/pdf/aitraining.pdf.

The AGREE Collaboration (2003b). Development and validation of an international appraisal instrument for assessing the quality of clinical practice guidelines: The AGREE project. *Quality & Safety Health Care, 12*, 18-23.

The Center for Case Management, Inc. (n.d.). Retrieved October 22, 2007, from http://www.cfcm.com

The Chartered Society of Physiotherapy (1998). Guidelines for the management of soft tissue (musculoskeletal) injury with protection, rest, ice, compression and elevation (PRICE) during the first 72 hours. [On-line].

US Department of Health and Human Services (Public Health Service, A. f. H. C. P. a. R. (1995). Post-stroke rehabilitation: clinical practice guidelines, number 16. Retrieved October 18, 2007, from http://www.ncbi.nlm.nih.gov/books/bv.fcgi?rid=hstat6.chapter.27305

US Department of Health and Human Services (Public Health Service, A. f. H. C. P. a. R. (1996). Urinary incontinence in adults: acute and chronic management. Clinical practice guidelines. Retrieved October 18, 2007, from http://www.ncbi.nlm.nih.gov/books/bv.fcgi?rid=hstat6.chapter.9995

van der Sanden, W. J., Mettes, D. G., Plasschaert, A. J., Grol, R. P., & Verdonschot, E. H. (2004). Development of clinical practice guidelines: Evaluation of 2 methods. *Journal of the Canadian Dental Association, 70*, 301.

Vanhaecht, K., De Witte, K., Depreitere, R., Sermeus, W. (2006). Clinical pathway audit tools: A systematic review. *J Nurs Manag, 14*(7), 529-537.

Vlayen, J., Aertgeerts, B., Hannes, K., Sermeus, W., Ramaekers, D. (2005). A systematic review of appraisal tools for clinical practice guidelines: Multiple similarities and one common deficit. *Int J Qual Health Care, 17*(3), 235-242.

Whittle, C. L., McDonald, P., Dunn, L. (2004). Developing the integrated care pathways appraisal tool: A pilot study. *Journal of Integrated Care Pathways, 8*(2), 77-81.

Zander, K., & Hill, M. (1995). *Managing outcomes through collaborative practice: Integration of CareMap tools into the documentation system* (pp. 149-163). South Natick, MA: American Hospital Association.

BIBLIOGRAPHY

Alberta Health and Wellness. (2006). Alberta Wellnet. Alberta NetCare Site [On-line]. Retrieved October 18, 2007, from www.health.gov.ab.ca

Burgers, J., Grol, R., Klazinga, N., van der, B. A., Makela, M., & Zaat, J. (2003). International comparison of 19 clinical guideline programs--a survey of the AGREE Collaboration. Zeitschrift fur Arztliche Fortbildung und Qualitatssicherung, 97, 81-88.

Cancer Care Ontario Practice Guidelines Initiative: Care Paths in Oncology. (1999). Information from the Program in Evidence-Based Care (PEBC). Retrieved October 18, 2007, from http://www.cancercare.on.ca/index_practiceGuidelines.tml

Center for Case Management (2002). The new definition. The Center for Case Management [On-line]. Retrieved October 18, 2007, from http://www.cfcm.com/.

StrokeNet. (2006). StokeNet Information resources. StrokeNet [On-line]. Retrieved October 18, 2007, from http://www.strokenet.info/index.html.

Guide for the Uniform Data Set for Medical Rehabilitation (including the FIMTM Instrument), Version 5.1 (1997). Retrieved October 18, 2007, from http://www.udsmr.org/brochures.php

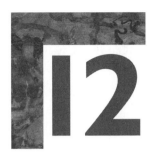

Communicating Evidence to Clients, Managers, and Funders

Linda Tickle-Degnen, PhD, OTR/L, FAOTA

LEARNING OBJECTIVES

After reading this chapter, the student/practitioner will be able to:
- Recognize the role that effective communication about evidence plays in being an evidence-based practitioner.
- Understand the various clinical roles of potential decision makers.
- Critically evaluate the body of evidence on a clinical situation, including distinguishing between different types of evidence.
- Use appropriate communication techniques to discuss the evidence and make treatment decisions based on the persons involved.

Imagine that next Monday you have your first appointment with Mr. Davis, a man with Parkinson's disease. As an evidence-based practitioner, you would seek recent research evidence on the daily lives of persons with this disease to supplement the knowledge you have accrued through your clinical experience and training. One important clinical outcome of gathering this evidence is that you would become a more knowledgeable practitioner. The evidence hopefully would inform your own practice actions. For example, during the appointed meeting time, you might have a list of issues to discuss with Mr. Davis and his family that is expanded beyond what you normally would have addressed. More importantly, beyond informing your own practice actions, you would possibly be able to expand Mr. Davis' knowledge in a manner that would enable him to become a collaborative partner in the clinical process. The more Mr. Davis knows about how his own life relates to others with similar circumstances, the more he can make reasoned choices that work for him.

The point of the above scenario is to demonstrate that the purpose of evidence gathering does not stop with the personal edification of the practitioner. The evidence is put to use to achieve many purposes, some of which require direct communication with others about the content of the evidence. A collaborative relationship requires this direct communication so that the client and family members become informed clinical partners. They are active rather than passive (i.e., they act with as much autonomy as possible and the least amount of dependency); clients and those acting on their behalf must be informed rather than uninformed or misinformed.

As an expert consultant, the therapist must directly communicate about evidence with other decision makers besides clients and their family members. The therapist talks about evidence with managers and funders of services so that management and funding decisions are informed. The focus of this chapter is on communicating about research evidence so that decision makers can make informed decisions that relate to clients' lives and the provision of rehabilitation services.

EFFECTIVELY COMMUNICATING EVIDENCE

Talking about evidence alone will not guarantee that decision makers will become more informed. The therapist must take steps to effectively communicate about the evidence. An effective communication regarding clinical evidence is one in which a message has not only been sent but also received, understood, and acted upon, a process called *knowledge utilization* (National Center for the Dissemination of Disability Research, 2005). A therapist may talk about evidence, but if the message is irrelevant, not framed in a manner that enables decision making and action, or incomprehensible, it will not be listened to, comprehended, and acted upon. Messages that are relevant, framed to enable decision making and action, and comprehensible are most effective for making a communication bridge between sender and receiver. Although the terms sender and receiver are used here, this is not to suggest that the information travels in a unidirectional path from therapist to the decision maker. Rather, as stated by the National Center for the Dissemination of Disability Research (1996), "...knowledge is not an inert object to be 'sent' and 'received,' but a fluid set of understandings shaped both by those who originate it and by those who use it" (p. 4). With this bidirectionality of knowledge construction as the underlying premise, this chapter describes four steps on the path to effective evidence-based communication:

1. Identify the clinical role of the decision maker with respect to the therapist.
2. Identify the decisions that the decision maker will be involved in making with the therapist.
3. Gather and interpret research evidence that is guided by the information needs of the decision maker and the clinical population of interest.
4. Translate the evidence into a comprehensible communication to facilitate an informed discussion with the decision maker.

Identify the Clinical Role of the Decision Maker With Respect to the Therapist

This chapter addresses three types of decision makers with whom therapists are likely to communicate—client or family member, manager, and funder. Effective communication begins with identifying the distinctions between the communication recipients' clinical roles and the contexts surrounding the performance of those roles. Different clinical roles generate different perspectives and needs. People are more likely to understand and respond to communication messages that are consistent with their own experiences and perspectives and based on their own needs, objectives, and preferences (National Council on Disability, 2003; Wills & Holmes-Rovner, 2003).

The clinical role of clients and family members is to receive therapy services to improve their lives. Communication with clients and family members often occurs face-to-face in periodic and repeated appointments. The clinical role of managers is to develop therapy programs; allocate resources, such as space, budget, materials, and staff support; and guide the therapist's provision of services. Managers must work within a set of multiple and complex organizational objectives (e.g., provide effective and efficient services to a particular population), initiatives (e.g., increase client satisfaction while increasing therapists' caseload), and constraints (e.g., limited building space). Communication with managers may occur frequently and informally, or infrequently and formally, and is often face-to-face. The clinical role of funders is to decide whether to fund the development of future clinical programs and the provision of current clinical services from an array of possible services and programs. Communication with funders is often formal and in written form.

Identify the Decisions That the Decision Maker Will Be Involved in Making With the Therapist

Communication is a two-way street. The therapist has a clinical role that intersects with the decision maker's clinical role, and together these roles determine what types of decisions will be important to communicate about. In rehabilitation, the therapist and client are concerned with helping the client to participate more competently and with more satisfaction in daily living and valued activities that occur in the home, community, and society at large. Throughout the chapter, the term *participation* is used to mean this activity and societal participation. The therapist and decision maker engage in three decision making tasks with respect to client participation outcomes:

1. *Description task*: Determine and describe participation issues that are relevant to a particular client population.

2. *Assessment task*: Select assessment procedures to measure client attributes related to participation.

3. *Intervention task*: Plan and implement intervention to maintain or improve client participation.

There are other tasks as well; however, these central ones are useful as a basis for demonstrating what types of information, or evidence, therapists will be most likely to communicate with decision makers. Decision making is required around all of these tasks, whether the decision making occurs in the context of direct service provision to clients, in the context of program development or resource allocation discussions with managers, or in the context of written communication with funders around program funding and service compensation.

- Clients and their family members need *descriptive* information from the therapist about the importance of participation in their lives. With this information they can begin to understand and give voice to their life experiences and begin to plan an adaptive course of action in response to their own rehabilitation needs. They need *assessment* and *intervention* information to make informed decisions related to choosing assessment and intervention procedures.

- Managers need *descriptive* information about participation from the therapist in order to develop and support clinical programs that are likely to be responsive to client rehabilitation needs. They need *assessment* and *intervention* information to decide which assessment and intervention procedures should be supported and provided by the organization.

- Funders need *descriptive* information about participation from the therapist in order to determine whether or not a clinical program addresses or will address, if in the planning

Table 12-1

ORGANIZING THE SEARCH FOR DESCRIPTIVE EVIDENCE TO DISCUSS WITH DIFFERENT DECISION MAKERS

Decision Maker	Decision Maker's Use of Evidence	Question That Guides the Search for Evidence
Client and family members	To understand and give voice to one's own life experience and to begin to plan an adaptive course of action.	What factors are associated with high quality of life and life satisfaction among 75-year-old men with Parkinson's disease?
Manager	To develop and support clinical programs that are likely to be responsive to client rehabilitation needs.	What factors are associated with high quality of life and life satisfaction among persons with Parkinson's disease?
Funder	To determine whether a clinical program will address important client rehabilitation needs.	Same question as for Manager.

phase, important client rehabilitation needs. They need to determine if there is a reasonable rationale for funding. They need *assessment* information to determine whether or not assessment procedures currently or will effectively document important attributes of clients and their responses to rehabilitation intervention. Finally, they need *intervention* information to decide whether or not the current or predicted level of effectiveness and feasibility of a clinical intervention program is worth funding.

Gather and Interpret Research Evidence That Is Guided by the Information Needs of the Decision Maker and the Clinical Population of Interest

Steps 1 and 2 provide a general conceptual territory for the kind of evidence that the therapist will have to gather to meet the needs of decision makers. At step 3, the therapist begins to narrow this territory to address the specific and unique needs of decision makers and the client population that is involved in the decisions. The therapist creates a clinical question to guide the retrieval of information (Sackett, Strauss, Richardson, Rosenberg, & Haynes, 2000). (See Chapter 5 for more information on this topic.) As the therapist gathers and interprets information, the therapist formulates possible answers to the question. The therapist then presents these possible answers to the decision maker for discussion.

Tables 12-1 through 12-3 show sample questions for organizing the gathering and interpretation of descriptive, assessment, and intervention evidence, separately for different types of decision makers. Each question is composed of at least three elements: the type of evidence that is being sought, an attribute related to participation, and a description of a clinical population.

Table 12-2

ORGANIZING THE SEARCH FOR ASSESSMENT EVIDENCE TO DISCUSS WITH DIFFERENT DECISION MAKERS

Decision Maker	Decision Maker's Use of Evidence	Question That Guides the Search for Evidence
Client and family members	To make informed decisions about participating in assessment procedures.	Is Goal Attainment Scaling a reliable and valid method for assessing personally meaningful goal achievement among 75-year-old men with Parkinson's disease?
Manager	To decide which assessment procedures should be supported and provided by the organization.	What are the most reliable and valid methods for assessing personally meaningful goal achievement among persons with Parkinson's disease?
Funder	To determine whether or not assessment procedures will effectively document important attributes of clients and their responses to rehabilitation intervention.	Same question as for Manager.

Keeping in mind this chapter's opening clinical scenario involving Mr. Davis, all of the questions in the tables are about the clinical population with Parkinson's disease.

The questions that guide the search for evidence for communicating with clients and their family members are written with the specific attributes of the client in mind (e.g., age and gender are specified). The questions that guide the search for evidence for communicating with managers and funders are written with a more general clinical population in mind. Based on the particular context and timing of decision-making activities, the therapist can develop the wording of the questions independently or in collaboration with the decision maker. The questions can be written with as much specificity or generality as is needed for decision making, as long as two conditions are met. The questions cannot be written so specifically that the evidence will be extremely restricted and hard to find (e.g., a question about quality of life [QOL] for 75-year-old men with Parkinson's disease who live in Minnesota and are retired business executives). Nor can they be written so generally that they would require lengthy evidence searching and synthesizing and be of no particular consequence to the decision makers (e.g., a question about concerns of patients in hospitals).

The questions vary across the three tables in terms of the type of evidence and the attribute of interests that are involved. The descriptive questions in Table 12-1 involve evidence about associations and attributes related to QOL and life satisfaction. The assessment questions in Table

Table 12-3

Organizing the Search for Intervention Evidence to Discuss With Different Decision Makers

Decision Maker	Decision Maker's Use of Evidence	Question That Guides the Search for Evidence
Client and family members	To make informed decisions about participating in intervention procedures.	What are the most effective and feasible occupational therapy interventions for achieving participation in successful and safe meal preparation among 75-year-old men with Parkinson's disease?
Manager	To decide which intervention procedures should be supported and provided by the organization.	What are the most effective and feasible occupational therapy interventions for achieving personally meaningful goals among persons with Parkinson's disease?
Funder	To decide whether or not the predicted level of effectiveness and feasibility of a clinical intervention program is worth funding.	Same question as for Manager.

12-2 involve evidence about reliability, validity, and attributes related to personally meaningful goal achievement. The intervention questions in Table 12-3 involve evidence about effectiveness, feasibility, and attributes related to meal preparation and, more globally, goal achievement. The attributes in all of these questions are the measured or outcome variables of interest in the research studies that the therapist retrieves in the literature search.

The emphasis in this chapter is on communicating about information from published research articles. This source of information is particularly important when the therapist does not have readily available data that have been systematically collected in his or her own setting. It should be noted, however, that in actuality, therapists will most likely draw upon a variety of information sources for meeting the decision-making needs of clients, managers, and funders. They can gather information by talking to clinical experts and clients, recalling their own clinical experience and training, and systematically collecting data in their clinical setting (Sackett et al., 2000).

Using key words or related words and synonyms in the questions to search the literature, the therapist retrieves research articles. Table 12-4 shows some possible terms that could be used to search for evidence relevant to the sample questions in Tables 12-1 through 12-3. The most effective and efficient use of the therapist's time is to first search for research syntheses and meta-analyses (with "synthesis" or "meta-analysis" as key words). These types of research articles

Table 12-4

SEARCH TERMS FOR THE SAMPLE QUESTIONS IN TABLES 12-1, 12-2, AND 12-3

Table	Type of Evidence		Participation Attribute		Client Population	
	Key Words	Related Words	Key Words	Related Words	Key Word	Related Words
12-1	Association	Correlation Regression Descriptive Qualitative Cross-sectional Longitudinal	Quality of life Life satisfaction	Well-being Coping Happiness Time use Daily activities Depression	Parkinson's Disease	Neurological Older adult Gerontology Geriatric Rehabilitation
12-2	Reliability Validity	Consistency Trustworthiness Assessment Outcome mea- sure Instrument Development	GAS Personally Meaningful Goal Achievement	Self-report Value Attainment Quality of life Personal Projects	Same as above	Same as above
12-3	Effectiveness Feasibility Occupational therapy interven- tion	Efficacy Outcome Rehabilitation Treatment Experiment Randomized trial Quasi-experiment	Same as above and Meal preparation	Same as above and cooking aids Food Activities of daily living	Same as above	Same as above

describe a whole body of research that might be relevant to answering a clinical question. Their strength is that they amass evidence in one location; however, this strength is the limitation of the research synthesis in that it may provide evidence that is highly summarized and general. Therefore, it is often useful to supplement synthesis and meta-analytic articles with research articles that report the findings from single studies to find detailed evidence about situations and issues related to the clinical population of interest. Once retrieved, the therapist must interpret the findings before communicating about them. The later section in this chapter, "Examples of Interpreting and Communicating Evidence," (see p. 273) gives details about how to interpret findings from sample research articles found in response to the questions in Tables 12-1 through 12-3. Chapter 7 also provides more information about systematic reviews of the evidence.

Translate the Evidence Into a Comprehensible Communication to Facilitate an Informed Discussion With the Decision Maker

Once the therapist has gathered and interpreted the evidence, it is time to have the direct face-to-face or written communication. By following steps 1 through 3, the therapist has assured that the evidence collected is important and relevant to the decision maker. Now the therapist must help make the evidence comprehensible. Individuals understand and retain information better when the content and presentation of the communication has the following attributes:

- Nontechnical, simple, and concrete language with simple grammatical structure, and words with few syllables, presented orally if possible.

- Terms that cross cultures and perspectives. The words and images have the same meaning for the sender and receiver of the communication. The communication is tailored to the decision maker's own words, messages, context, and preference for information format (e.g., words, pictures, or numbers).

- Brevity, with just enough detail for decision making. Limit the number of ideas expressed in the communication to three or less.

- Checks for confusion or lack of comprehension, perhaps by having the decision maker repeat back the information in his or her own words.

- Suggestions for concrete actions or choice options related to the information.

These attributes are discussed in the patient education literature (Davis et al., 1996; Doak, Doak, & Root, 1996; Griffin, McKenna, & Tooth, 2006; Redman, 1997; Schillinger et al., 2003; Wills & Holmes-Rovner, 2003; Wilson, 2003) and health literacy Web sites (Ebeling, 2003; Rudd, 2005; and links found at www.hsph.harvard.edu/healthliteracy). They apply to persons regardless of their level of education or comprehension. Although it is always best to use common, everyday language and simple phrasing, the therapist should be prepared to give a detailed report of synthesized evidence should the listener ask for this information.

For clients who have comprehension disabilities, limited education, or a primary language other than the therapist's, the therapist adjusts the language and concepts appropriately. In these cases, pictures and visual images are helpful supplements. It is important to keep distractions at a minimum and create a comfortable communication environment. Despite the listener's level of comprehension and scientific background, the therapist should allow enough time for the listener to absorb and discuss the communicated information before engaging in any decision making.

The most important attribute of the communication to keep in mind is that the therapist is providing possible answers, not the one correct answer, to a clinical question. Research with human beings is based on a model of tendencies and variations in living organisms and complex events, not upon determined facts. As a result, the therapist offers information to discuss, not to dictate. Examples for how to communicate about a body of evidence are given in the sections that follow.

EXAMPLES OF INTERPRETING AND COMMUNICATING EVIDENCE

Using a clinical case of a person with Parkinson's disease is useful for communicating about evidence because evidence relevant to this disease is not found easily in the rehabilitation literature. Such is the case with many of the clinical populations with whom therapists work. Despite this challenge, there is hope for the evidence-based therapist who works with populations about which there is seemingly little research evidence. There is a growing body of research on QOL and life satisfaction descriptions, assessments, and interventions for persons with chronic illness and disability. The terms *QOL* and *life satisfaction* tap into aspects of persons' lives related to their everyday participation in activities and satisfaction with their activities. Knowledge that these terms are highly relevant to therapists is one of the first steps in bridging the communication gaps that face the evidence-based therapist. In the next few sections, the case of Mr. Davis as an individual client and Parkinson's disease as a clinical population is used to demonstrate how the research literature is interpreted and communicated to clients and their family members, managers, and funders. Three types of evidence are discussed: descriptive, assessment, and intervention. There are two illustrations for each of these areas of evidence: one from an article that is a synthesis of more than one study and one from an article on a single study.

To begin interpreting the evidence given in each article, the therapist—let us call him or her Therapist Foster—must first determine if the research participants are relevant to Mr. Davis or the general population of clients with Parkinson's disease with whom he or she works at the clinic. For the findings to be highly relevant for discussion with Mr. Davis and his family, some of the research participants should be similar to him with respect to important attributes that could affect the answers to the clinical questions. These attributes of interest may be disease severity, gender, age, cultural background, marital status, and socioeconomic status. For the findings to be relevant for discussions with managers and funders, the participants should be similar to the Parkinson's disease population seen in Therapist Foster's own clinic. Table 12-5 summarizes the fictional characteristics of the case of Mr. Davis, as well as the therapist's Parkinson's disease caseload and the actual characteristics of research participants in six research articles that are reviewed in the sections below. Second, the therapist should determine what possible answers this study gives to the clinical questions that guided the search for the evidence. Therapist Foster will be concerned with answering those questions listed in Tables 12-1 through 12-3. Table 12-6 shows the types of data analytic findings that would most likely provide answers to the questions. Third, and finally, the therapist should determine the strength of the evidence in answering the questions by evaluating the quality of the study design, procedures, and measures.

Evidence That Describes the Lives and Needs of Clients With Parkinson's Disease

Interpretation of a Synthesis of Descriptive Studies

Using the clinical questions in Table 12-1 to organize a literature search, Therapist Foster found an article by Pinquart and Sörensen (2000) that reported the findings of a meta-analysis on subjective well-being in later life. Subjective well-being is a construct that encompasses QOL and life satisfaction concepts. The meta-analysis combined the findings of 286 research studies that examined well-being in relation to socioeconomic status; quantitative and qualitative aspects of older persons' social networks; and competence, defined as skills to manage basic, instrumental, and leisure daily life activities.

Therapist Foster begins the interpretation of this meta-analytic study by determining how relevant it is to Mr. Davis' case and to Therapist Foster's larger Parkinson's disease caseload. Table 12-5 shows that the meta-analysis included studies that had research participants similar to Mr.

Table 12-5

CHARACTERISTICS OF THE THERAPIST'S CLINICAL POPULATION AND THE REVIEWED STUDIES' RESEARCH PARTICIPANTS

Characteristic	Mr. Davis	Therapist Foster's Parkinson's Caseload	Pinquart & Sörensen (2000)	Koplas et al. (1999)	Stolee et al. (1999)[a]	Yip et al. (1998)	Murphy & Tickle-Degnen (2001)	Kondo et al. (1997)
Disease	Parkinson's	Parkinson's	Well and ill	Parkinson's	Diverse illnesses	Diverse illnesses	Parkinson's	Diverse illnesses
Degree of disability	Moderate	Mild to severe, inpatient and outpatient rehabilitation	None to severe	Mild to severe	Diverse, inpatients of geriatric rehabilitation unit	Diverse, inpatients of geriatric rehabilitation unit	Mild to severe	Fine/gross motor or vision disability
Age (in years)	75	≥50	≥55	51 to 87	61 to 96	Average of 77	Average of 70	62 to 92
Gender	Male	60% male 40% female	Male and female	59 males 27 females	40 males 133 females	55 males 88 females	Male and female	4 females 1 male
Race and ethnicity	Black, United States	Diverse races, United States	Race NR, N. America, Europe	79 White 5 Black 2 other	Race NR, Canada	Race NR, Canada	Race NR, N. America, Europe	Race NR, U.S.

Note: NR = not reported or unable to infer from article.
[a] This article presents three studies but the participant characteristics are from the third study. The authors did not report specific participant characteristics for the first two studies; however, those studies occurred in settings similar to the third study.

continued

Table 12-5, continued

CHARACTERISTICS OF THE THERAPIST'S CLINICAL POPULATION AND THE REVIEWED STUDIES' RESEARCH PARTICIPANTS

Characteristic	Mr. Davis	Therapist Foster's Parkinson's Caseload	Pinquart & Sörensen (2000)	Koplas et al. (1999)	Stolee et al. (1999)a	Yip et al. (1998)	Murphy & Tickle-Degnen (2001)	Kondo et al. (1997)
Work status	Retired banker	Retired	Diverse	75 retired 8 working 2 unemployed 1 homemaker	NR	NR	NR	Retired
Socio-economic status	Upper middle	Diverse	Diverse	Diverse	NR	NR	NR	NR

Note: NR = not reported or unable to infer from article.
a This article presents three studies but the participant characteristics are from the third study. The authors did not report specific participant characteristics for the first two studies; however, those studies occurred in settings similar to the third study.

Table 12-6

STUDY RESULTS THAT PROVIDE PROBABLE ANSWERS
TO DIFFERENT TYPES OF QUESTIONS

Type of Question	Data Analytic Results
Descriptive	General and unique qualitative themes, categories Means, medians, modes Frequency distributions, ranges, variances Sgn and magnitude of measures of association (e.g., r) and difference (e.g., d).
Assessment[a]	Reliability coefficients Validation coefficients and measures of difference (e.g., d, t, F)
Intervention	Mean and variation of change scores Magnitude of difference between intervention change and control change (e.g., r or d)[b] Confidence intervals Tests of significance (e.g., t, F)

[a] See Tables 12-7, 12-8, and 12-9 for more detail.
[b] See Table 12-10 for detail.

Davis in many respects. Although the meta-analysis included studies with participants who were chronically ill, it did not report information about specific diseases. However, some findings were reported separately for males and females and separately for participants of different age groups. Therefore, Therapist Foster could pay attention to the findings for males and the oldest adults for communicating with Mr. Davis.

Therapist Foster, having determined that the meta-analytic report is relevant, turns to locating the findings that will help to answer the clinical questions. Table 12-6 shows the types of findings that are often important to descriptive evidence. In the case of Pinquart and Sörensen's report (2000), correlations are the primary findings of interest. It was found that the higher the participants' socioeconomic status, the higher their life satisfaction (r = 0.17), but this association was smaller for adults who were 75 years and older (r = 0.10). The quality of social contacts had a higher association with life satisfaction (r = 0.22) than quantity of contacts (r = 0.12). The quality of contacts association was highest for participants over the ages of 70 (r = 0.29). Finally, the higher the participants' competence in basic and instrumental daily living skills, the higher their life satisfaction (r = 0.23) regardless of age. In general, the differences between genders in the associations appeared to be less relevant to Mr. Davis' case than the differences between different ages, so gender differences are not discussed here.

Two important pieces of evidence to note from the correlations described above are their signs and magnitude (i.e., how big they are). The signs are positive, indicating that on the average participants tended to have higher life satisfaction when they had higher socioeconomic status, stronger social networks, and more competence in performing daily living activities. As far as magnitude is concerned, Cohen (1988) suggests that correlations with absolute values of about 0.10 are of a small magnitude, of about 0.30 are of a moderate magnitude, and of about 0.50 or higher are of a large magnitude. Using these criteria, the magnitude of the correlations in the meta-analytic report of Pinquart & Sörensen (2000) were of a small to moderate magnitude. Another way of thinking about these magnitudes is that it was a small to moderate majority of people, not a large majority, that fell within the pattern of having high life satisfaction with high socioeconomic status, strong social networks, and competent performance, or of having low life satisfaction with low status, weak networks, and less competent performance. Another important piece of evidence is the statistical significance of the findings. The correlations and comparisons between correlations reported in the above paragraph were reported to be statistically significant below the traditional level of 0.05. This statistical significance indicates that the findings were strong enough, given the sample size, to feel confident in ruling out chance as the factor responsible for the strength. Studies that have large sample sizes, such as meta-analyses (this one having thousands of research participants represented), often have significant findings, thus effectively ruling out chance as an explanation for the magnitude of the findings.

Therapist Foster can take away from this examination of the Pinquart and Sörensen (2000) meta-analysis the following possible answer to the questions in Table 12-1: high quality of social contacts, continued competence in daily living activities, and socioeconomic status may be important aspects of life satisfaction for clients with Parkinson's disease. For Mr. Davis, in particular, socioeconomic status may not be an important factor unless he has financial concerns at this time. This possibility is based upon the meta-analytic findings that socioeconomic status was not an important QOL factor for participants who were at least 75 years old, the age of Mr. Davis.

Descriptive evidence, unless it is derived from experimental or, sometimes, from longitudinal studies, does not usually give strong indication of causality. The associations found in the Pinquart and Sörensen (2000) meta-analysis are not causal patterns despite the authors' questionable use of the word *influence* in the title and throughout the text, a word that implies causality.[1] The quality of social contacts could affect a person's life satisfaction, but the reverse could be true as well. A person who feels satisfied may engender high-quality social interactions. There may be a different, unmeasured factor that may explain why both life satisfaction and quality of contacts are high together or low together—perhaps, good physical and mental health. Descriptive evidence helps the therapist to understand possible patterns that exist in human behavior and experience, but it does not provide definitive prescriptions for intervention. Intervention decisions require evidence of a causal nature, as when individuals are randomly assigned to intervention and control conditions or when interventions are systematically provided and withdrawn. Descriptive evidence, on the other hand, helps a therapist to recognize potentially important client issues and to have a language for discussing and exploring these issues with clients, managers, and funders.

Interpretation of a Single Descriptive Study

There is a growing body of research that describes QOL issues for people with Parkinson's disease. Take for example a study by Koplas et al. (1999) that examined the association between QOL and the following factors: physical disability, depression, self-perceived mastery, and health locus of control. Table 12-5 shows that the participants in this study were similar to Mr. Davis and Therapist Foster's broader Parkinson's disease caseload in many respects. The associations between QOL and these factors were demonstrated with a multiple regression analysis and a multivariate analysis of variance. Many quantitative descriptive studies of QOL issues use complex statistical association analyses since QOL itself is a complex construct and there are many factors associated with it. The therapist, however, need not be an expert in multivariate analysis to glean evidence from the article.

One of the primary findings of this study was that mastery, which was defined as the degree to which an individual believes that his or her behavior can influence important personal outcomes, was found to have the largest association with QOL, with all the other measured factors being statistically controlled in the regression analysis. The association was statistically significant. No other association with QOL was found to be statistically significant in the regression model; however, this lack of significance may be an artifact of high correlations between mastery and the other factors, a possibility that the authors failed to discuss. Unfortunately, the authors did not present simple correlations, which would give a clearer picture of the findings. Nonetheless, Therapist Foster would still learn from the article, primarily through the text, the direction of the associations, and the relatively high magnitude of the mastery association relative to the other factors' associations. The higher the participants' mastery beliefs, the higher their self-reported QOL. The statistical significance suggests that the magnitude of the findings was not attributable to chance.

The authors provide some basic means and standard deviations that are informative. For example, they show the distribution of mastery scores separately for the early, middle, and late stages of the disease. Individuals in the middle stage group, who would be most similar to Mr. Davis in disease severity, had an average mastery score of 25.5 (on a possible scoring range of 10 through 40) with a standard deviation of 3.7. One property of a normal distribution of scores, described in any statistics textbook (e.g., Portney & Watkins, 2000), is that 68% of the sample's scores fall within one standard deviation, in either direction, of the average score. Another property is that 95% of the sample's scores fall within two standard deviations. Assuming that the scores are distributed normally, then 95% of the scores of individuals in the middle stage of the disease fall within the range of 25.5 − (2 x 3.7) = 18.1 to 25.5 + (2 x 3.7) = 32.9. This range of 18.1 to 32.9 indicates that there is variation from a relatively low mastery score to a relatively high mastery score among people in the middle stage of the disease.

Just as Pinquart and Sörensen (2000) suggest that the factors they describe "influence" subjective well-being, so do Koplas et al. (1999) draw indefensible causal implications from their correlational study. They infer from their findings that health care professionals may be able to improve their Parkinson's disease clients' QOL by trying to optimize clients' perceptions of control. A more appropriate take-into-the-clinic message would be to think of QOL as a multidimensional phenomenon that, for clients with Parkinson's disease, is likely to include feelings related to mastery.

Koplas et al. (1999) did not examine social networks as a possible factor associated with QOL; however, they did note that when participants were asked to discuss aspects of Parkinson's disease that were most difficult for them, the participants "frequently" (no statistical evidence given) discussed the loss of the ability to effectively communicate in speech and writing, difficulty in the workplace, loss of emotional control, and concerns with the progression of the disease.

Therapist Foster can take away from this examination of the Koplas et al. (1999) findings the following possible answer to the questions in Table 12-1: high feelings of mastery may be an important component of QOL among clients with Parkinson's disease. Mr. Davis and other clients currently may have low or high feelings of mastery. Other quality-of-life factors may be related to communication ability, workplace factors, emotional control, and thoughts about the progression of the disease.

Communication Examples for Descriptive Evidence

Therapist Foster would probably want to peruse other research articles about QOL and Parkinson's disease, but the two reviewed in this section provide enough evidence to compose initial communications to Mr. Davis, managers, and funders. The following example might be a way to begin a discussion with Mr. Davis:

> *I would like to get to know you better by discussing what it is like for you to go about your daily life while living with Parkinson's disease. It may be helpful for us to discuss*

some recent research findings about older people and people with Parkinson's disease. It has been found that people are more satisfied with life when they can continue to be with their friends and family members, have loving and good times with them, and give one another useful support and help. [Discuss]. It has also been found that being able to keep doing activities independently and skillfully is important for feeling satisfied with life for many people. [Discuss.] One study of people with Parkinson's disease found that many people are more satisfied with their lives when they feel in control over things that happen in their lives. Have you thought about whether or not you feel in control and whether or not this matters to you? [Discuss.] Communication can be a problem for people with Parkinson's disease. Is this a concern for you? [Discuss, and raise other remaining issues in a similar fashion]. We've talked a lot about what makes life satisfying and worth living for you today. Are there any changes in your day-to-day life that would make your life more satisfying to you, your wife, and others who are important to you?

The wording in this communication example may be too complex or too simple for Mr. Davis. One way to assess the complexity of this example, as suggested by health literacy experts (Griffin et al., 2006; Rudd, 2005) is to type out the communication and score its readability using Microsoft Word's readability calculations under its speller and grammar check tool. Using this tool, the above example contains 229 words, has 16.3 words per sentence on the average, and requires a comprehension level at the eighth-grade level in the United States. In comparison, a study of written occupational therapy education material for older clients found that this material required clients to have a reading level between the ninth and tenth grades (Griffin et al., 2006). Therefore, the communication example is simpler than what is generally found in occupational therapy. However, health literacy advocates advise that oral and written patient education material be presented at no more than the fifth-grade level, even for individuals who have higher comprehension ability (Wilson, 2003). The example below is a modified and less complex version of the previous example. It contains 150 words, 10 words per sentence on the average, and requires a fifth-grade comprehension level:

I would like to get to know you better by talking about your daily life. Let's start by talking about some studies of older people. These studies find that people feel good about life when they have loving and good times with family and friends. [Discuss]. People also feel good about life when they can do things by themselves and do them well. [Discuss.] One study found that many people with Parkinson's disease feel better when they feel in control over things in their lives. Do you feel in control over things? Does this matter to you? [Discuss.] Communication can be a problem for people with Parkinson's disease. Is this a concern for you? [Discuss, and raise other remaining issues in a similar fashion]. We've talked about what makes you feel good. Are there any changes in your life that would that would make you and your family feel better?

A communication with a manager or funder could be stated more formally. It could be used to start a discussion about the development of an evidence-based rehabilitation program for a Parkinson's disease population. If the communication is in written form, it is appropriate to include research literature citations and to have more complex wording. The example that follows contains 140 words (not including the citations), has an average of 35 words per sentence, and requires very high comprehension ability (20.7):

A research synthesis [Pinquart & Sörensen, 2000] found that older people, including those with chronic illnesses, had higher life satisfaction when they had active and high quality relationships with friends and family members, were able to perform their daily living and leisure activities competently, and were of a higher socioeconomic status. A study [Koplas et al., 1999] of people with Parkinson's disease, in particular, found that people with high feelings of mastery were more likely to report having a high quality of life than people with low feelings of mastery, regardless of their level of disability or depression. Further quality-of-life concerns in this Parkinson's disease sample were the ability to communicate in speech and writing, difficulties in the workplace, loss of emotional control, and concerns about disease progression. These quality-of-life factors should be taken into consideration when developing a rehabilitation program for people with Parkinson's disease.

Evidence That Guides the Choice and Use of Assessment Tools for Clients With Parkinson's Disease

Every score or conclusion drawn from an assessment procedure is a measure of several simultaneous elements; the client's performance is only one of those elements. Other elements are called error and include the context of the assessment, the attributes of the therapist, and the testing tool itself. For example, a measure of a client's dressing performance could also be a measure of the client's familiarity with the room in which the dressing is performed and with the clothing used; a measure of the therapist's emotions, expectations, and behavior with the client; and a measure of the scale used in scoring. Imagine a client putting on an unfamiliar blouse, in an unfamiliar environment, with a harried therapist who was using a two-point rating scale (0 = dependent, 1 = independent) to judge the performance. Now imagine this client putting on a familiar blouse, in a familiar environment, with a relaxed therapist who was using a five-point scale (graduated from 0, requires another to perform every step to 4, able to perform every step with no assistance) to judge the performance. This client may receive two very different recommendations based upon these two testing situations; perhaps a recommendation for further rehabilitation in the first situation and for immediate discharge home in the second. Standardized assessment procedures that are reliable and valid are, by definition, less likely to result in inconsistent and incorrect conclusions compared to unstandardized, low reliability or low validity procedures. Obviously, therapists, clients, funders, and managers do not want to waste the client's and therapist's time and resources in assessments that will result in incorrect conclusions. More importantly they want assessments to generate correct clinical recommendations that have the potential for improving client outcomes.

The challenge of the evidence-based practitioner is to use assessment procedures that have demonstrated reliability and validity, are feasible in the therapist's clinical context, and are the right fit for the client. The research literature on the measurement properties of assessment procedures uses a dizzying array of terminology to discuss and report reliability and validity findings. What is most crucial to the selection of an assessment tool is whether or not that tool has been tested for the particular forms of reliability and validity most pertinent to the purpose of the assessment. See Tables 12-7, 12-8, and 12-9 for common forms, methods, and standards derived from a quantitative paradigm that are used with many assessments relevant to rehabilitation.

Interpretation of a Synthesis of Assessment Studies

Using the clinical questions in Table 12-2 to organize a literature search, Therapist Foster found an article by Stolee et al. (1999) that reviewed two previous studies by their research group and a newly completed one. The researchers studied the measurement properties of Goal Attainment Scaling (GAS) with a geriatric rehabilitation population. Table 12-5 shows that there were participants in this study that were similar to Mr. Davis and Therapist Foster's broader Parkinson's disease caseload with respect to age and disability. Let us assume that

Table 12-7

A RELIABILITY PRIMER

Form of Reliability	Tested when the score or assessment conclusion is expected to be consistent across different ...	Examples of assessments that should demonstrate an adequate degree of this form of reliability	The degree of reliability is commonly summarized with a coefficient that represents the consistency between different raters, times, or items, such as...	What is an "adequate" degree of reliability?
Interrater	Therapists or raters.	Therapist's judgment of ADL independence from observing client's performance. Therapist's summary of a client's feelings or experiences.	Correlation (e.g., intra-class). Cohen's kappa. Percentage agreement.	>0.70 >0.40 > 80%
Test-retest	Testing times, as long as the client has not changed.	Client's ADL performance before receiving intervention. An interest checklist.	Correlation (e.g., intra-class). Difference in standard deviation units (e.g., d).	>0.70 <0.20
Internal Consistency	Items of a measure.	A 20-item short-term memory test. A 10-item self-esteem questionnaire	Correlation. Cronbach's alpha.	>0.40 >0.70

Note: Reliability testing methods and standards vary across different research areas. See a research methods textbook (e.g., Portney & Watkins, 2000) for general and common methods and interpretation standards.

Table 12-8

A VALIDITY PRIMER I

General Form of Validity	Tested when the score or assessment conclusion is expected to be a valid (true) measure of...	Why Tested?	Specific Forms of Validity Testing (See Table 12-9)
Descriptive	Current client attributes at one point in time, such as current ADL performance or feelings about self.	To see if the measure differentiates between clients who have different attributes.	Content Criterion-related Construct
Predictive	Client attributes in the future, such as ability to successfully perform work activities or to adjust to disability.	To see if the current measurement predicts future attributes.	Content Criterion-related Construct
Evaluative	Change over time in client attributes, such as change in ADL performance, change in feelings of self-efficacy.	To see if the measure is responsive to change in the client.	Content Criterion-related Construct

Note: Validity testing terminology, methods, and standards vary across different research areas (see Portney & Watkins, 2000).

Mr. Davis is coming to Therapist Foster as an outpatient, whereas the participants in the study were inpatients. Stolee et al.'s research participants were predominantly female, unlike Mr. Davis and Therapist Foster's caseload, but males were represented in the sample. Finally, the participants were in Canada rather than the United States, but Canada and the United States are similar in that they are Western cultures that put strong values on individual goal achievement. The research participants were of unknown race and socioeconomic status, so they cannot be compared to the therapist's caseload in this respect.

With GAS, clients and therapists create individualized goals and then measure the achievement of the goals against a graded set of behavioral outcomes. Even though the goals can be different for every client, the score derived from the GAS can be compared and averaged across different clients in a meaningful way. The higher the score, the more successfully the client and therapist achieved the goals. For example, suppose Mr. Davis wanted to be able to cook more quickly and with less spilling. His meal preparation activities have declined in quality and efficiency as his tremors, bradykinesia, and fatigue have increased. A goal for Mr. Davis' meal

Table 12-9

VALIDITY PRIMER II

Specific Form of Validity	Addresses the Question…	Example	How This Form of Validity is Assessed	What is an "Adequate" Degree of Validity?
Content	Does the content of the measure cover all aspects or elements of the attribute being measured?	Does a basic ADL instrument measure all important self-care activities?	Documented expert opinion. Comparison with relevant theory.	Relative congruence between content and expert opinion. There is a logical direct relationship between the measure and theory.
Criterion-related	Does the score or conclusion drawn from the measure relate to a score or conclusion drawn from a valid criterion?	Does the score from a new ADL instrument (the one that is yet to be validated) lead to the same conclusions as a score from an established ADL instrument?	Administration of both new and established measure to clients and calculation of correlation between the two measures.	A level of association that should theoretically exist between the two (e.g., r > 0.60).
		Do clients with brain damage have a different score on a cognitive test than clients without brain damage?	Administration of the test to different populations of clients and comparison of the scores.	A difference that should theoretically exist between the two (e.g., d > 0.30).
		Do clients who are known to have improved their ability to drive show this improvement in a new driving test?	Administration of a test before and after an intervention and comparison of the two scores.	A difference that should theoretically exist between the two (e.g., d > 0.80).

continued

Table 12-9, continued

VALIDITY PRIMER II

Specific Form of Validity	Addresses the Question...	Example	How This Form of Validity is Assessed	What is an "Adequate" Degree of Validity?
Construct (convergent and discriminant)	Does the score or conclusion drawn from the measure relate more to validated measures of the same attribute than to validated measures of a different attribute?	Does a dementia test relate more to another dementia test than it does to a test of depression?	Administration of measures designed to measure similar and different attributes and comparisons of the relationships between the various measures.	Larger correlations between similar measures compared to smaller correlations between different measures.

Note: Validity is not normally determined by comparison to one absolute standard. It is established through a variety of means that make scientific and theoretical sense and is best determined by comparison with standards in a specific field of research.

preparation activities would be scaled from −2, the worst plausible outcome, such as the home delivery of meals, to +2, the best plausible outcome, such as the efficient and safe preparation of nutritious and pleasant meals.

Stolee et al. (1999) found that interrater reliability of the GAS outcome score was high, ranging from intraclass correlations of 0.87 to 0.93 across the three studies. An earlier study had found beginning evidence of adequate interrater reliability for the development of the goals. In addition to reliability findings, Stolee et al. reported evidence related to several types of descriptive and evaluative validity. A descriptive form of content validity was supported through an analysis of the content of individualized goals. The goals were found to fall into 10 primary categories (including mood/motivation and cognition, but predominantly activities of daily living (ADL), future care, and mobility), all of which were appropriate for geriatric inpatient rehabilitation needs. Descriptive and evaluative forms of criterion-related validity were reported as well. In terms of descriptive validity, the GAS outcome scores were highly correlated with outcome scores on the Barthel Index (r's ranging from .59 to .86) and with scores on the Older Americans Resources and Services (OARS) Index of Instrumental Activities of Daily Living (r = 0.54). These correlations suggest that the GAS can be used to measure goal achievement related to ADL. Evaluative criterion-related validity was demonstrated on change scores, from before to after rehabilitation. Change on the GAS correlated with change on the Barthel (r = 0.60) and the OARS (r = 0.48). In addition, the standardized response mean, a measure of the magnitude of the change in the score in standard deviation units, was 1.73 for the GAS compared to 0.97 and 0.80 for the Barthel and the OARS. This finding means that participants' scores increased by more than one standard deviation on the GAS, whereas their scores increased by almost one standard deviation on the two ADL measures. All of these magnitudes are considered large (> 0.80 according to Cohen, 1988). Other validity tests consistently suggested the GAS to adequately describe differences in goal achievement among the participants and to adequately evaluate changes in goal-related behaviors from before to after rehabilitation.

Stolee et al. (1999) also began an investigation of the descriptive and evaluative construct validity of the GAS scores. They found that the GAS outcome and change scores correlated more highly with the ADL outcome and change scores than with scores on a QOL measure. This finding was unexpected but several explanations are possible. Stolee et al. noted that ADL and mobility problems were the most prevalent presenting problems in the research participants, and possibly goals addressing these problems are not QOL goals, or at least, not a comprehensive representation of QOL goals. Alternatively, there may have been a validity problem with the QOL measure given that many of the participants reported that the questions on the measure were inappropriate for their situation (no details given).

Together these findings suggest a possible answer to the questions in Table 12-2: GAS is a reliable and valid method for assessing goal achievement among individuals in a geriatric rehabilitation program. It is one possible method to be compared against others for determining which is the most reliable and valid one for assessing goal achievement in a Parkinson's disease population.

Interpretation of a Single Assessment Study

The GAS may be an appropriate tool for measuring goal achievement; however, the traditional form of GAS takes extra work compared to simpler rating scales or checklists. The extra work and time needed to make meaningful, measurable, and consistently set goals for each client in a busy clinical setting may not be feasible. Therapist Foster might continue to search the literature to determine if there were other individualized goal achievement measures with acceptable measurement properties. The therapist might find a study by Yip et al. (1998) that tested a simpler, less time-consuming version of GAS. The research participants in this study were similar to that of Stolee et al.'s (1999), as shown in Table 12-5. Yip et al. reported the development of a standardized menu to use with GAS. This menu, which operates as a checklist, retains the primary elements of GAS. The authors reported the new form of the GAS to be feasible, with goal setting taking 10 to 15 minutes per client and subsequent attainment discussions taking 2 to 3 minutes. These steps were completed during team conferences with the client and family members' preferences in mind but not with these individuals present. Yip et al. did not report interrater reliability for the menu. They reported the standardized menu to have acceptable content validity, with content similar to that reported by Stolee et al. In addition, Yip et al. found that evaluative criterion-related validity coefficients were supportive of sufficient validity but were of a slightly lower magnitude than those found with the traditional GAS in Stolee et al.'s study. The correlation between the GAS menu form outcome score and the changes on standardized ADL measures (including the Barthel and OARS) ranged from 0.43 to 0.45, compared to the 0.48 to 0.60 found in Stolee et al.'s study. This is probably not a meaningful validity difference. The standardized response mean, a measure of the magnitude of the change in the score in standard deviation units, was 1.56 for the menu GAS compared to 0.82 and 0.72 for the Barthel and the OARS, respectively. This finding was similar to that for the more traditional GAS.

This study builds the repertoire of possible answers to the questions in Table 12-2: the measurement properties of the menu GAS suggest that it would be an equally adequate, yet more feasible, measure of goal attainment than the traditional GAS in a busy clinical setting.

Communication Examples of Assessment Evidence

Therapist Foster would probably want to find syntheses and study reports about other goal attainment and client-centered assessments (McColl & Pollock, 2005), but the two reviewed in this section provide enough evidence to compose initial communications to Mr. Davis, managers, and funders. The following example might be a way to begin a discussion with Mr. Davis and his wife, who comes with Mr. Davis to every rehabilitation appointment. It includes 84 words, has 10.4 words per sentence on the average, and requires a fifth-grade comprehension level. The terms *validly* and *reliably* have not been included in this example because they require a high level of technical understanding and are not needed to convey the information necessary for decision making. Rather the term *good* is used to convey the quality of the assessment procedure.

> One of the first steps of rehabilitation is to determine your needs and goals. One good method is to talk about goals together and then write them down. [Discuss examples based upon some needs already identified with Mr. Davis.] Then we work together to meet these needs and goals. First we work on the easiest goals. [Give examples.] We can write the goals ourselves or check off goals that are already written on a checklist. Would you like to try writing the goals ourselves?

A communication with a manager or funder could be stated more formally, as in the example below, to start a discussion about the development of assessment tools in rehabilitation with a Parkinson's disease population. If the communication is in written form, it is appropriate to include research literature citations. The example that follows contains 186 words (not including the citations), has 13.7 words per sentence on the average, and requires a college sophomore comprehension level:

> The geriatric rehabilitation literature has demonstrated that Goal Attainment Scaling is one reliable and valid procedure for writing rehabilitation goals with clients like those with Parkinson's disease [Stolee et al., 1999]. One form of the scaling is to identify goal areas, such as dressing, mobility, or visiting friends, that are important

for an individual client, and then to write a series of concrete behavioral objectives related to each goal area. Usually five objectives are written and graded from the worst to best possible outcome for the client. Because the development of objectives can be somewhat time-consuming, another form of doing the scaling has been created [Yip et al., 1998]. This form involves a behavioral outcome checklist that is completed for each client. This form, like the other one, has been found to demonstrate good interrater reliability as well as descriptive and evaluative validity. The scaling has been used effectively to both plan the intervention programs for individual clients as well as to evaluate their progress in response to intervention. Both forms yield scores that can be entered into a database for tracking outcomes of therapy. [Describe and compare other client-centered assessment tools.]

Evidence That Guides the Choice of Interventions Used With Clients With Parkinson's Disease

Suppose that Mr. Davis decides to try GAS with the therapist to develop and track the achievement of his rehabilitation goals. Through discussion with Mr. and Mrs. Davis, Therapist Foster finds that successfully and safely preparing meals is a major concern for the couple. Since Mrs. Davis' stroke some years back, Mr. Davis has assumed primary responsibility in preparing meals. He derives satisfaction from his ability to prepare nutritious and delicious meals. Over the years, as his symptoms of bradykinesia and tremors have increased, he has found it fatiguing and inefficient to prepare meals. He also worries that he will burn himself or spill cooked food as he pulls it out of the oven, which is at knee level. Both he and his wife are concerned that the meals are not as nutritious or satisfying as they once were because Mr. Davis has reduced the amount and type of food that he prepares. With the therapist, Mr. Davis and his wife write goal attainment levels aimed at improving the success and safety of Mr. Davis' meal preparation activities. Next, based on the clinical question in Table 12-3, the therapist searches for the latest evidence on interventions for improving meal preparation performance among individuals like Mr. Davis. Table 12-3 also shows a broader question for communication with managers and funders that addresses client-centered intervention designed to achieve clients' personally meaningful goals.

Interpretation of a Synthesis of Intervention Studies

To start to develop possible answers to these questions, Therapist Foster retrieves a meta-analysis published in the rehabilitation literature that examined the effectiveness of rehabilitation-related interventions for persons with Parkinson's disease (Murphy & Tickle-Degnen, 2001). Table 12-5 demonstrates that the participants in the studies included in the meta-analysis are similar to the therapist's Parkinson's disease population in many respects. After determining that the meta-analysis is relevant to this population, the therapist looks for the major meta-analytic result, which is the average effect size estimate. Meta-analysts convert every relevant statistical finding to an effect size that can be averaged across all studies. Tests of significance (such as t or F and their p values) cannot be compared across studies because their magnitudes are a function of both the size of the effect and the sample size (Rosenthal & Rosnow, 1991). The most common estimates of effect size used in the rehabilitation and psychological literature are the effect size r and the effect size d. Table 12-10 shows interpretations and calculations for these effect sizes. The magnitude of the effect size (i.e., how big it is) is an estimate of the degree to which two conditions (such as intervention versus control) differ in terms of their therapeutic effectiveness. Alternatively, the magnitude is the degree to which involvement in intervention had a more successful or beneficial outcome for research participants than involvement in a control condition. Better average outcomes for the intervention versus control conditions are indicated by a positive

Table 12-10

EFFECT SIZES AND SUCCESS RATES

d Success Rates

Magnitude of Effect[a]	d	Control	Intervention	Change
Zero	0	50%	50%	0
Small	.20	46%	54%	8%
Medium	.50	40%	60%	20%
Large	.80	34%	66%	32%
Very Large	2.00	16%	84%	68%

r Success Rates

Magnitude of Effect[a]	r	Control	Intervention	Change
Zero	0	50%	50%	0
Small	.10	45%	55%	10%
Medium	.24	38%	62%	24%
Large	.37	32%	69%	37%
Very Large	.71	15%	86%	71%

Notes: [a] Based on Cohen (1988) and Rosenthal & Rosnow (1991). See Tickle-Degnen (2001) for calculation details.

effect size, equal average outcomes by a 0 effect size, and worse average outcomes by a negative effect size, regardless of whether the effect size is measured as an r or a d.

Murphy and Tickle-Degnen (2001) found the average effect size of 16 studies was $r = 0.26$. The effect size was statistically significant ($p < 0.0001$), indicating chance was not a reasonable explanation for the effect. The magnitude of effect was essentially the same regardless of whether the measured outcome of the intervention was change in a capacity, such as motor coordination or depression, or an activity performance, such as ADL or functional mobility. This r of 0.26 can be compared to the r column in Table 12-10. In that column, there is an r of 0.24, which is very close to 0.26. Such a magnitude of r is considered to be of "medium" or "moderate" size for intervention effects (Cohen, 1988; Rosenthal & Rosnow, 1991).[2]

The effect size r is a point-biserial correlation or partial correlation coefficient that indicates the degree to which the independent variable (intervention versus control) is associated with the outcome scores. Rosenthal and Rubin (1982) have shown that the magnitude of the r, when multiplied by 100%, can most easily be understood as an estimate of the change in success rates across two conditions. They created a practical tool, called the Binomial Effect Size Display, for translating the effect size r into intervention success rates. Success is defined here as receiving a score that is higher than the combined average of both conditions, and failure as receiving a lower than average score. Table 12-10 shows that for a moderate size r of 0.24, 62% of the participants who received intervention had a successful outcome relative to 38% of the participants in the control condition who had a successful outcome. Since 62% minus 38% is equal to 24%, the success rate increases by 24% from the control to the intervention conditions. These success rates, which are essentially equivalent to those for r = 0.26, indicate that rehabilitation intervention was successful for more people with Parkinson's disease than was the control condition, and the failure rate was lower for the intervention than control condition.

The other common effect size in the rehabilitation literature is d, which can be directly converted to or from r (see Tickle-Degnen, 2001 for details) or can be calculated directly from the means and standard deviations of reported outcome findings. The effect size d is the difference between the mean outcomes for two conditions in standard deviation units. A d of 0.50 means that the average intervention outcome was one-half of a standard deviation higher than the average control outcome. Table 12-10 shows that a d of 0.50 is equivalent to an r of 0.24. For the same magnitude of intervention effect, the d-related success rates are slightly different from the r-related rates, but either one gives a useful approximation of the difference in success rates. If Therapist Foster made a practice of noting or calculating effect sizes from research reports, he or she would know that an intervention effect of d = 0.50 or r = 0.24 is of a magnitude often found in effective rehabilitation interventions with older adults (Carlson, Fanchiang, Zemke, & Clark, 1996; de Goede, Keus, Kwakkel, & Wagenaar, 2001), including client-centered ones in which clients are involved in developing their own goals (Clark et al., 1997). It is important to note that the effect size found in these studies as well as that found by Murphy and Tickle-Degnen (2001) indicates that there was still a number of older clients, approximately 40%, for whom rehabilitation intervention was not successful, and a number of clients, also approximately 40%, for whom the control condition was successful.

The findings of the meta-analysis offer possible answers to the second question in Table 12-3, the one posed for communication with managers and funders: it is likely that it would be beneficial for Therapist Foster's population of Parkinson's clients to take part in rehabilitation. However, as with many forms of intervention, there is no guarantee that rehabilitation will provide a greater benefit to all clients than no treatment or other forms of treatment.

Interpretation of a Single Intervention Study

Therapist Foster may continue to search the literature for evidence specifically related to Mr. Davis' desire to improve functioning in meal preparation. A study by Kondo et al. (1997) examined the use of microwave ovens as an intervention to improve meal preparation functioning among five older adults with disabilities. Although none of the participants had Parkinson's disease, they were disabled and living in the community like Mr. Davis, as shown in Table 12-5. Participants kept a daily log of their frequency of using cooking appliances, number of food items they prepared, and duration of meal preparation during four systematically applied phases of intervention and nonintervention, each of 3 weeks duration. During the first phase, there was no intervention; the participants used their normal cooking appliances. Then they were given a microwave oven and trained in its use. The second phase consisted of having the microwave oven available for use in their homes. In the third phase, the microwave oven was withdrawn, and in the fourth phase it was replaced. The researchers presented the findings with means and standard deviations at each phase, as well as frequency graphs that showed changes in the outcome variables within and across each phase.

This type of study and data presentation can be very useful for evidence-based therapists because the therapist is given access to qualitative and quantitative details about each participant. As a result, the therapist can directly examine similarities and differences in responses across different clients. Therapist Foster would see that, overall, the participants were able to cook more easily and with less time when the microwave oven was available to them than when it was not. In terms of meal preparation time, for example, a visual inspection of the means and graphs shows that cooking time decreased from phases 1 to 2 and 3 to 4, each time with the introduction of the microwave oven. For example, participant 3 took an average of 41 minutes in meal preparation during phase 3 without the microwave oven and 29 minutes with the reintroduction of the appliance. This 12-minute change is a 29% reduction in time. In terms of the effect size d, the average time in the fourth phase was 1.26 standard deviations below the average time in the third phase. Therapist Foster calculated this effect size by dividing the 12-minute difference by the standard deviation of meal preparation time during the nonintervention third phase. This large effect size d is the magnitude of the time decrease relative to participant 3's own normal variation in preparation time.

Among the five participants in general, there was a decrease in preparation time of 17 minutes on the average, ranging from an 8- to 30-minute decrease. The average of the participants' d's was 1, a large effect. On the average, the participants had a preparation time with the microwave that was one standard deviation below their preparation time without a microwave. From these findings, Therapist Foster can derive a possible answer to the first question in Table 12-3, the one addressed specifically to Mr. Davis' goal: a microwave may help Mr. Davis to meet his meal preparation goal.

Communication Examples of Intervention Evidence

The therapist might begin the communication with Mr. Davis about the intervention evidence in the manner below. This communication involves 74 words, has an average of 14.8 words in a sentence, and requires almost a seventh-grade comprehension level.

> *Studies show that some clients with Parkinson's disease do fine without therapy. These studies also suggest that therapy helps the majority of clients do things easier and better. One study found that it was helpful to give people microwave ovens and teach them how to use them. People ate more variety of foods and cooked faster when they used these ovens. Let's talk more about how to meet your goal to make good meals.*

Health literacy experts suggest that clients receive both an oral presentation about information as well as supplementary materials written in plain language (Rudd, 2005). One recommended "plain language" Web site, and one appropriate for Mr. Davis' needs, is that developed by the U.S. Food and Drug Administration located at www.fda/gov/opacom/lowlit/englow.html. It contains a brochure called Eating Well as We Age (FDA 00-2311) that might be a useful supplement to Therapist Foster's oral communication.

In all of the client communication examples in this chapter, no numbers have been used. Clients vary in their level of understanding of percentages, proportions, and graphical representations of data (Wills & Holmes-Rovner, 2003). It is important to remember that some clients may prefer to know the numbers and the therapist should be comfortable with providing statistical information or gathering it for the client if the client desires it.

On the other hand, for a communication to managers or funders, a more statistical frame for the communication is appropriate typically. In the example that follows, there are 167 words (not including the citations), with an average of 27.8 words per sentence, and the required educational level for comprehension of the message is a 4-year undergraduate college degree:

> *Recent meta-analyses of rehabilitation intervention with older clients in general and Parkinson's disease clients in particular have found intervention to have a larger positive outcome relative to control interventions [Carlson et al., 1996; de Goede et al., 2001; Murphy & Tickle-Degnen, 2001]. The effect is of a moderate magnitude, such that 62% of research participants who received intervention had a successful outcome relative to 38% of the participants in the control condition who had a successful*

outcome. There are many types of individualized interventions that may be effective for clients, dependent upon their own needs and goals. For example, a study with a small sample single-subject design [Kondo et al., 1997] found a large and positive effect of microwave ovens on the meal preparation activities of older individuals with physical disabilities. The meals of these participants had more variety and took less time to prepare when they had a microwave oven available, for which they had received training, compared to when they used their standard cooking appliances. The research evidence supports the provision of rehabilitation services to older individuals with Parkinson's disease.

EVIDENCE-BASED COMMUNICATION IN THE FACE OF UNCERTAINTY

When the search for evidence has turned up a recent and high-quality published literature review or meta-analysis, the integration that is needed has already been completed by the published author. The therapist need only translate the technical language and presentation of these reviews into language understandable to decision makers. However, if no such review has been found, the therapist must make an accurate integration him- or herself. Such integration takes skill, which develops with the study of research methods and the practice of having to communicate clearly about a body of evidence. Among the guidelines to follow when making an integrated interpretation of a body of evidence are the following two (Tickle-Degnen, 2000):

- Give heavier emphasis to studies that provide more accurate (stronger) evidence than to those studies with potentially less accurate (weaker) evidence. The therapist should refer to the sections of standard research methods textbooks (Portney & Watkins, 2000) that address how to evaluate the internal and external validity, or accuracy, of studies.

- When examining statistics, do not rely solely on significance tests and their p-values for determining what the study found unless the study involved a large sample size, roughly about 60 or more participants. Studies that have large sample sizes have more power to detect a statistically significant effect than studies with small sample sizes (Ottenbacher & Maas, 1999).

It is possible that the findings of two studies may appear to be different. For example, one claims to support the effectiveness of an intervention and the other claims to not support it. The study that claims to fail to support the effectiveness, typically represented as $p > 0.05$, may have had a small sample size, possibly making it a low power study. The study that claimed to support the effectiveness, with a $p < 0.05$, may have had a large sample size, enhancing its power to detect a statistically significant effect. Despite the difference in the p-values of the two studies, the actual mean scores of the participants may show that participants in both studies derived benefit more from the intervention than the nonintervention condition. Therefore, the p-value findings may have led to different conclusions about effectiveness, simply because of power issues, not because of underlying differences in true effectiveness. The integrated interpretation of these two studies would be that they appear to support the effectiveness of the intervention.

When the findings from two, high-quality, large-sample studies are in opposite directions, the therapist will find the task of integration to be more challenging. In this case, the therapist must report to the decision makers that the body of evidence gives conflicting answers to the clinical question. This conflicting evidence will be one factor that therapist and decision makers consider as they discuss the evidence. Conflicts in evidence call upon the therapist to use the highest level of clinical reasoning skills. There is much uncertainty in therapy because every human being is unique and responds to therapy in an individual manner. Nevertheless, there is a great deal of predictable and systematic behavior in human beings as well. The therapist uses reasoning that brings uniqueness and predictability together to make decisions in the face of uncertainty (Mattingly & Fleming, 1994).

Conflicts in evidence call upon therapists to not only tap into their clinical reasoning skills but also to start developing research questions for an onsite research study. This chapter has addressed how the therapist collects and talks about evidence from published research studies undertaken by researchers other than the therapist. The next logical step in EBP is to design an on-site study for collecting evidence about one's own clinical population and to use that evidence to help resolve the conflicting findings found in the body of published evidence.

EVIDENCE-BASED COMMUNICATION OPPORTUNITIES IN EVERYDAY PRACTICE

EBP requires therapists to keep current in the research findings that are relevant to their clinical populations. To keep current, the therapist must incorporate time for literature searching and reading into clinical practice. The communication about evidence with others will not be an additional time burden if the therapist learns to turn everyday communication opportunities into evidence-based ones.

Communication opportunities with clients arise at the first meeting, at assessment and intervention planning sessions, during the provision of treatment, and discharge planning sessions. Whenever the therapist is giving recommendations or involving the client in decision making, there is an opportunity for incorporating evidence into the message. Even if the client is not interested in hearing evidence-based information, the therapist can communicate about it in an indirect manner to support the client's development of knowledge and active involvement in decision making. For example, using evidence from research on the effectiveness of microwave ovens in enhancing participation in meal preparation activities, the therapist might say, "Some people similar to you have found it easier to make meals with a microwave oven. Do you want to try a microwave oven in therapy to see if it works for you?"

With managers and colleagues, group meetings are an ideal forum for disseminating research evidence because the message is discussed among several people at one time in one location. Appropriate types of meetings are team conferences about clients, staff education sessions, and departmental meetings directed at program planning, budget review, and quality assurance. Journal clubs, in which members take turns in reviewing and presenting a summary of a body of research literature, can reduce the individual burden of searching and reading literature. Discussions at journal clubs are relatively unfettered by day-to-day clinical demands. This type of context supports brainstorming and creative thinking that can stimulate the evidence-based modification or development of assessment and intervention procedures.

Any communication with a funder can be an opportunity for the discussion of research evidence, whether it be face-to-face, via telephone, or written documentation. One of the more formal communications might be a funding proposal, which requires tight organization and scholarly citations. The more comfortable therapists become with the published research evidence in their area of clinical expertise, the more skillfully they will be able to communicate about that evidence in a brief and understandable format. There is no need to tell the client, the manager, or the funder everything that is known about the evidence, unless asked to do so. The therapist communicates enough evidence for informed decision-making, yet is prepared to communicate about evidence in a more detailed manner.

TAKE HOME MESSAGES

Communicating Evidence Effectively

✔ Message must be relevant, framed to enable decision making and action, and comprehensible.

✔ Four steps to evidence-based communication:

1. Identify clinical role of decision maker: client/family member, manager, and funder are all potential decision makers.

2. Determine the decisions to be made: describe relevant client participation issues, select assessment procedures, and choose and plan intervention. The types of information are descriptive, assessment, and intervention.

3. Gather/interpret evidence: formulate clinical question and research possible answers. Type of evidence being sought; attribute of interest; description of clinical population. Most efficient to search for research synthesis and meta-analysis.

4. Communicate the evidence: for communication with clients use simple language, terms that cross cultures and perspectives, brevity with appropriate amount of detail, repetition and checks for confusion, suggestion for concrete action related to the information.

Interpretation

✔ Assessment tool should have been tested for the particular form of reliability and validity that is needed.

✔ Studies that provide access to both quantitative and qualitative details help in examining similarities and differences in responses.

Uncertainty

✔ If no meta-analysis is available, therapist can perform this function, but it takes a great deal of skill.

✔ Give heavier emphasis to studies that provide more accurate evidence than those with potentially less accurate evidence (internal and external validity).

✔ Do not rely solely on statistical significance tests and their p-values unless there are more than 60 participants in the study; studies with a larger size have more power to detect a statistically significant effect.

✔ When findings are in contradictory directions, report on conflict and use reasoning skills; opportunity to develop research questions for on-site study.

Everyday Practice

✔ Incorporate time for literature searching and reading.

✔ Take advantage of opportunities for communicating evidence to clients and for utilizing group meetings as a forum for disseminating research evidence.

✔ Therapists maintain balance of communicating just enough evidence for informed decision making while being prepared to communicate about evidence in a more detailed manner.

LEARNING AND EXPLORATION ACTIVITIES

The purpose of this chapter is to demonstrate the important role that effective communication plays in incorporating evidence into practice. The following exercise builds upon the process developed in the chapter to assist the student interpreting research studies and relating them to the individual.

1. Research and Communication

To complete the following exercises, create a case scenario or think of an actual client in your area of clinical interest. Write down a description of the client. Be sure to specify the diagnosis or presenting reasons for coming to the therapist and other attributes of interest about the client, such as those in Table 12-5.

   a. Create a descriptive, an assessment, and an intervention clinical question for guiding the search for evidence and the development of possible answers to discuss with the client or the client's family members.

   b. Create a table like Table 12-5 and, using the following template, include columns for describing the client and research participants from each of the three types of studies: a descriptive, assessment, and intervention study. Complete a preliminary literature search based upon the three clinical questions, and locate three studies that appear relevant from their titles. Retrieve and read the articles. Fill in the table by summarizing the research participants' attributes.

   c. Interpret the results from the study that you judge to be most relevant for generating possible answers to one of the clinical questions. Based upon the results, what is the possible answer to the clinical question? Is the study of a quality that makes you feel confident that the possible answer is justifiable? Explain.

2. Clinical Role of Decision Makers

As presented in this chapter, there are different individuals involved in clinical decisions with whom a therapist is likely to communicate. Gather in a group of four to five colleagues using the same scenario as created for question 1. Have each group member take on the role of therapist, client (and/or family member), manager, and funder. Discuss the scenario from these perspectives, keeping the following in mind:

- Goals for treatment
- Relevant participation issues
- Types of evidence available to each player
- Possible background forces influencing communication

How did each of the players affect communication? What were some of the barriers surrounding communication in this scenario? What were some of the supports?

Template for Research and Communication Exercise

Client Identity	Case Description	Study #1 (Descriptive)	Study #2 (Assessment)	Study #3 (Intervention)
Disease				
Degree of Disability				
Age				
Gender				
Race and Ethnicity				
Family and Living Context				
Work Status				
Socioeconomic Status				

ENDNOTES

1. It is possible to defend the authors' use of causality language on a couple of grounds, however. First, from a theoretical perspective, the factors studied in the meta-analysis are predicted to have a causal influence on subjective well-being. Second, some of the studies may have had designs that were supportive of a causal explanation, but the meta-analytic authors did not report information about designs in such a manner as to determine the validity of making a causal interpretation. A perusal of the titles on their reference list suggests that most of the designs were correlational in nature.

2. Cohen (1988) gave two different sets of standards for interpreting the magnitude of r and d. Rosenthal and Rosnow (1991) pointed out that the two sets of standards do not match when r is converted to d and that Cohen applied a stricter criterion to r than d. The d standards are used in this chapter to interpret intervention effect r's since Cohen intended d to be used for comparing the means of treatment and control groups. On the other hand, Cohen's stricter r standards are used in this chapter to interpret descriptive associations since Cohen intended his r standards to be applied primarily to descriptive associations.

REFERENCES

Carlson, M., Fanchiang, S., Zemke, R., & Clark, F. (1996). A meta-analysis of the effectiveness of occupational therapy for older persons. *American Journal of Occupational Therapy, 50,* 89-98.

Clark, F., Azen, S. P., Zemke, R., Jackson, J., Carlson, M., Mandel, D., et al. (1997). Occupational therapy for independent-living older adults: A randomized controlled trial. *Journal of the American Medical Association, 278,* 1321-1326.

Cohen, J. (1988). *Statistical power analysis for the behavioral sciences* (2nd ed.). Hillsdale, NJ: Lawrence Erlbaum.

Davis, T. C., Bocchini, J. A., Fredrickson, D., Arnold, C., Mayeaux, E. J., Murphy, P. W., et al. (1996). Parent comprehension of polio vaccine information pamphlets. *Pediatrics, 97*, 804-810.

de Goede, C. J. T., Keus, S. H. J., Kwakkel, G., & Wagenaar, R. C. (2001). The effects of physical therapy in Parkinson's disease: A research synthesis. *Archives of Physical Medicine and Rehabilitation, 82*, 509-515.

Doak, C. C., Doak, L. G., & Root, J. H. (1996). *Teaching patients with low literacy skills* (2nd ed.). Philadelphia, PA: J. B. Lippincott.

Ebeling, S. (2003). Lessons and tips for addressing health literacy issues in a medical setting. Harvard School of Public Health: Health Literacy Website. Retrieved May 31, 2006, from http://www.hsph.harvard.edu/healthliteracy/insights.html

Griffin, J., McKenna, K., & Tooth, L. (2006). Discrepancy between older clients' ability to read and comprehend and the reading level of written educational materials used by occupational therapists. *American Journal of Occupational Therapy, 60*, 70-80.

Kondo, T., Mann, W. C., Tomita, M., & Ottenbacher, K. J. (1997). The use of microwave ovens by elderly persons with disabilities. *American Journal of Occupational Therapy, 51*, 739-747.

Koplas, P. A., Gans, H. B., Wisely, M. P., Kuchibhatla, M., Cutson, T. M., Gold, D. T., et al. (1999). Quality of life and Parkinson's disease. *Journal of Gerontology: Medical Sciences, 54A*, M197-M202.

Mattingly, C., & Fleming, M. H. (1994). *Clinical reasoning: Forms of inquiry in a therapeutic practice.* Philadelphia, PA: F. A. Davis.

McColl, M. A., & Pollock, N. (2005). Measuring occupational performance using a client-centered perspective. In M. Law, C. Baum, & W. Dunn (Eds.), *Measuring occupational performance: Supporting best practice in occupational therapy* (2nd ed.). Thorofare, NJ: SLACK Incorporated.

Murphy, S., & Tickle-Degnen, L. (2001). The effectiveness of occupational therapy-related treatments for persons with Parkinson's disease: A meta-analytic review. *American Journal of Occupational Therapy, 55*, 385-392.

National Center for the Dissemination of Disability Research (1996). A review of the literature on dissemination and knowledge utilization. Retrieved October 19, 2000, from http//www.ncddr.org/du/products/review/index.html

National Center for the Dissemination of Disability Research (2005). Focus: What is knowledge translation? Technical Brief Number 10. Southeast Educational Development Laboratory. Retrieved May 31, 2006, from http//www.ncddr.org/du/products/focus/focus10

National Council on Disability, Cultural Diversity Initiative. (2003). Outreach and People with Disabilities from Diverse Cultures: A review of the literature. Retrieved May 31, 2006, from http://www.ncd.gov/newsroom/advisory/cultural/cdi_litreview.htm#Executive

Ottenbacher, K. J., & Maas, F. (1999). How to detect effects: Statistical power and evidence-based practice in occupational therapy research. *American Journal of Occupational Therapy, 53*, 181-188.

Pinquart, M., & Sörensen, S. (2000). Influences of socioeconomic status, social network, and competence on subjective well-being in later life. *Psychology and Aging, 15*, 187-224.

Portney, L. G., & Watkins, M. P. (2000). *Foundations of clinical research: Applications to practice* (2nd ed.). Upper Saddle River, NJ: Prentice Hall Health.

Redman, B. K. (1997). *The practice of patient education* (8th ed.). St. Louis, MO: Mosby.

Rosenthal, R., & Rosnow, R. (1991). *Essentials of behavioral research: Methods and data analysis* (2nd ed.). New York, NY: McGraw-Hill.

Rosenthal, R., & Rubin, D. B. (1982). A simple general purpose display of magnitude of experimental effect. *Journal of Educational Psychology, 74*, 166-169.

Rudd, R. E. (2005). How to create and assess print materials. Harvard School of Public Health: Health Literacy Website. Retrieved May 31, 2006, from http://www.hsph.harvard.edu/healthliteracy/materials.html

Sackett, D. L., Strauss, S. E., Richardson, W. S., Rosenberg, W., & Haynes, R. B. (2000). *Evidence-based medicine: How to practice and teach EBM* (2nd ed.). New York, NY: Churchill Livingstone.

Schillinger, D., Piette, J., Grumbach, K., Wang, F., Wilson, C., Daher, C., et al. (2003). Closing the loop: Physician communication with diabetic patients who have low health literacy. *Archives of Internal Medicine, 163,* 83-90.

Stolee, P., Stadnyk, K., Myers, A. M., & Rockwood, K. (1999). An individualized approach to outcome measurement in geriatric rehabilitation. *Journal of Gerontology: Medical Sciences, 54A,* M641-M647.

Tickle-Degnen, L. (2000). Evidence-based practice forum—Communicating with clients, family members, and colleagues. *American Journal of Occupational Therapy, 54,* 341-343.

Tickle-Degnen, L. (2001). From the general to the specific: Using meta-analytic reports in clinical decision-making. *Evaluation & the Health Professions, 24,* 308-326.

Wills, C. E., & Holmes-Rovner, M. (2003). Patient comprehension of information for shared treatment decision making: State of the art and future directions. *Patient Education and Counseling, 50,* 285-290.

Wilson, J. F. (2003). The crucial link between literacy and health. *Annals of Internal Medicine, 139,* 875-878.

Yip, A. M., Gorman, M. C., Stadnyk, K., Mills, W. G. M., MacPherson, K. M., & Rockwood, K. (1998). A standardized menu for goal attainment scaling in the care of frail elders. *The Gerontologist, 38,* 735-742.

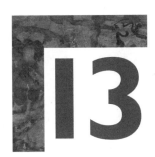

Research Dissemination and Transfer of Knowledge

Mary Law, PhD, OTReg(Ont), FCAOT and Jessica Telford, BA

LEARNING OBJECTIVES

After reading this chapter, the student/practitioner will be able to:

- Distinguish between the various models of research transfer.
- Identify effective research transfer dissemination models.
- Recognize the differences between knowledge-driven models and problem-driven models of evidence-based policy.
- Characterize the roles and challenges of evidence-based policy within EBP.

Transferring research into practice seems to be the very reason for the existence of EBP, and it would be reasonable to assume that it is something at which evidence-based practitioners would be skilled. Despite the need for research transfer, however, the best methods for doing it still remain a mystery for many who embrace EBP. Traditionally, "transfers of health care information" took place through either the undiscriminating distribution of print media (such as a bulletin or a journal article) or through large group seminars. For a long time, this was thought to be enough; however, practitioners have recently realized that these methods are inadequate. The problems were substantial—either the information was not reaching those who needed it, it was not convenient for the practitioners who wanted to learn, or the format of the material alienated the participants. In the past decade, there have been major efforts made to create organizations that will ensure effective research transfer.

Perhaps one of the most important points is the complexity involved in research transfer. There are many more considerations than just the fact that the research has been done correctly. We must also examine the characteristics of the different pieces in the research transfer equation. What are the characteristics of the scientific evidence used? Who are the decision makers who will be examining it? In what organizational context do we expect this research information to be used? There are a rich variety of variables that must be considered, and their interplay is discussed in the chapter on evidence-based policy. Effective research transfer can sometimes be more of an art than a science.

MODELS OF KNOWLEDGE TRANSFER AND EXCHANGE

Let us begin by examining models about how research/knowledge transfer works in health care and other fields. Some research theories about how to transfer knowledge into practice have centered on changing the behavior of individual practitioners while others have centered more on changing the organizations in which practitioners work.

The Readiness to Change (The Transtheoretical Model) by Prochaska and DiClemente is an example of a model that looks specifically at the individual. It incorporates features of a variety of behavior models and suggests that change in behavior is modulated by a person's readiness to make changes at the time the information is provided (Dalton & Gottlieb, 2003; Kerns & Habib, 2004; Miller & Spilker 2003). This model is useful to understand how clinicians respond to knowledge translation. The stages of change in this model, as outlined by Sherman & Carothers (2005), are as follows:

- Precontemplation (no awareness of or intention of taking action toward an idea)
- Contemplation (awareness of idea and consideration of changing)
- Preparation (making plans to change behavior)
- Action (engaging in a new behavior)
- Maintenance (continuing the behavior and making it part of routine)

There are also processes of change, which are as follows (Prochaska, Norcross, & DiClemente, 1995, p. 33, as cited in Sherman & Carothers, 2005):

- "Consciousness-raising ("increasing information about self and problem")
- Emotional arousal ("experiencing and expressing feelings about one's problems and solutions")
- Commitment ("choosing and committing to act, or belief in ability to change")
- Reward ("rewarding self, or being rewarded by others, for making change") .
- Environmental-re-evaluation ("assessing how one's problem affects the physical environment") (Prochaska et al., 1992, p. 1108, as cited in Sherman & Carothers, 2005).

Knowledge translation strategies can be tailored using this information about how people respond to change. For example, providing information that increases conscious thoughts about an intervention is more effective for those at the consciousness raising or emotional arousal stages while behavioral interventions such as rewards are more effective for the action and maintenance stages (Sherman & Carothers, 2005).

Some research has shown that interventions influencing individuals have not had a large impact on knowledge translation (Davies & Nutley, 2002). Researchers such as Rogers (1995) have taken a more combined or "diffusion of innovations" approach (Teplicky, 2005)—one that focuses on both the individual and the organization. Rogers (1995) proposed a model entitled the "Innovation Decision Process Model." He defined diffusion as "the process by which an innovation is communicated through certain channels over time among the members of a social system." In short, his model looks at how individuals and organizations change over time, how they become familiar with new research information, how they use this information, and the types of information that are most effective within a given stage of the process. This model has been used in health research and in other disciplines and other models have built upon it (Teplicky, 2005). The five stages of the model are as follows:

1. Knowledge (learning about a new idea)
2. Persuasion (forming an opinion about the idea)
3. Decision (deciding whether to use the idea or not)

4. Implementation (trying out the new idea)

5. Confirmation (evaluating the implementation of the idea to determine if it is producing the desired outcome— continuing to seek out information along the way) It is important to note that these stages may not always have to occur in the order presented above.

Rogers (2005) also discusses a two-pronged strategy for communication and knowledge transfer. He refers to two types of "communication channels" within the Innovation Decision Process Model: mass media channels and interpersonal channels. In other words, he suggests that the way information is delivered should differ depending on the stage of the model the individual or organization is working through. The use of mass media channels such as TV, radio, peer-reviewed journals, and teleconferences is most effective during the knowledge and awareness phase whereas interpersonal channels (face-to-face communications) such as interactions between colleagues, small group discussions, and knowledge brokering work best within the persuasion and decision stages (Teplicky, 2005).

Another model for research transfer comes from researcher Maureen Dobbins and colleagues (2002). They break the research transfer process into the same five key stages as Rogers (knowledge, persuasion, decision, implementation, and confirmation) but build on the model by applying it to health care research (Teplicky, 2005). Dobbins et al.'s (2002) model extends to evidence-based policy, as do many larger models of research transfer activities, since the two (research transfer and policy making) interact. Each of Dobbins et al.'s five phases has a specific purpose. The knowledge stage begins when research is complete and attempts to identify the best ways for presenting that knowledge to others (discussed later in this chapter). The persuasion stage is twofold—it includes persuading other practitioners and policy makers of the merits of one's research. Third, the decision stage leads to evidence-based decision making on whether or not this innovation will be put to use. The fourth and fifth stages, implementation and confirmation, deal more specifically with evidence-based policy.

On a smaller level, how is research best transferred to individual practitioners? A good systems theory model for research transfer comes from an older article (Goode, Lovett, Hayes, & Butcher, 1987) from the *Journal of Nursing Administration*. It describes the research transfer process as a three-pronged mechanism consisting of input, throughput, and output, and Goode et al. (1987) set out a series of eight steps to research transfer. They are as follows:

1. Identifying problems occurring in the clinical area.

2. Gathering information from research studies that add knowledge regarding the problems.

3. Assuring that the (practitioners) have adequate knowledge to read the research studies critically and understand their implications.

4. Determining if the research is relevant to the type of patients and clinical setting in which it was to be used.

5. Devising ways to transform knowledge so that it can be used in clinical practice.

6. Defining what patient outcomes are expected.

7. Providing education and training that is needed to get the practice change into the system.

8. Evaluating and adjusting or modifying the new practice protocol.

Goode et al.'s (1987) model builds upon the realization that research transfer cannot be a passive endeavor. Once practitioners finish their formal training, health "authorities" dictating what should and what should not be learned underestimate the abilities of individual clinicians. Of course, large agencies will distribute clinical guidelines and evidence-based policy; however, it will be up to individuals to assimilate much of the knowledge on their own. The strategy of teaching practitioners the process and having them perform short, self-directed inquiries into subjects is better than distributing information that will not be used. More important, perhaps, than even the content of the evidence being transferred is the method of transfer. Choosing a research transfer flow that accords practitioners respect for their experience and makes them enthusiastic to use their own critical appraisal skills, while simultaneously encouraging researchers when they see that the fruits of their labor put to good use, is the ultimate goal. Returning to Goode et al.'s model, the input, throughput, and output stages encompass the eight steps quite well.

Input—Steps 1 to 3

At this point of the research transfer process, the emphasis is on preparing the practitioners to gather and assimilate new knowledge. When the research transfer process is started, it begins with a topic that is a current clinical problem in the practitioners' everyday setting. The surest way to alienate new inductees to EBP is to make them work on esoteric, theoretical cases because they will soon lose interest and respect for the evidence-based process. If practitioners are set to work on improving care in an area that is known to be a clinical problem, however, they will respond much more positively and will see it as a chance to test themselves against real clinical challenges. One must ensure that practitioners feel supported and capable of working with the evidence they have gathered, and if not, they have recourse to experienced help.

Throughput—Steps 4 to 6

The throughput stage is a crucial one and will be discussed again later in this chapter. Especially important is step 5, which concerns transforming knowledge to practice. This can mean interpreting knowledge useful for individuals, but it also includes the practitioner preparing to teach others about what he or she has found. Research and findings into this topic will be discussed later in this summary. Throughput generally encompasses the making of critically appraised topics (CATs) (and possibly systematic reviews) and preparing them for use with clients in a clinical setting.

Output—Steps 7 and 8

In this last step of the model, the findings of the research inquiry are collated, and research has effectively been transferred into practice. At this stage, reflection on the entire process should occur, and thoughts on how research transfer can be improved or further tested should be recorded. The evaluation of the entire process follows a feedback loop and returns to the input step of the process. In this way, Goode et al.'s (1987) research transfer strategy is like a self-cleaning machine: Each time this strategy is used by a practitioner, it is further integrated into his or her thinking and becomes open to his or her insights and modifications.

KNOWLEDGE TRANSFER NEEDS THE INVOLVEMENT OF ALL STAKEHOLDERS

While the above model describes a top-down flow of information from researcher to practitioner, Ho, Bloch, et al. (2004) describe more of a push down and pull up system ("knowledge translation cycle") in which all stakeholders work together. They describe three key groups in the health care system that possess different types of valuable information and, therefore, must work together as a system to pass knowledge along:

1. Knowledge producers (the community of researchers)
2. Knowledge consumers (the community of practice—clinicians)
3. Knowledge beneficiaries (the community of patients)

Although research can inform practice, the reverse is also very important whereby patients inform research about the most relevant issues. Practitioners are in the middle linking the two ends together. Knowledge transfer strategies need to keep in mind the needs of patients at all times (Ho, Bloch, et al., 2004, p. 92):

> *Factors influencing the process of knowledge transfer can be conceptualized in a matrix model. knowledge transfer is initiated either by knowledge producers or the system in a push configuration or by knowledge consumers and beneficiaries in a pull operation. In the former case, practitioners remain in a passive role as information receivers. In the latter case, the practitioner is actively seeking specific information.*

SPECIFIC RESEARCH TRANSFER STRATEGIES

As was mentioned before, when a practitioner is undertaking a research transfer project, he or she will need to be able to teach others what he or she has found when finished. It was also stated at the beginning of this summary that conventional speech and print methods were found to be inadequate for effective, long-lasting research transfer. Research transfer dissemination strategies, which are more effective, are those that conform to the personal learning needs of the researcher and utilize two or more different approaches simultaneously.

Evidence from RCTs and systematic reviews, which examined practitioners' habits, indicates that there is no one optimal way to disseminate research to other practitioners. In their powerful article, "No Magic Bullets: A Systematic Review of 102 Trials of Interventions to Improve Professional Practice," Oxman, Thomson, Davis, and Haynes (1995) conclude that "there are no 'magic bullets' for improving the quality of health care, but there are a wide range of interventions available that, if used appropriately, could lead to important improvements in professional practice and patient outcomes" (p. 142). Table 13-1 is a list of research transfer strategies from Oxman et al.'s article.

Much of Oxman et al.'s (1987) article examines each type of intervention and its particular individual or combined effectiveness. Specific combinations of research transfer dissemination strategies must be made to suit the content being disseminated. Strategies such as "local opinion leaders," "audit and feedback," and "reminders" are discussed in this article as well as later articles by Oxman and show that research transfer works well when personalized to individuals practitioners' needs (Jamtvedt et al., 2006; O'Brien, Oxman et al., 1999; Oxman et al., 1987).

The Provincial Centre of Excellence for Child and Youth Mental Health at the Children's Hospital of Eastern Ontario, Canada has published a toolkit for knowledge transfer entitled, "Doing more with what you know: A toolkit on knowledge exchange" (2006). This toolkit is an excellent source of knowledge and includes frameworks for knowledge transfer, checklists to follow, scenarios, and several suggested vehicles for knowledge transfer. The overall message of the toolkit is that knowledge translation "takes innovative and creating thinking." Five key strategies for knowledge transfer that can all include the production of lay summaries, introducing online forums, inviting media, linking researchers with patients/clinicians (and which may overlap with Table 13-1) are as follows:

1. Cultural approach: Using artifacts or symbols to get information across. For example, storytelling and socializing can be a great way to affect tacit knowledge.

2. Multi-sector partnerships: Bring different organizations/strengths together.

3. Conferences/conference leverage: Good place to push out and pull in knowledge.

4. Research summaries: Specific to a wide range of stakeholders.

Table 13-1

RESEARCH TRANSFER TEACHING STRATEGIES FOR PRACTITIONERS

Educational Materials

Distribution of published or printed recommendations for clinical care, including clinical practice guidelines, audiovisual materials, and electronic publications.

Conferences

Participation of health care providers in conferences, lectures, workshops, or traineeships outside their practice settings.

Outreach Visits

Use of a trained person who meets with providers in their practice setting to provide information, which may include feedback on the provider's performance.

Local Opinion Leaders

Use of providers explicitly nominated by their colleagues to be "educationally influential."

Patient-Mediated Interventions

Any intervention aimed at changing the performance of health care providers for which information was sought from or given directly to patients by others (e.g., direct mailings to patients, patient counseling delivered by others, or clinical information collected directly from patients and given to the provider).

Audit and Feedback

Any summary of clinical performance of health care over a specified period, with or without recommendations for clinical action. The information may have been obtained from medical records, computerized databases, or patients or by observation.

Reminders

Any intervention (manual or computerized) that prompts the health care provider to perform a clinical action. Examples include concurrent or intervisit reminders to professionals about desired actions such as screening or other preventive services, enhanced laboratory reports, or administrative support (e.g., follow-up appointment systems or stickers on charts).

Marketing

Use of personal interviewing, group discussion (focus groups), or a survey of targeted providers to identify barriers to change and the subsequent design of an intervention.

Multifaceted Interventions

Any intervention that includes two or more of the last six interventions described above.

Local Consensus Process

Inclusion of participating providers in discussion to ensure agreement that the chosen clinical problem is important and the approach to managing it appropriate.

"No magic bullets: a systematic review of 102 trials of interventions to improve professional practice." Reprinted from *Canadian Medical Association Journal*, 15-Nov-95; 153(10), Page(s) 1423-1431 by permission of the publisher. © Canadian Medical Association.

5. Supportive infrastructures within organizations.

The article also summarizes necessary processes that effective knowledge transfer. Working together in partnerships, building capacity, writing in plain language, and evaluating knowledge transfer approaches are highlighted.

Specific types of interpersonal channels that have shown some positive effects on knowledge uptake in practice settings are as follows:

- Two-way communications (like interactive workshops) where clinicians are actively involved as opposed to one-way sessions (which have not shown positive change).

- Information presented by local opinion leaders.

- Educational outreach visits by trained people to clinicians.

- Problem-based learning groups (clinicians work together to solve problems).

A further application of research transfer dissemination strategies is through organizations known as journal clubs. Long popular with physicians, journal clubs are a group of practitioners who split up the literature to be read, with each person focusing on one particular article, journal, or group of journals. When the journal club convenes, practitioners summarize and present what they have garnered from their reading to the other participants, thereby cutting down the amount of slogging through the medical literature that must be done by each practitioner. Jaan Siderov (1995) recently wrote an article in which he meta-analyzed the habits of 131 journal clubs for medical residents. His main conclusions were that the crucial elements that make a good journal club include mandatory attendance from participants, meetings with the provision of food, fewer full staff attending (thus giving students the feeling of greater freedom to debate and discuss without being evaluated), and a modest size to preclude feelings of exclusion.

Finally, technology enabled knowledge translation (TEKT) or information and communication technology has been shown to be an effective method of pushing out evidence (Davis et al., 2003; Ho, Bloch, et al., 2004; Ho, Lauscher, et al., 2004). Examples are handheld PDAs that give physicians immediate access to knowledge, and technologies that provide summaries of evidence. Ho, Lauscher, et al. (2004) state that the use of technology as vehicle for knowledge transfer may be extremely useful because technology:

- Can assist practitioners with access and uptake of information.

- Can improve the uptake of research in policy making since it speeds up the knowledge transfer process.

- Can facilitate the transfer of public data (e.g. national health surveys) to policy makers more quickly.

- Can support communities of practice where groups share knowledge and information regarding a specific topic(s) of interest.

In their article "Technology-enabled knowledge translation: Frameworks to promote research and practice," Ho, Bloch, et al. (2004) discuss a framework for implementing TEKT as well as evaluation and dissemination methodologies. The framework focuses on measuring the effectiveness of knowledge transfer across several dimensions—structural, subjective, cognitive, behavioral, and systemic use. Although the importance of TEKT has been recognized and will likely be the way of the future, few innovative technologies have been developed in general and none have been developed for rehabilitation.

Information from a conference organized by the Canadian Research Transfer Network (CRTN; 2001) is useful in helping therapists and researchers focus the most effective strategies for knowledge transfer. These strategies, as outlined below, center on engaging the audience, constructing a clear message, and ensuring effective delivery. In terms of the audience, it is important to focus on the information they want or need, tailor messages according to the

Figure 13-1. The evidence-informed policy and practice pathway. (Reprinted with permission from Bowen, S. & Zwi, A.B. (2005). Pathways to evidence informed policy and practice: A framework for action. *PLos Medicine, 2(7)*, e166.)

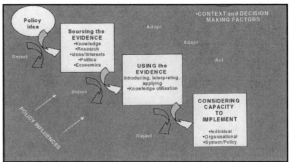

group you are trying to reach and according to the values that are important to that group, and speak in terms of what you think they "need to know" rather than what they "ought to know." A good way to achieve these goals is to involve members of the audience in each step of the knowledge translation process. The message also needs to be valuable to the audience. It should be tangible, compelling, and clear. It is wise to spread the message to different groups so that "word of mouth" will continue to pass the information along to people or areas you may not have considered. When delivering the message, a fellow stakeholder that is trusted is the best type of messenger. The messenger should speak the same language as the audience (do not use too much jargon or technical wording) and listen to the audience. It is important to go at their pace and remember that policy-making takes time.

EVIDENCE-BASED POLICY

Evidence-based policy is a relatively new field of study in the realm of EBP. EBM and the work of Archie Cochrane were the inspirations for the movement; however, all of the evidence gathered and analyzed for EBM was concentrated on better patient care. The idea that evidence could be used on policy successes and failures could be gathered in the same way did not initially pique the same outpouring of interest and work, but it is becoming increasingly important. Hanney, Gonzalez, Block, Buxton, and Kogan (2003) state that "Policy-making can be viewed as involving the 'authoritative allocation of values,' and when interpreted broadly can include people making the policy as government ministers and officials, as local health service managers, or as representatives of a professional body" (p. 3). Nutley, Davies, and Walter (2002) note that "policy making is always inherently political" (p. 1).

Bowen and Zwi (2005) in an article entitled "Evidence-informed policy and practice pathway," discuss the place of evidence in the policy-making process. Figure 13-1 details their framework for the various political and "rapidly changing" factors that go into the decision-making process.

There are reasons why evidence-based policy has been slow to catch on. The material we have covered in EBP up to this point has been primarily logical, rational processes. This makes sense, since EBP is an attempt to introduce a more systematic approach to the use of health care knowledge. When entering into the realm of evidence-based policy, however, logic cannot always be trusted. The creation of policy from research findings is a fundamentally different exercise than the careful synthesis and analysis of academic data. EBP, as a process, is based on individual or small group consideration of knowledge and research information. In contrast, evidence-based policy is based on the consideration of health care research by large groups that must come to a consensus and by those who may not be experts in the field, namely managers and policy makers. As such, processes that worked in EBP cannot necessarily be completely replicated in the creation of policy.

MODELS OF KNOWLEDGE TRANSFER INTO POLICY

One of the major obstacles to policy being made along evidence-based lines is the fact that the two contributors to policy—scientists and managers—perceive and value research differently. A good example of this problem is given by Dr. Francois Champagne, a researcher at Quebec's Université de Montréal. Presenting at a 1999 conference in Toronto, Dr. Champagne discussed the differences by proposing that evidence-based policy making can be perceived through two fundamentally different models (Champagne, 1999).

The first, which Champagne calls the "knowledge-driven model," is one that makes sense in a rationally determined environment. It follows five steps:

1. Research (basic, then applied)

2. Technological development

3. Use (adoption of technology)

4. Quality of implemented actions

5. Outcome

This model is the view most commonly held by scientists, who work primarily in the first steps of the model, doing research that could be directed toward certain ends. This model is built on several inherent assumptions. The knowledge-driven model assumes that once new knowledge exists, it will naturally be pressed toward use. In evidence-based policy making, however, this is not necessarily the case. "Perfect knowledge" would be required for policy making to work in this way.

"Perfect knowledge" implies that all evidence is applied in exactly the most beneficial way. This rests on the idea that policy makers and scientists are able to omnisciently see exactly where basic and applied research could be put to use. Furthermore, it assumes that all relevant knowledge will be adopted in its field without impediments. Unfortunately, however, there are many factors standing in the way of research being used in this manner. Basic and applied research is distributed in health care journals, which grow in number and size each month. Scientists and policy makers are not able to sort through all of the new knowledge, nor see how it could be applied to their work; thus, new findings sometimes go unused. Even when evidence and research findings are identified as important, the process of implementing them into policy is often a long and rocky one. Even the best evidence can be doomed by hasty decision making, poor presentation, or political reasons. There are often reasons other than evidence that support implementation of specific policies. This leads to an important truth of evidence-based policy making: management, or the creation of new policies from research, is inherently based in its context. The environment in which policy is made has a strong hand in shaping its eventual outcome.

A second model of evidence-based policy making, known as the "problem-driven model," takes an alternative approach to the process and avoids some of the idealism of the knowledge-based model (Champagne, 1999). Realizing the contextual nature of health care policy, this model does not begin with research but rather with a problem or question.

This model, a view more commonly held by managers, suggests that evidence-based policy is made according to the following logic:

- Definition of problem

- Identification of missing knowledge

- Acquisition of knowledge, various possible channels

- Interpretation for the problem situation

- Use (adoption of technology)

In the problem-driven model, once a problem or information need has been understood, policy makers decide which evidence they will require and use various channels to obtain it. Furthermore, both of the channels by which the model suggests that research knowledge is obtained take note of realities. In the problem-driven model, research findings will generally come from either a pool of knowledge already available to policy makers or through commissioned research into a specific problem. This understanding of the realities of how research findings come to practice acknowledges the fact that evidence distribution is not always perfect and that policy makers do tend to draw upon knowledge already available to them. Once policy makers have the research they require, they will interpret it for the situation at hand and finally use it.

The problem-driven model approximates the "real" processes of policy making better than the knowledge-driven model, but why is that? Why do scientists tend to believe that evidence will be used in a different way than managers do? Investigation into this problem has shown that different groups perceive how research should be used in different ways. In a 1981 article, Weiss and Weiss posed the question, "What is meant by using research for policy making?" (p. 846). While seemingly simple, this question is central to the issue, as it highlights the differences of opinion between groups (researchers and policy makers) and reasons why misunderstandings to occur.

What Weiss and Weiss found is that researchers see the use of evidence in policy as a fundamentally rational, linear process. When new evidence is published, they feel it should, and will be, expediently put to use in the most applicable field. Decision makers, on the other hand, see a greater and more varied number of ways to use research and are less willing to act on specific pieces of research alone. Much more is required than just top-notch research for policy makers to implement evidence into policy. They see evidence-based policy making as a holistic, multifaceted, nonlinear process. Champagne (1999) summarizes that "researchers and decision makers belong to separate communities with different values and different ideologies and [thus] these differences impede utilization."

Decision making in complex situations is not necessarily a rational process; decision makers and managers draw in a great deal of evidence and assess it in a holistic manner. Instead of affording evidence weight based purely on its methodology and scientific rigor, policy makers are much more apt to take in and consider a great deal of evidence simultaneously, sometimes placing more emphasis on proximate sources, the opinions of local experts, etc. They also generalize the results of many studies together, working with this accumulated evidence. Finally, managers may not always use research purely for the purposes of making the best policy. As Champagne (1999) says, they may use knowledge "deliberately, politically, tactically, and conceptually" to manipulate or work within the context of their policy environment.

Table 13-2, from Charlotte Waddell's (2002) article, shows the differences in the types of evidence that the various decision making groups prefer. In Table 13-3, Bowen and Zwi (2005) also list the different types of evidence that policy makers use.

CHALLENGES OF MOVING EVIDENCE INTO POLICY

Does the complexity of the policy-making process mean that EBP fundamentally breaks down during its final stage? Not necessarily. Although evidence-based policy making is not necessarily a linear exercise, it can still yield valid and useful conclusions. Therefore, is there anything that health care professionals can do to influence policy makers to use our high-quality evidence? Dobbins et al. (2002) suggests that "tailoring" evidence to fit the needs and desires of policy makers is a good way to get evidence heard. They looked specifically at systematic

Table 13-2

CONTEXTUAL/SYSTEMATIC DIFFERENCES FOR RESEARCHERS, CLINICAL PRACTITIONERS, AND ADMINISTRATIVE AND LEGISLATIVE DECISION MAKERS

Context Setting	*Types of Evidence Preferred*	*Communication Formats Used*
Researchers: Universities; private sector; discipline oriented; long-term time frames	Original research; peer reviewed; scientific > qualitative; basic > applied research	Academic journals; academic meetings; Internet
Clinical: Community practice; clinical management; patient oriented; short-term time frames	Practical summaries; clinical applications; patient preferences; applied > basic research	Colleagues/conferences; summaries/reviews; audit/feedback; professional journals
Administrative: Public agencies; program oriented; population oriented; varying time frames	Practical summaries; program evaluations; cost effectiveness; applied > basic research	Summaries/reviews; personal contacts; conferences/meetings; Internet, journals, media
Legislative: Elected fora; problem oriented; responsiveness to crises; varying time frames	Problem summaries; policy solutions; cost effectiveness; anecdotal > scientific	Staff briefings; personal contacts; polls; constituents; media

Reprinted with permission from Waddell, C. (2002). So much research evidence, so little dissemination and uptake: Mixing the useful with the pleasing. *Evidence Based Nursing, 5*(38), 38-40.

overviews of research and how to get decision makers to agree to them. Decision makers, it must be remembered, have specific needs for the evidence they use. Among these, as Champagne (1999) says, is the need for data to be available, accessible, and valid. Without these characteristics even the most methodically rigorous study is liable to be given less importance than it may deserve:

Even when the evidence about outcomes and effectiveness is clear, local circumstances dictate how that evidence is translated into practice. Opportunities have recently emerged to share evidence globally about the outcomes and effectiveness of health care (globalization) and then translate that evidence into improved heath care at the local level (localization). To succeed in globalizing the evidence, policymakers must realize that opportunities to do so will be tempered by three competing core values: choice, efficiency, and equity (Elsenberg, 2002, p. 166).

Chunharas (2006) discusses the complexity of the knowledge chain and states that knowledge translation for policy works best if a "learning organization" is built within the health services and policy field. Their definition of a learning organization is an environment "structured in such as way as to facilitate learning as well as the sharing of knowledge among members or employees" (p. 652). Characteristics of a learning organization include the regular sharing of information

---

Table 13-3

TYPES OF EVIDENCE AND HOW THEY ARE USED IN POLICY MAKING

Types of Evidence	Information and Influence on Decision Making
Research	Empirical evidence from RCTs and other trials
	Analytic studies such as cohort or case control studies
	Time series analyses
	Observations, experiences, and case reports
	Qualitative studies
	Before and after studies
Knowledge and information	Results of consultation processes with networks/groups
	Internet
	Published documents/reports (including policy evaluations and statistical analyses)
Ideas and interests	Opinion and view—"expert knowledge" of individuals, groups, networks (shaped by past personal and professional experiences, beliefs, values, skills)
Politics	Information relevant to the agenda of government
	Political risk assessment and saleability
	Opportunity
	Crises
Economics	Finance and resource implications
	Cost effectiveness and other forms of economic evaluation
	Opportunity cost

Reprinted with permission from Bowen, S. & Zwi, A.B. (2005). Pathways to evidence informed policy and practice: A framework for action. *PLos Medicine, 2*(7), e166.

---

amongst colleagues, ensuring that the environment of the organization is considered in the transfer of knowledge, and a focus on developing a "problem-solving cycle" as the best means to use knowledge for management and policy decisions.

The author states the following types of knowledge that are used by health services decision makers:

- Information from their own organization via policies and guidelines about how to deal with and decide upon certain issues.

- Information from their own personal experience, knowledge, or discipline.

- Information from research evidence. (According to Chunharas [2006], this type of information is relied upon least often by decision makers. Reasons for this are similar to the reasons clinicians find it difficult to use EBP as discussed in Chapter 10).

Nuyens and Lansang (2006, p. 590) wrote an editorial that summarizes "lessons from knowledge translation initiatives" at the country level. The five lessons that they refer to are: (1) the systems context is extremely important; (2) continuity between past, current, and future research is important; (3) "complexity should be considered"—knowledge translation messages need to be modified for the intended recipient; (4) the various stakeholders should be involved in the knowledge transfer process (knowledge brokers can be used to aid this process); and (5) knowledge translation efforts need to pay more attention to increasing the skills and competencies needed to transfer the information ("capacity strengthening") and not just pay attention to the information itself.

In addition to macrolevel work on evidence-based policy, which attempts to understand the entire system, there are also smaller steps that have been taken toward moving research into policy. By examining the literature on evidence-based policy, common trends of the field can be understood. The first article to consider appeared in the journal Health Policy and discusses "practice guidelines." The authors (Lohr, Eleazer, & Mauskopf, 1998) contend that practice guidelines are the main format of evidence-based policy today. A practice guideline consists of a series of clinical recommendations or dictates on an issue that has been assembled from the best possible evidence. Practice guidelines are distributed by national clearinghouses to avoid conflict between them and to allow care to be standardized to one high standard. The foremost clearinghouse for evidence-based guidelines is the U.S. Agency for Health Care Policy and Research (AHCPR), which distributes a large volume of information on health care and EBP on the World Wide Web at www.ahcpr.gov. A more recent article by Gartlehner, et al. (2004) stresses the importance of keeping clinical practice guidelines up to date so that guidelines themselves remain "current and evidence based." This is an expensive process so the purpose of the article was to compare two different methods for updating guidelines.

Guidelines, like any health care documents, are subject both to practitioner bias and clinical error. Despite possible flaws, they are and can prove to be a strong initial link between research and policy. Lohr et al. (1998) present suggestions about guidelines themselves. Their suggestions are that guides should be systematic, logical, defensible (i.e., reliable and valid), practical, feasible, clear, and understandable to experts and laypersons alike (within reason). By making guidelines accessible, clients who take an interest in their care can begin to inform themselves as well. Lohr et al. also list benefits or goals of practice guidelines. A good practice guideline should do the following:

Improve knowledge by making clinicians aware of the recommendations.

- Change attitudes about standards of care.
- Shift practice patterns.
- Enhance patient outcomes.

In their article "Clinical practice guidelines: Between science and art," authors Battista and Hodge (1998) also discuss practice guidelines. As they see it, guidelines serve six principal roles:

1. Cost control
2. Quality assurance
3. Enhancing access to care
4. Patient empowerment
5. Safeguarding professional autonomy and medical liability
6. Resolving management issues (i.e., rationing, competition, micromanagement)

Once again, we can see that guidelines are expected to fulfill a variety of roles. The pressure put on clinical practice guidelines to fill all of these needs sometimes precludes them being very useful in any one area, and they may end up being only partially useful in many. Chapter 11 of this book discusses guidelines in detail.

In order to be able to form the best possible practice guidelines, Davis and Howden-Chapman's (1996) article, "Translating research findings into health policy," suggests several insights into the policy-making process. Foremost amongst their report is the admission that "the [decision making] process is more one of incremental adjustment to competing pressures than the rational formulation and pursuit of a single goal" (p. 867). Davis and Howden-Chapman suggest that research formed with the express goal of becoming a practice guideline and planned by policy makers as such is much more likely to be used.

As a word of warning, Davis and Howden-Chapman (1996) raise a very important point about the universality of practice guidelines. Although a practice guideline sanctioned by a body such as the AHCPR is a testament to the clinical knowledge that has been accumulated in the field, it runs the risk of segregating smaller local communities from the health care loop. Smaller centers and rural practitioners may feel that the currents of evidence, policy, and research have passed them by and since they had no hand in crafting this strange guideline, they will not heed it. Guidelines must be rigid enough to make some suggestions on the issue in question while simultaneously allowing flexibility for individual interpretation and adaptation to local surroundings. This is concordant with the goals of EBP: to take the best available evidence from the health sciences literature and policy and to integrate it into local practices.

A final word on practice guidelines comes from Stephen Birch (1997) at McMaster's Centre for Health Policy Analysis (CHEPA). In a detailed paper entitled, "As a matter of fact—Evidence-based decision making unplugged," Birch lucidly outlines how RCTs, systematic reviews, and EBP guidelines can all "lie." By failing to consider the socioeconomic class of study participants, for example, the "best evidence" for one population may be totally different from that for another. Practice guidelines can be dangerous, however, if they are used too universally. This speaks to the need for the holistic policy-making process and the contribution and input of local decision makers who attempt to draw many factors into a decision.

In a recent article in the Bulletin of the World Health Organization, Tugwell, Robinson, Grimshaw, and Santesso (2006) discuss this issue on a more global scale—trying to achieve equitable heath care through appropriate knowledge transfer to poor and disadvantaged countries or areas of the world. They propose a framework called "cascade for equity oriented knowledge translation" in which steps are to be followed to "assess and prioritize barriers and thus choose effective knowledge translation interventions that are tailored for relevant audiences" (Tugwell et al., 2006, p. 643). The authors suggest that the model can also be used by policy makers and health-care managers within practice their practice settings. Within the framework, the authors define six "Ps":

1. Public (community)
2. Patient
3. Press
4. Practitioner
5. Policy maker
6. Private sector

The five steps for knowledge translation into policy are as follows (Tugwell et al., 2006, p. 645):

1. Barriers and facilitators: Assess values, awareness, resources (e.g., skills, financial, human) for six Ps by socioeconomic status (SES).
2. Prioritize modifiable barriers across six Ps by SES.
3. Choose KT interventions to address key barriers: adapt evidence-based actionable messages, tailored for relevant audiences by SES.
4. Knowledge transfer effectiveness: Evaluate both process and health outcomes using appropriate study designs by SES.

5. Knowledge management and sharing: dissemination, diffusion, and application to other clinical conditions for six Ps.

Birch's article (1997) also raises another interesting point: Are there any characteristics of organizations themselves that can make them more open to considering new policies? Champagne (1999) has worked on the question and suggests that there are. Organizations that have an informal atmosphere, specialize in a particular field of knowledge, and participate in interorganization networks of knowledge sharing are most likely to adopt new innovations and recommendations with greater ease. In conventional institutions, problems with adopting new ideas may arise, such as the resistance of established health care professionals to new ideas due to their familiarity with the old. In more informal and less hierarchical systems, however, practitioners are more apt to feel as if they have a stake in shaping the use of a policy for their institution; therefore, they may be more willing to follow it.

A comprehensive discussion of EBP guidelines can be found in Gray and colleagues' (1997) article, "Transferring evidence from research into practice." Evidence-based policy and clinical guidelines, however, will be most apparent when examined on a case-by-case basis in which the blend of research and politics is evident. A good rule of thumb for all evidence-based policy making is that policies must apply to a wide range of people, be adaptable to the needs of local practitioners, and keep the best evidence at hand while spurring on toward future research.

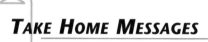

TAKE HOME MESSAGES

Research Transfer into Practice

✔ New innovations to replace usual transfer of research using widespread print media and large conferences.

✔ Research transfer model as three-pronged mechanism:

1. Input—Emphasis on preparing practitioners to gather and assimilate new information.

2. Throughput—Interpreting knowledge to be useful for individuals, preparing to teach others the knowledge.

3. Output—Reflection on research process and improvements; feedback loop.

✔ Effective research transfer dissemination strategies conform to personal learning needs of the researcher and utilize at least two different strategies simultaneously.

Evidence-Based Policy

✔ Not always a logical process, but based on the considerations of health care policy research and the consensus of a group who may not always be experts.

✔ Knowledge-driven model—Requires "perfect knowledge" and assumes knowledge will be adopted without impediment; unrealistic.

✔ Problem-driven model—Alternative approach; begins with a problem rather than research; acknowledges that evidence distribution is not always perfect and that policy makers tend to draw upon previously available information.

✔ Practice guidelines—Consist of series of clinical recommendations that have been assembled from the best possible evidence.

✔ Researchers see evidence in policy as a fundamentally linear and rational process; decision makers see more variety and are less likely to act on a single piece of evidence.

LEARNING AND EXPLORATION ACTIVITIES

The purpose of this chapter is to build upon the previous methods of organizing evidence in order to demonstrate the methods for transferring that evidence into practice and policy. These exercises highlight various sections of the chapter through leading the student through exercises both as an individual and as a group, which allow opportunities to utilize this understanding of the different types of evidence.

1. Research Transfer into Practice

a. What methods work best when transferring research findings? Oxman et al.'s (1995) chart suggests a number of ways of transferring research. Can you think of any more? Why would some be better than others? Which kind of learners are they primarily aimed at? Is there a way to make research transfer strategies which speak equally well to many different learning styles?

b. Try out your own research transfer. Choose a field, and find a piece of previously (to your knowledge) unapplied research. Through careful examination of the research conclusions, determine which parts of the research can be transferred into practice, and develop ways to do this (again, Oxman et al.'s [1995] methodologies will help here). If working in a group, each participant may attempt this exercise, and all can take turns at teaching others what they have found. Whose research transfer strategy worked "the best" (was memorable for the most people)? Why is this?

2. Evidence-Based Policy

a. This exercise will take some preparation and is best attempted in a group. Choose a topic of clinical interest and find a current clinical policy related to it. In the reference list of the policy should be a list of articles and academic sources used in its creation. Find two or three of the articles on this list, and assign one to each group member. Have each person read both the policy and their assigned article, and then convene together as a group. How was each person's article reflected in the policy? Which articles received more or less weight? Why might this have been? Does this policy make good use of current knowledge?

b. Attempt the same exercise in reverse: Find a number of articles on a subject and convene a "policy conference" around them. You will probably want to assign one article to each person and have them argue for it in the conference, as well as designating some nonaligned administrators and decision makers. Even more complex (and interesting) would be if every member of the group was given a specific interest that they were to support during the meeting, but which they could not directly reveal to others. After you have finished the exercise, evaluate your performance. How did you interact in the conference? What forms of discussion worked best? Were everyone's needs met to their satisfaction? Who "won"?

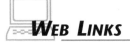

WEB LINKS

- *United States Agency for Health Care Policy and Research*
  www.ahcpr.gov
  This site has a great deal of information on health care policy, as well as a list of practice guidelines, which can be downloaded and examined.

- *Centre for Health Economics and Policy Analysis*
  www.chepa.org
  CHEPA, home of author Stephen Birch (mentioned previously in the chapter), does a great deal of work on health policy analysis and is on the forefront of new knowledge in the field.

- *Canadian Health Services Research Foundation*
  www.chsrf.ca
  Contains information on knowledge transfer as well as research summary info/ways to access "research-based evidence." Resources (conference reports, etc.) for knowledge transfer located at www.chsrf.ca/knowledge_transfer/resources_e.php

- *The Provincial Centre of Excellence for Child and Youth Mental Health at CHEO*
  www.onthepoint.ca
  Toolkit to support KT as well as online forum.

REFERENCES

Battista, R. N., & Hodge, M. J. (1998). Clinical practice guidelines: Between science and art. *Health Policy, 46*, 1-19.

Birch, S. (1997). As a matter of fact—Evidence-based decision making unplugged. *Health Economics, 6,* 547-559.

Bowen, S., & Zwi, A. B. (2005). Pathways to evidence informed policy and practice: A framework for action. *PLos Medicine, 2*(7), e166.

Canadian Research Transfer Network. (2001). Knowledge transfer: Looking beyond health. Retrieved October 16, 2006, from http://www.chsrf.ca/knowledge_transfer/resources_e.php

Champagne, F. (1999). *The use of scientific evidence and knowledge by managers: Closing the loop.* Toronto, ON: Third International Conference.

Chunharas, S. (2006). An interactive and integrative approach to translating knowledge and building a "learning organization" in health services management. *Bulletin of the World Health Organization, 84*(8), 652-657.

Dalton, C. C., & Gottlieb, L.N. (2003). The concept of readiness to change. *Journal of Advanced Nursing, 42*(2), 108-117.

Davis, D., Evans, M., Jadad, A., Perrier, L., Rath, D., Ryan, D., et al. (2003). The case for knowledge translation: shortening the journey from evidence to effect. *British Medical Journal, 327*(7405), 33-35.

Davis, P., & Howden-Chapman, P. (1996). Translating research findings into health policy. *Social Science & Medicine, 43*(5), 865-872.

Davies, H. T. O., & Nutley, S. M. (2002). Evidence-based policy and practice: Moving from rhetoric to reality. Discussion Paper 2. St Andrews: Research Unit for Research Utilisation, University of St. Andrews.

Dobbins, M., Ciliska, D., Cockerill, R., Barnsley, J., & DiCenso, A. (2002). A framework for the dissemination and utilization of research for health care policy and practice. *Online Journal of Knowledge Synthesis for Nursing, 9*(7).

Elsenberg, J. M. (2002). Globalize the evidence, localize the decision: Evidence-based medicine and international diversity. *Health Affairs, 21*(5), 166-168.

Gartlehner G., West, S. L., Lohr, K. N., Kahwati, L., Johnson, J. G., Harris, R. P., et al. (2004). Assessing the need to update prevention guidelines: A comparison of two methods. *International Journal for Quality in Health Care, 16*(5), 399-406).

Goode, C. J., Lovett, M. K., Hayes, J. E., & Butcher, L. A. (1987). Use of research based knowledge in clinical practice. *Journal of Nursing Administration, 17*(2), 11-18.

Gray, J. A., Haynes, R. B., Sackett, D. L., Cook, D. J., & Guyatt, G. H. (1997). Transferring evidence from research into practice: 3. Developing evidence-based clinical policy. *Evidence-Based Medicine, 2*(2), 36-8.

Hanney, S. R., Gonzalez-Block, M. A., Buxton, M. J., & Kogan, M. (2003). The utilization of health research in policy-making: concepts, examples and methods of assessment. Health Research and Policy Systems, 1(2). Retrieved October 16, 2006, from http://www.health-policysystems.com.libaccess.lib.mcmaster.ca/content/1/1/2)

Ho, K., Bloch, R., Gondocz, T., Laprise, R., Perrier, L., Ryan, D., et al. (2004). Technology enabled-knowledge translation: frameworks to promote research and practice. *Journal of Continuing Education in the Health Professions, 24*(2), 90-99.

Ho, K., Lauscher, H.N., Best, A., Jervis-Selinger, S., Fedeles, M., & Chockalingam, A. (2004). Dissecting technology-enabled knowledge translation: Essential challenges, unprecedented opportunities. *Clinical and Investigative Medicine, 27*(2), 70-78.

Jamtvedt, G., Young, J. M., Kristoffersen, D. T., O'Brien, M. A., & Oxman, A. D. (2006). Audit and feedback: Effects on professional practice and health care outcomes. Cochrane Database of Systematic Reviews, Issue 2. Art. No.: CD000259. DOI: 10.1002/14651858.CD000259.pub2.

Kerns, R. D., & Habib, S. (2004). A critical review of the pain readiness to change model. *Journal of Pain, 5*(7), 357-367.

Lohr, K. N., Eleazer, K., & Mauskopf, J. (1998). Health policy issues and applications for evidence-based medicine and clinical practice guidelines. *Health Policy, 46,* 1-19.

Nutley, S., Davies, H., & Walter, I. (2002). Evidence Based Policy and Practice: Cross Sector Lessons From the UK. Research Unit for Research Utilisation Department of Management, University of St. Andrews. ESRC UK Centre for Evidence Based Policy and Practice: Working Paper 9.

Nuyens, Y., & Lansang, M. A. D. (2006). Knowledge translation: linking the past to the future. *Bulletin of the World Health Organization, 84*(8), 590-591.

O'Brien, M. A., Oxman, A. D., Haynes, R. B., Davis, D. A., Freemantle, N., & Harvey, E. L. (1999). Local opinion leaders: Effects on professional practice and health care outcomes. Cochrane Database of Systematic Reviews, Issue 1. Art. No.: CD000125. DOI: 10.1002/14651858.CD000125.

Oxman, A. D., Thomson, M. A., Davis, D. A., & Haynes, R. B. (1995). No magic bullets: A systematic review of 102 trials of interventions to improve professional practice. *Canadian Medical Association Journal, 153*(10), 1423-1431.

Prochaska, J. O., Norcross, J. C., & DiClemente, C. C. (1995). *Changing for good.* New York: Morrow, William & Co.

Rogers, E. M. (1995). *Diffusion of innovations* (4th ed.). New York: The Free Press.

Sherman, M. D., & Carothers, R. A. (2005). Applying the readiness to change model to implementation of family intervention for serious mental illness. *Community Mental Health Journal, 41*(2), 115-127.

Siderov, J. (1995). How are internal medicine residency journal clubs organized and what makes them successful? *Archives of Internal Medicine, 155,* 1193-1197.

Teplicky, R. (2005). *Facilitating the use of family-centred service in a children's rehabilitation centre.* Hamilton, ON: McMaster University.

The Provincial Centre of Excellence for Child and Youth Mental Health at CHEO. (2006). Doing more with what you know. Ottawa, ON. www.onthepoint.ca

Thomson-O'Brien, M. A., & Moreland, J. (1998). Evidence-based practice information circle. *Physiotherapy Canada, 50*(3), 184-189, 205.

Tugwell, P., Robinson, V., Grimshaw, J. & Santesso, N. (2006). Systematic reviews and knowledge translation. *Bulletin of the World Health Organization, 84*(8), 643-651.

Waddell, C. (2002). So much research evidence, so little dissemination and uptake: mixing the useful with the pleasing. *Evidence Based Nursing, 5*(38), 38-40.

Weiss, C. H., & Weiss, J. A. (1981). Social scientists and decision makers look at the usefulness of mental health research. *American Psychologist, 36*(8), 837-847.

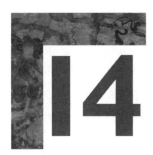

14

A Knowledge Transfer Example

Getting the Word Out: Disseminating Evidence About Children With Developmental Coordination Disorder

Cheryl Missiuna, PhD, OTReg(Ont); Robin Gaines, PhD, SLP(C), CASLPO, CCC-SLP; and Nancy Pollock, MSc, OTReg(Ont)

LEARNING OBJECTIVES

After reading this chapter, the student/practitioner will be able to:
- Gain insight into the application of knowledge transfer principles in a clinical context.
- Identify processes and specific strategies that may be useful in the development of educational materials for different target audiences.

It is your third referral this month for a school-aged child who has handwriting problems. Your wait-list is 15 months long and your manager has suggested that you consider eliminating those "fine motor kids" as one way of decreasing the load. From past experience, you know that most of the children referred with handwriting difficulties turn out to have a lot more going on. In fact, you believe that many children have developmental coordination disorder (DCD), even though none have been diagnosed with it. Your manager has never heard of DCD and does not understand why you are so concerned.

RECOGNIZING AND RESPONDING TO A PROBLEM

This scenario is one that is frequently faced by rehabilitation practitioners who work with school-aged children. Children who have difficulty performing everyday activities such as handwriting, tying shoelaces, and catching balls have been recognized by the American Psychiatric Association (APA) (2000) as having a distinct and primary disorder of motor development called developmental coordination disorder (DCD). DCD was first included in the Diagnostic and Statistical Manual of Mental Disorders in 1989 (APA, 1989), yet more than 15 years later, few health care providers know about it. Consistent prevalence estimates of 5% to 6%, tell us that this is an extremely common condition (APA, 2000). Why do so few health care and educational professionals know about it? What can be done to increase recognition and understanding of these children?

This was the situation that we faced in 2000. The problem was clear. A lot of research was accumulating about children with DCD but the evidence was not being translated into clinical practice. It was time to focus efforts on increasing awareness of children with DCD and disseminating the knowledge that was available.

What Did We Know?

In the past, children with DCD have been called "clumsy" (Gubbay, 1975), physically awkward (Wall, McClements, Bouffard, Findlay, & Taylor, 1985), or said to have developmental dyspraxia (Cermak, 1985) or sensory integrative dysfunction (Ayres, 1972). In 1994, however, an international consensus decision was reached that all of these types of children would be called children with *developmental coordination disorder* (Polatajko, Fox, & Missiuna, 1995). Many years spent researching the underlying difficulties of children with DCD and possible therapeutic interventions had led us to be able to make some strong statements.

- DCD is present from birth, yet most children are not recognized as having problems until behavioral and academic problems began to emerge during the school years (Fox & Lent, 1996).

- Children do not outgrow DCD. It is a chronic physical health condition and the motor problems persist (Cantell & Kooistra, 2002; Losse et al., 1991).

- Children's coordination difficulties are associated with the subsequent development of mental health difficulties, including the following:
  - Poor social competence (Cantell, Smyth, & Ahonen, 1994; Geuze & Borger, 1993)
  - Low self-esteem (Piek, Dworcan, Barrett, & Coleman, 2000; Skinner & Piek, 2001)
  - Anxiety (Sigurdsson, Van Os, & Fombonne, 2002);
  - Academic failure (Dewey, Kaplan, Crawford, & Wilson, 2002; Gillberg & Gillberg, 1989).
  - Decreased fitness, endurance, and participation in physical activity (Cairney, Hay, Faught, & Hawes, 2005; Raynor, 2001).

- Prevention of serious secondary physical and mental health issues is possible if parents, teachers, and children are educated about the disorder. This understanding allows the child and others to learn strategies to compensate for the motor difficulties (Cantell et al., 1994; Hamilton, 2002).

How Do You Approach a Problem of This Magnitude?

When planning this program of dissemination, we conceptualized new evidence from health care research about children with DCD as an "innovation" that could be transferred to family members, physicians, and service providers using methods that are appropriate to each individual or group (Dobbins, Cockerill, & Barnsley, 2001). This way of thinking about knowledge transfer comes from Roger's *Diffusion of Innovations* model (Rogers, 1995) and will be described in more detail later in this chapter. Information about other knowledge transfer models and methods was outlined in Chapter 13.

The purpose of this systematic program of knowledge translation was two-fold: 1) to facilitate earlier identification of children with DCD; and 2) to prevent the secondary consequences of DCD. Each objective had to be approached differently.

Dissemination Designed to Facilitate Early Identification

A large study conducted in 1998 by the Dyspraxia Foundation had shown that parents often recognized their children's motor difficulties at quite an early age (Dyspraxia Foundation, 2006). Typically, they would ask their physician or another health professional about their concerns and would be told not to worry (Fox & Lent, 1996; Hamilton, 2002). We recognized that the optimal approach would be to educate family physicians and pediatricians; however, DCD was still largely unknown, particularly in the medical community. It seemed reasonable to begin to increase awareness among other health professionals who might be receptive to the information. Children with DCD were being seen for other reasons by allied health care practitioners, such as speech-language pathologists and optometrists, when they were toddlers and preschoolers. Physical and occupational therapists, although having more general knowledge about childhood movement disorders, also seemed to be unfamiliar with DCD. We needed to figure out what information was needed for these practitioners to be able to recognize the early signs of DCD from their individual perspectives.

A series of flyers was developed that describe the *"Role of the _____ in Recognizing Children with DCD"* (Missiuna, 2004; Missiuna & Gaines, 2003; Missiuna & Pollock, 2001, 2005, 2006; Missiuna & Rivard, 2003). Literature was reviewed and clinical experts were identified within each profession (optometry, speech-language pathology, medicine, psychology, physiotherapy, occupational therapy) who could outline the informational needs of their profession and who would be willing to participate either in writing the flyer or in providing feedback. In some cases, a small study was conducted to identify what particular service providers would be able to observe during typical treatment sessions. For example, we learned through videotape observation of preschool speech-language sessions that speech-language pathologists need to pay attention to which children they are giving extra help with self-care and table top activities; these are the children who are most likely to have DCD (study described in Missiuna, Gaines, & Pollock, 2002).

Using the principles of keeping materials attractive, easy to read, evidence based, and to the point, each professional flyer followed the same format. Page 1 outlined the specific role of that health professional in recognizing the young child with DCD. Pages 2 and 3 provided more information about DCD, geared to the interests of that profession and describes the types of observations they might be able to make. Page 4 was written for parents so it could be photocopied and distributed directly. This latter page introduced the idea of DCD to the parent and recommended referral for further motor and/or medical assessment. Once each flyer was drafted, it was circulated for feedback to other members of that profession; typically, feedback was requested from practitioners who knew quite a bit about DCD and those who did not. Revisions were made and flyers were then posted on the *CanChild* Centre for Childhood Disability Web site at McMaster University, Canada at www.canchild.ca. Whenever possible, a lengthier, evidence-based and profession-specific article was also written and published (e.g., DeLaat, 2006 [psychology]; Missiuna, Gaines, & Soucie, 2006 [MD]; Missiuna, Pollock, DeLaat, Egan, Gaines & Soucie, 2007 [OT]; Missiuna, Rivard, & Bartlett, 2003 [PT]; Missiuna et al., 2002 [SLP]) for practitioners who were interested in learning more. An example of one of these flyers is provided in Appendix K).

Preventing the Secondary Consequences of Developmental Coordination Disorder

The second objective of preventing the physical and mental health deterioration that so often accompanies DCD required quite a different approach. If one accepted the research evidence that suggested that the underlying motor impairment in DCD would not go away, then the

---

M.A.T.C.H. the Activity to the Child

Modify the task
This involves changing aspects of an activity that are too difficult for the child to perform. The important thing about modifying a task is that the child can still experience success if they make a genuine effort to participate in the activity.

Alter your Expectations
Consider what the ultimate goal of an activity is and then think about where you can be flexible. Allowing extra time or alternate methods of completing a task can make the difference between a lesson learned and an experience of failure for a child with DCD.

Teaching Strategies
Children with DCD have full capacity to learn with their peers, but may require a slightly different teaching approach. Investigate alternate teaching strategies designed for children with special needs.

Change the Environment
Pay attention to what is going on around a child when he/she is experiencing success or difficulty (i.e. noise, level of activity, visual distractions). Minimize the environmental factors that make performance difficult for the child.

Help by Understanding
Understanding the nature of DCD will help you to problem solve and provide all of your students with rich learning experiences. If children feel supported and understood, they are more likely to attempt new activities and to persevere until they achieve success.

Figure 14-1. Using a meaningful acronym to guide problem solving.

emphasis needed to be on helping people in the child's environment to understand the reasons for the child's daily challenges and to accommodate for them. The most important target audiences for this type of dissemination are the child's parents and teachers.

In 1992, a general information booklet was written for parents and teachers of school-aged children with DCD (Missiuna, 1992). Feedback was collected systematically from therapists, teachers, and parents across Canada and was used to revise it (Missiuna, 1995). The booklet seemed to be very useful, particularly for parents, and they have continued to provide input and suggestions since then. Changes to the booklet occurred over the next decade and it was posted on the *CanChild* Web site in 2003 (Missiuna, 2003). The booklet continues to be accessed frequently and has subsequently been posted in French and Portuguese; a translation into Mandarin is underway.

Teachers who were surveyed reported that the booklet was useful but it became apparent, from what parents were telling us, that very few teachers were aware of either the booklet or the condition of DCD. We decided to develop short flyers that were specific to the needs of busy teachers who are struggling with a particular child with DCD in their classroom. A series of flyers was developed to introduce teachers to a problem-solving method that can be used to "MATCH" a difficult task to the child's abilities rather than trying to change the child. The acronym M.A.T.C.H. reminds teachers that they can **M**odify the task, **A**lter their expectations, **T**each strategies, **C**hange the environment, or **H**elp the child by understanding their difficulties (Figure 14-1). Grade-specific examples of each of these steps are then provided so teachers can relate the information directly to the specific difficulties being observed in their classroom. The background and rationale for this particular problem-solving method is outlined in the article by Missiuna and colleagues (Missiuna, Rivard, & Pollock, 2004). The flyers were subsequently posted on the *CanChild* Web site and parents are often the ones who access the flyer appropriate to their child's grade and provide it to his or her teacher.

In response to other needs identified by parents, flyers were developed that were also designed to prevent the secondary consequences of DCD through increased awareness and understanding of the condition. Simple short flyers (Appendix L) were written to give coaches, sports instructors, and community leaders (e.g., Scouts, faith-based groups, art instructors) a quick overview of the issues they might see in a leisure program and some suggestions of things that might be able to support the child's participation. Another flyer was developed to help parents understand the types of organized sports that will be easier/more difficult for their child with DCD so they can increase the likelihood of success (Rivard & Missiuna, 2004). Handwriting difficulties are a very common issue, and both parents and teachers frequently ask when to introduce keyboarding: "To type or to write, that is the question!" (Pollock & Missiuna, 2005) systematically addresses these concerns. An annotated bibliography rounds out this set of flyers by providing parents with guidance about where they can find books about DCD for themselves, for teachers, and for the child who has DCD (Pollock, 2004).

RESEARCHING KNOWLEDGE TRANSFER AND EXCHANGE

Although the flyers and booklets were evidence based and developed with consumers and stakeholders, their effectiveness in meeting the objectives of improving identification and management of children with DCD had not been systematically tested. By 2004, we were ready to undertake a research study that would directly examine knowledge transfer about DCD. This type of study is called a *research utilization* study and is defined as "the process of transferring research-based knowledge into clinical practice" (Dobbins, Ciliska, Cockerill, Barnsley, & DiCenso, 2002, p. 2). Evidence-based information is translated into a form that is useful to the user and then implemented into practice (Dobbins et al., 2002). So, the first question was, who should the target audience be?

A qualitative study that we had conducted with parents of children with DCD had shown clearly that parents related concerns about their child's motor difficulties to their family physicians when their children were still young. In some cases, they also provided information suggesting that their child might have DCD, yet most physicians had never heard of it; hence, families traveled from one health provider to another, looking for answers (Missiuna, Moll, Law, King, & King, 2006). With the support of representatives of the College of Family Physicians of Ontario, a research project was developed to examine the transfer of information to physicians about how to listen for and diagnose DCD (Gaines, Missiuna, Egan, & McLean, 2006). Family physicians are in an ideal position to identify children with DCD as they have frequent contact with them as young children and are viewed by parents as their primary health service and referral source for interdisciplinary care. Also, these physicians have the skills to rule out related disorders such as cerebral palsy and degenerative neurological conditions, a step that is necessary in providing a diagnosis of DCD.

Many approaches to enhance research utilization within health care are now informed by Roger's *Diffusion of Innovations* model (Rogers, 1995). In this study, knowledge about DCD and its diagnosis, prognosis, and appropriate intervention was viewed as the "innovation" and primary care family physicians as the "adopters" of the innovation. The process involved in adopting new knowledge consists of learning about the innovation (in this case identifying children with DCD), being persuaded of its usefulness, deciding to use it, implementing it, and continuing its use in clinical practice.

There is a lot to be learned about children with DCD so it was important to focus the type of knowledge that was going to be introduced. We decided to focus on screening techniques and a model that would involve the physician identifying children as having "probable DCD" and then requesting further assessment of the children's motor abilities. Identification and subsequent diagnosis of DCD would occur following collaborative discussion between the physician and an occupational therapist. This process helped to confirm the physician's uptake and application of knowledge. This emphasis was based on consideration of Rogers' principles (Rogers, 1995) for ensuring rapid adoption of knowledge into practice. The specific type of knowledge that is to be disseminated needs to have the following (Berwick, 2003; Rogers, 1995):

- *Compatibility*—Be compatible with the values, beliefs, and current needs of individuals.
- *Relative advantage*—Be perceived as beneficial by the user.
- *Simplicity*—Have a message that is relatively easy to understand and communicate to others.
- *Trialability*—Able to be tested by the user on a small scale before trying to implement it more broadly.
- *Observability*—Potential users can watch others try out the new knowledge first.

Early identification of DCD has a high level of *compatibility* with primary care physicians' beliefs in the importance of early identification and prevention of associated disorders. We anticipated that family physicians would appreciate the *relative advantage* of having rapid access to interdisciplinary information that assisted them in the identification and management of children with DCD. Third, there was *simplicity* regarding integration of knowledge into practice because screening for DCD could occur during annual office visits. Also, the physicians' role in referring children for confirmatory assessment was easy to understand. Fourth, there was *trialability*; primary care physicians would receive feedback on the appropriateness of their referrals for assessments by discussing the child's profile with the occupational therapist. Finally, there was the potential for *observability* because physicians who were early adopters of this knowledge would share their experience of learning about DCD and referring children with other members of their group practices.

The next decision was about which particular knowledge translation methods to use for this audience and this innovation. Systematic reviews of methods to transfer knowledge to physicians had shown that passive dissemination strategies such as the distribution of written materials were largely ineffective (Davis, Thomson, Oxman, & Haynes, 1992). Education sessions that included an interactive component and involved face-to-face contact had shown positive results in the literature with a variety of health care practitioners so that was certainly one possibility (Davis et al., 1999; Oxman, Thomson, Davis, & Hayes, 1995; Thomson et al., 2001). The most promising approach for the type of innovation that we had in mind, however, was referred to as educational outreach or "academic detailing" (Albert, Ahluwalia, Ward, & Sadowsky, 2004)

Educational outreach is a knowledge translation intervention designed to improve clinical practice through face-to-face training of health professionals in their practice setting (Albert et al., 2004). One study that used educational outreach to improve physicians' detection and management of intimate partner violence had shown that this approach significantly improved screening and documentation by physicians (Edwardson, Pless, Fiscella, Horwitz, & Meldrum, 2004). In a systematic review of studies on the effectiveness of educational outreach visits on professional practice and health care outcomes, O'Brien et al. (1997) had concluded that the evidence strongly supported outreach visits as an effective knowledge translation intervention especially when combined with any other intervention (including educational materials, conferences, reminders, audit and feedback, opinion leaders, and marketing strategies).

Multiple knowledge translation methods were used in our study; however, the novel emphasis in the family physician study was the educational outreach provided by occupational therapists who went into the community and met with individual or small groups of family physicians. These occupational therapists provided short talks over breakfast or lunch that included showing and discussion of a DVD. The DVD was created to illustrate typical children and children with DCD performing screening activities that a physician could administer in the office setting (for description and example items, see Missiuna, Gaines, & Soucie, 2006).

The occupational therapist responded to each physician's level of awareness and knowledge of DCD, tailoring educational opportunities based upon the physician's learning needs and interests. In some cases, a physician might review the DVD with the occupational therapist highlighting key observations of children's movement. Another physician might ask the occupational therapist to demonstrate the use of screening tools designed for physicians so that he or she would learn to administer them in a consistent way. In other cases, the physician would refer a child and would then observe the occupational therapist conducting a complete assessment and discuss the observations. In all instances, the learning needs and interests of the individual physician was respected.

In order to maximize the likelihood of uptake of knowledge about DCD, we used other multifaceted interventions as recommended by Oxman and colleagues (1995). In this study, these included the following:

- *Educational materials:* An attractive and user-friendly binder (DCD PACK, see description later in this chapter) and access to a Web site that covered the same information were provided to each physician who participated.

- *Interactive workshops:* Presentations were given at local research rounds and pediatric update days.

- *Workshops/inservices:* Educational sessions were given to allied health and educational professionals in the community who provided grass roots support and encouragement to physicians to identify children with movement difficulties.

- *Audit:* The occupational therapists reviewed charts with any physician who was wondering about whether a child might have DCD.

- *Feedback:* After the occupational therapist assessed a child who was referred, he or she met with the physician to review the findings. This served to provide feedback to the physician about the accuracy of the referral.

- *Reminders:* Laminated folders were produced that outlined the screening activities that the physician was to use. A tear-off pad was created with a short questionnaire for parents to complete.

The family physician project was very successful. In just over a year, 147 doctors participated in the project, learning ways to interview parents and screen for DCD while collaborating with an occupational therapist in the primary care setting. A *shared care* model was implemented as the occupational therapist identified and assessed specific coordination difficulties while the doctor ruled out other possible causes. Physicians were asked to provide feedback about the ways in which they accessed or used different types of knowledge translation methods. Physicians reported that the individualized educational outreach by the occupational therapist was extremely valuable and enhanced their service to families and children. Finally, the physician and occupational therapist disseminated to the families the educational materials described earlier in this chapter so the family could become the provider of information to teachers and others. Families reported a high level of satisfaction with the information and method of delivery of service to their child.

What Have We Learned Along the Way?

A few tips and strategies are outlined in this section that have emerged throughout our knowledge transfer and exchange program and that may be useful, regardless of the content that you wish to disseminate.

Work With Your Target Audience to Develop Materials That Meet Their Needs, Not Yours

Each of our educational materials, from the allied health professional flyers to the booklet and workshop for parents, has been developed in partnership with one or more representatives from the target audience. The first step is to identify what information they already have and what they identify as important for them to know. Then, materials are developed based on existing evidence. The next stage is to obtain feedback from target users who were not involved in the preliminary phases; this feedback is used to revise the material. Ideally, materials are then tested more formally with a broader audience. Feedback is again solicited and used to revise the final product.

The *DCD Physician Allied Health Collaboration Kit* (DCD PACK) (Missiuna & Gaines, 2004) is a good illustration of this process. A binder of information was developed in collaboration with representatives from the College of Family Physicians of Ontario who identified the type of knowledge that physicians already had and what new information was needed and gave feedback about the presentation of each section. The binder was then disseminated to 10 practicing family physicians who provided individual feedback. It was then revised and reprinted, and 200 hundred copies were shared. Written feedback was solicited by questionnaire from the physicians who used the binder clinically. The final version has now been posted as a physician Web site at www.dcdpack.ca (username: dcdpack; password: dcdchild) and is available to physicians who did not participate in the study.

Keep It Short and User-Friendly!

The information that you have to convey is usually grounded in clinical and research evidence but not all users are interested in knowing as much as you do about it. Following a 1-3-25 page approach may be helpful (Fooks, Cooper, & Bhatia, 1995). Produce a one-page summary of the key points and bottom line messages that you want people to remember. Produce a slightly longer version, perhaps three to four pages, that provides more detail for interested users but is not overwhelming. In each of these short documents, refer people to a longer peer-reviewed article (written by you or someone else) that is a good summary of the research evidence. Readers will quickly come to learn that your materials are evidence based but will appreciate the effort that you have put into summarizing the material and making it accessible.

Give Them a "Hook" to Hang It On

While new information may be of interest to your target audience, it is often unfamiliar and, therefore, may be hard for them to remember. Information needs to be synthesized into key points that will be recalled easily by the user.

Alliteration or meaningful acronyms can be used to help organize information in a way that makes it accessible. For example, the key points that family physicians need to remember about children with DCD were summarized as the 5 Cs of DCD (Figure 14-2). Children with DCD are *Clumsy*. It is a *Common* and *Chronic* disorder that doesn't go away. DCD is *Comorbid* with a number of other developmental conditions and, if left unrecognized, there are *Consequences*. These key points were laminated with screening activities on the back, creating a simple reminder that could be placed in each examining room.

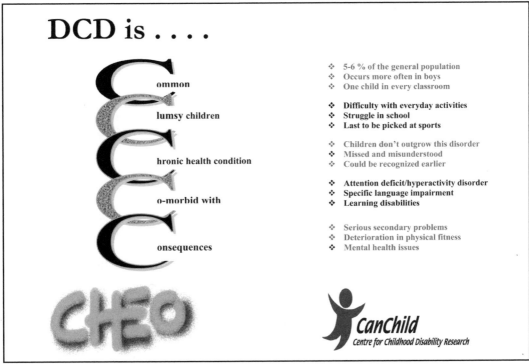

Figure 14-2. Using alliteration to facilitate recall of key messages.

Acronyms can also be useful, particularly if they have inherent meaning. The M.A.T.C.H. flyers (see Figure 14-1) were designed to remind teachers to "match" the task to the child with DCD. The *DCD PACK* is a "pack" of materials and the words **P**hysician **A**llied health **C**ollaboration **K**it remind physicians that the key message is to collaborate with allied health professionals in identifying, diagnosing and managing children with DCD.

Translations Need to Be Developed With Care

Given the bilingual nature of Canada, and clients from multiethnic backgrounds in many countries, many therapists find it useful to have educational materials translated into other languages. Purchasing the services of a professional translator is always recommended but can be costly. If materials are translated by a nonprofessional volunteer, it is important to ensure that you get at least two back translations—one from a user who knows something about the content and one from a user who is unfamiliar with the content.

Miscommunication can occur due to differences in the language itself or in the cultural background and assumptions of the user. As an example, an interesting difficulty arose when we tried to translate the teacher M.A.T.C.H. flyers into French. The equivalent term in French could not be translated easily into words that would still cue teachers to recall the five-step problem-solving strategy. Our solution was to use the word A.D.A.P.T.E., which altered the order but retained the concept that we were trying to illustrate:

- **A**dapter la tache
- **D**éfinir de nouvelles attentes
- **A**ider en comprenant mieux

- **Pr**êter son appui et se montrer compréhensive
- **T**ransformer l'environnement
- **E**nseigner des stratégies

As another, rather humorous example, cultural differences became evident when the DCD parent booklet was being translated into Mandarin. A suggestion in the DCD booklet to *photocopy pages from a math text book* (to reduce the child's need to copy from the board) was translated in Mandarin into a recommendation to have the child *copy math pages many times*. The point was clearly lost in translation as this is the worst thing you could ask a child with fine motor problems to do!

Do Not Assume: Demonstrate Effectiveness!

Rehabilitation professionals are in a key position to develop and share information and skills with other professionals and with caregivers. All too often, however, educational materials are provided to clients, or workshops are delivered to other professionals, with an assumption that simply providing evidence-based information will be sufficient. Even when you develop materials with a representative from your target population, you still need to check the effectiveness of your knowledge transfer with the larger audience. In the family physician project, change in the knowledge and empowerment of both the physicians and the families, as well as their sharing of educational materials with others, were measured. This is obviously easier to do in a research project, but service providers can enhance and check the impact of knowledge translation by discussing how key concepts impact on a client's current issues; pointing to diagrams, charts of tips, or strategies to demonstrate use of educational materials; asking the client about whether they have shared the materials with others; tracking rates and appropriateness of referrals and so on. Information needs to be applicable to the *current* needs of your target audience or it will not be used and applied.

BRINGING IT ALL TOGETHER:
A SYSTEMATIC PROCESS OF DISSEMINATION

In summary, the "innovation," or knowledge that was being disseminated, was rooted in evidence about DCD from the research literature but also in the observations and experiences that parents have shared with us (Missiuna, Moll, & Law et al., 2006; Missiuna, Moll, King, King, & Law, 2006, in press), in the experiences of service providers and, most recently, in experiences shared with us by young adults with DCD (Missiuna, Moll, Stewart, King, & Macdonald, 2007). As new evidence emerges from any of these sources, the innovation will develop and change. The branches, or targets, of the DCD dissemination program have been illustrated in Figure 14-3. Each branch was identified based upon either the ability of a target audience to contribute to earlier identification or their need for knowledge that would facilitate better understanding and management of the children. As knowledge grows and educational materials expand, initial target audiences such as families begin to become the primary disseminators of knowledge—to teachers, extended family members, and the community. Rooted in research and a solid trunk of knowledge, the limbs and branches have now reached many target groups and, in the process, have hopefully made a difference in the lives of children and families.

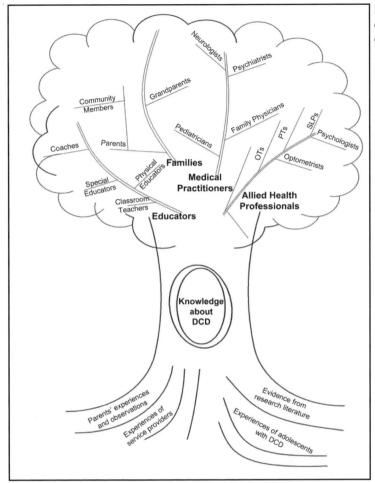

Figure 14-3. Rooted in evidence—disseminating knowledge about DCD.

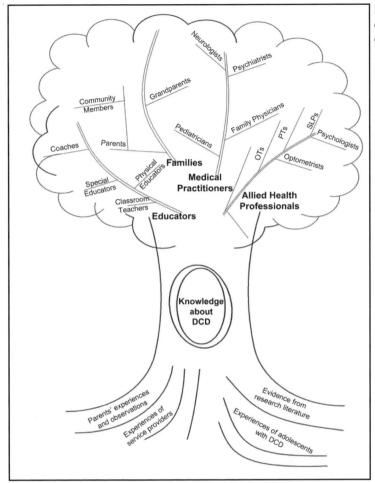

TAKE-HOME MESSAGES

✔ To be effective, knowledge transfer materials should be based in evidence, easy to read, and provide practical strategies.

✔ Knowledge exchange is a two-way street that works best when the target audience is involved in identifying the knowledge that is needed and the way that it is presented.

✔ Creative use of techniques such as pictures, alliteration, or acronyms can facilitate retention and application of new knowledge.

✔ Whenever possible, the impact of knowledge transfer materials should be evaluated.

LEARNING AND EXPLORATION ACTIVITIES

The purpose of this chapter is to provide the students with a concrete example of how information about a condition can be transferred to the different stakeholders involved.

1. In this chapter, the author describes key components of disseminated knowledge which can lead to greater understanding. These are:
   - Compatibility
   - Relative advantage
   - Simplicity
   - Trialability
   - Observability

   What are characteristics of each of these components? What is the most constructive way that each of these components can be presented? In what ways can the alteration of each component affect how the information is received?

2. In this chapter, several methods of knowledge dissemination are presented. These include educational materials, interactive workshops, in-services, audit, feedback, and reminders. In your class, choose a partner or small group. Discuss with your partner/group an instance where each method of knowledge dissemination would be appropriate. Discuss an instance where each technique would not be the most appropriate choice.

REFERENCES

Albert, D. A., Ahluwalia, K. P., Ward, A., & Sadowsky, D. (2004). The use of "academic detailing" to promote tobacco-use cessation counseling in dental offices. *Journal of the American Dental Association, 135*, 1700-1706.

American Psychiatric Association. (1989). *Diagnostic and statistical manual of mental disorders* (3rd ed., revised). Washington, DC: Author.

American Psychiatric Association. (2000). *Diagnostic and statistical manual of mental disorders* (4th ed., text rev.). Washington, DC: Author.

Ayres, A. J. (1972). *Sensory integration and learning disorders*. Los Angeles: Western Psychological Services.

Berwick, D. M. (2003). Disseminating innovations in health care. *Journal of the American Medical Association, 289*(15), 1969-1975.

Cairney, J., Hay, J. A., Faught, B. E., & Hawes, R. (2005). Developmental coordination disorder and overweight and obesity in children aged 9-14 y. *International Journal of Obesity, 29*(4), 369-372.

Cantell, M., & Kooistra, L. (2002). Long-term outcomes of developmental coordination disorder. In S. Cermak, & D. Larkin (Eds.), *Developmental coordination disorder* (pp. 23-38). Albany, NY: Delmar.

Cantell, M. H., Smyth, M. M., & Ahonen, T. (1994). Clumsiness in adolescence: Educational, motor and social outcomes of motor delay at five years. *Adapted Physical Activity Quarterly, 11*, 115-129.

Cermak, S. (1985). Developmental dyspraxia. In E. A. Roy (Ed.), *Neuropsychological studies of apraxia and related disorders* (pp. 225-248). Amsterdam: North-Holland.

Davis, D., O'Brien, M. A. T., Freemantle, N., Wolf, F. M., Mazmanian, P., & Taylor-Vaisey, A. (1999). Impact of formal continuing medical education: Do conferences, modules, rounds and other traditional continuing education activities change physician behavior or health care outcomes? *Journal of the American Medical Association, 282*(9), 867-874.

Davis, D. A., Thomson, M. A., Oxman, A. D., & Haynes, R. B. (1992). Evidence for the effectiveness of CME: A review of 50 randomized controlled trials. *Journal of the American Medical Association, 268*(9), 111-117.

De Laat, M. D. (2006). Developmental coordination disorder. In M. Mamen (Ed.), *Nonverbal learning disabilities and their clinical subtypes: A handbook for parents and professionals* (pp. 78-80). Ottawa, ON: Centrepointe Professional Services.

Dewey, D., Kaplan, B. J., Crawford, S. G., & Wilson, B. N. (2002). Developmental coordination disorder: Associated problems in attention, learning, and psychosocial adjustment. *Human Movement Science, 21*(5-6), 905-918.

Dobbins, M., Ciliska, D., Cockerill, R., Barnsley, J., & DiCenso, A. (2002). A framework for the dissemination and utilization of research for health-care policy and practice. *Online Journal of Knowledge Synthesis in Nursing, 9*, 7.

Dobbins, M., Cockerill, R., & Barnsley, J. (2001). Factors affecting the utilization of systematic reviews. *International Journal of Technology Assessment in Health Care, 17*, 203-214.

Dyspraxia Foundation. (2006). Article title? Retrieved June 5, 2006, from http://www.dyspraxiafoundation. org.uk

Edwardson, E. A., Pless, N. A., Fiscella, K. A., Horwitz, S. H., & Meldrum, S. C. (2004). Pilot educational outreach project on partner violence. *Preventive Medicine, 39*, 536-542.

Fooks, C., Cooper, J., & Bhatia, V. (1995). *Making research transfer work.* Toronto, ON: Institute for Clinical Evaluative Sciences.

Fox, A. M., & Lent, B. (1996). Clumsy children: Primer on developmental coordination disorder. *Canadian Family Physician, 42*, 1965-1971.

Gaines, R., Missiuna, C., Egan, M., & McLean, J. (2006). Promoting interdisciplinary identification and improved service delivery for children with developmental coordination disorder and their families. *Final Report to Ontario Ministry of Health and Long-Term Care and Health Canada.*

Geuze, R., & Borger, H. (1993). Children who are clumsy: Five years later. *Adapted Physical Activity Quarterly, 10*, 10-21.

Gillberg, I. C., & Gillberg, C. (1989). Children with preschool minor neurodevelopmental disorders. IV: Behaviour and school achievement at age 13. *Developmental Medicine and Child Neurology, 31*, 3-13.

Gubbay, S. S. (1975). *The clumsy child: A study of developmental apraxic and agnostic ataxia.* London: W. B. Saunders.

Hamilton, S. S. (2002). Evaluation of clumsiness in children. *American Family Physician, 66*(8), 1435-40, 1379.

Losse, A., Henderson, S. E., Elliman, D., Hall, D., Knight, E., & Jongmans, M. (1991). Clumsiness in children--do they grow out of it? A 10-year follow-up study. *Developmental Medicine and Child Neurology, 33*, 55-68.

Missiuna, C. (1992). *Management of children with developmental coordination disorder: At home and in the classroom. [booklet].* Hamilton, ON: Author.

Missiuna, C. (1995). *Management of children with developmental coordination disorder: At home and in the classroom. [booklet].* Hamilton, ON: CanChild Centre for Childhood Disability Research.

Missiuna, C. (2003). *Children with developmental coordination disorder: At home and in the classroom.* (5th ed.). *[booklet].* Hamilton, ON: McMaster University: CanChild Centre for Childhood Disability Research.

Missiuna, C. (2004). *Recognizing and referring children with developmental coordination disorder: The role of the medical practitioner.* Retrieved June 5, 2006 from www.canchild.ca

Missiuna, C., & Gaines, B. R. (2003). *Recognizing and referring children with developmental coordination disorder: The role of the speech-language pathologist.* Retrieved June 5, 2006 from www.canchild.ca.

Missiuna, C., & Gaines, R. (2004). *The DCD physician allied health collaboration kit (DCD PACK).* Hamilton, ON: Author.

Missiuna, C., Gaines, B. R., & Pollock, N. (2002). Recognizing and referring children at risk for developmental coordination disorder: Role of the speech-language pathologist. *Journal of Speech-Language Pathology & Audiology, 26*, 172-179.

Missiuna, C., Gaines, R. B., & Soucie, H. C. (2006). Why every office needs a tennis ball: A new approach to assessing the clumsy child. *Canadian Medical Association Journal, 175, 471-473.*

Missiuna, C., Moll, S., King, G., King, S., & Law, M. (2006). "Missed and misunderstood": Children with developmental coordination disorder in the school system. *International Journal of Special Education, 21*, 53-67.

Missiuna, C., Moll, S., Law, M., King, S., & King, G. (2006). Mysteries and mazes: Parents' experiences of children with developmental coordination disorder. *Canadian Journal of Occupational Therapy, 73,* 7-17.

Missiuna, C., Moll, S., King, G., King, S., & Law, M. (2007). A troubling trajectory: The impact of coordination difficulties on children's development. *Physical and Occupational Therapy in Pediatrics, 27,* 81-101.

Missiuna, C., Moll, S., King, G., Stewart, D., & Macdonald, K. (2007). Managing differences: Pathways to resilience for young adults with DCD. *Proceedings of the International DCD VII Conference* (p. 35). Melbourne, Australia.

Missiuna, C., & Pollock, N. (2001). *Role of the optometrist: A new perspective on school-aged children with visual motor difficulties.* Retrieved June 5, 2006 from www.canchild.ca.

Missiuna, C., & Pollock, N. (2005). *Recognizing and referring children with developmental coordination disorder: The role of the psychologist.* Retrieved June 5, 2006 from www.canchild.ca.

Missiuna, C., & Pollock, N. (2006). *Recognizing and referring children with developmental coordination disorder: The role of the occupational therapist.* Retrieved June 5, 2006 from www.canchild.ca.

Missiuna, C., Pollock, N., DeLaat, D., Egan, M., Gaines, R., & Soucie, H. (In press). Enabling occupation through facilitating the diagnosis of developmental coordination disorder. *Canadian Journal of Occupational Therapy.*

Missiuna, C., & Rivard, L. (2003). *Recognizing and referring children with developmental coordination disorder: Role of the physical therapist.* Retrieved June 5, 2006 from www.canchild.ca.

Missiuna, C., Rivard, L., & Bartlett, D. (2003). Early identification and risk management of children with development coordination disorder. *Pediatric Physical Therapy, 15,* 32-8.

Missiuna, C., Rivard, L., & Pollock, N. (2004). They're bright but can't write: Developmental coordination disorder in school aged children. *TEACHING Exceptional Children Plus, 1*(1). Article 3.

Moll, S., Missiuna, C., Stewart, D., King, G., & Macdonald, K. (2006). Young adults with developmental coordination disorder: From disability to resilience. [Abstract]. *Canadian Journal of Occupational Therapy, Conference Supplement.*

O'Brien, M. A., Oxman, A. D., Davis, D. A., Haynes, R. B., Freemantle, N., & Harvey, E. L. (1997). Educational outreach visits: Effects on professional practice and health care outcomes (review). *The Cochrane Database of Systematic Reviews, 4,* CD000409-DOI: 10.1002/14651858.CD000409.

Oxman, A. D., Thomson, M. A., Davis, D. A., & Hayes, J. E. (1995). No magic bullets: A systematic review of 102 trials of interventions to improve professional practice. *Canadian Medical Association Journal, 153,* 1423-1431.

Piek, J. P., Dworcan, M., Barrett, N., & Coleman, R. (2000). Determinants of self-worth in children with and without developmental coordination disorder. *The International Journal of Disability Development and Education, 47,* 259-271.

Polatajko, H., Fox, M., & Missiuna, C. (1995). An international consensus on children with developmental coordination disorder. *Canadian Journal of Occupational Therapy, 62,* 3-6.

Pollock, N. (2004). *Annotated bibliography.* Retrieved June 6, 2006 from www.canchild.ca

Pollock, N., & Missiuna, C. (2005). *To write or to type: That is the question!* Retrieved June 6, 2006, from www.canchild.ca.

Raynor, A. J. (2001). Strength, power and co-activation in children with developmental coordination disorder. *Developmental Medicine and Child Neurology, 43,* 676-684.

Rivard, L., & Missiuna, C. (2004). *Encouraging participation in physical activities for children with developmental coordination disorder.* Retrieved June 6, 2006 from www.canchild.ca.

Rogers, E. M. (1995). *Diffusion of innovations.* New York: Free Press.

Sigurdsson, E., Van Os, J., & Fombonne, E. (2002). Are impaired childhood motor skills a risk factor for adolescent anxiety? Results from the 1958 U.K. birth cohort and the national child development study. *The American Journal of Psychiatry, 159,* 1044-1046.

Skinner, R. A., & Piek, J. P. (2001). Psychosocial implications of poor motor coordination in children and adolescents. *Human Movement Science, 20*(1-2), 73-94.

Thomson, O., MA., Freemantle, N., Oxman, A., Wolf, F., Davis, D., & Herrin, J. (2001). Continuing education meetings and modules: Effects on professional practice and health care outcomes. *Cochrane Database of Systematic Reviews, 2*, CD003030.

Wall, A. E., McClements, J., Bouffard, M., Findlay, H., & Taylor, M. J. (1985). A knowledge-based approach to motor development: Implications for the physically awkward. *Adapted Physical Activity Quarterly, 2*, 21-42.

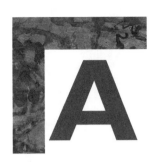

Appendix A:
Critical Review Form
Quantitative Studies

CITATION:

	Comments
STUDY PURPOSE: Was the purpose stated clearly? ○ Yes ○ No	Outline the purpose of the study. How does the study apply to occupational therapy and/or your research question?
LITERATURE: Was relevant background literature reviewed? ○ Yes ○ No	Describe the justification of the need for this study.
DESIGN: ○ randomized (RCT) ○ cohort ○ single case design ○ before and after ○ case-control ○ cross-sectional ○ case study	Describe the study design. Was the design appropriate for the study question (e.g., for knowledge level about this issue, outcomes, ethical issues, etc.)? Specify any biases that may have been operating and the direction of their influence on the results.

Comments

SAMPLE: N = Was the sample described in detail? ○ Yes ○ No Was sample size justified? ○ Yes ○ No ○ N/A	Sampling (who; characteristics; how many; how was sampling done?) If more than one group, was there similarity between the groups? Describe ethics procedures. Was informed consent obtained?
OUTCOMES: Were the outcome measures reliable? ○ Yes ○ No ○ Not addressed Were the outcome measures valid? ○ Yes ○ No ○ Not addressed	Specify the frequency of outcome measurement (i.e., pre, post, follow-up). Outcome areas (e.g., self-care, productivity, leisure). List measures used.
INTERVENTION: Intervention was described in detail? ○ Yes ○ No ○ Not addressed Contamination was avoided? ○ Yes ○ No ○ Not addressed ○ N/A Cointervention was avoided? ○ Yes ○ No ○ Not addressed ○ N/A	Provide a short description of the intervention (focus, who delivered it, how often, setting). Could the intervention be replicated in occupational therapy practice?

Comments

RESULTS: Results were reported in terms of statistical significance? ○ Yes ○ No ○ N/A ○ Not addressed	What were the results? Were they statistically significant (i.e., $p < 0.05$)? If not statistically significant, was study big enough to show an important difference if it should occur? If there were multiple outcomes, was that taken into account for the statistical analysis?
Were the analysis method(s) appropriate? ○ Yes ○ No ○ Not addressed	
Clinical importance was reported? ○ Yes ○ No ○ Not addressed	What was the clinical importance of the results? Were differences between groups clinically meaningful? (if applicable)
Drop-outs were reported? ○ Yes ○ No	Did any participants drop out from the study? Why? (Were reasons given and were drop-outs handled appropriately?)
CONCLUSIONS AND CLINICAL IMPLICATIONS: Conclusions were appropriate given study methods and results ○ Yes ○ No	What did the study conclude? What are the implications of these results for occupational therapy practice? What were the main limitations or biases in the study?

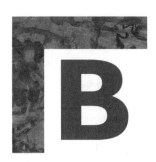

Appendix B:
Guidelines for
Critical Review Form

Quantitative Studies

© Law, M., Stewart, D., Pollock, N., Letts, L., Bosch, J., & Westmorland, M., 1998.

Introduction

- These guidelines accompany the Critical Review Form for Quantitative Studies developed by the McMaster University Occupational Therapy Evidence-Based Practice Research Group (Law et al. 1998). They are written in basic terms that can be understood by clinicians, students and researchers.
- Where appropriate, examples and justification for the guidelines/suggestions are provided to assist the reader in understanding the process of critical review.
- Guidelines are provided for the questions (left hand column) in the form, and the instructions/questions in the Comments column of each component.

Critical Review Components

Citation
- Include full title, all authors (last name, initials), full journal title, year, volume and page numbers.
- This ensures that another person could easily retrieve the same article.

Study Purpose
- <u>Was the purpose stated clearly</u>? The purpose is usually stated briefly in the abstract of the article, and again in more detail in the introduction. It may be phrased as a research question or hypothesis.
- A clear statement helps you determine if the topic is important, relevant, and of interest to you. Consider how the study can be applied to occupational therapy practice and/or your own situation before you continue. If it is not useful or applicable, go on to the next article.

Literature
- <u>Was relevant background literature reviewed</u>? A review of the literature should be included in an article describing research to provide some background to the study. It should provide a synthesis of relevant information such as previous work/research, and discussion of the clinical importance of the topic.
- It identifies gaps in current knowledge and research about the topic of interest, and thus justifies the need for the study being reported.

Design
- There are many different types of research designs. The most common types in rehabilitation research are included.
- The essential features of the different types of study designs are outlined, to assist in determining which was used in the study you are reviewing.

- Some of the advantages and disadvantages of the different types of designs are outlined to assist the reader in determining the appropriateness of the design for the study being reported.
- Different terms are used by authors, which can be confusing—alternative terms will be identified where possible.
- Numerous issues can be considered in determining the appropriateness of the methods/design chosen. Some of the key issues are listed in the Comments section, and will be described below. Diagrams of different designs, and examples using the topic of studying the effectiveness of activity programs for seniors with dementia, are provided.
- Most studies have some problems due to biases that may distort the design, execution or interpretation of the research. The most common biases are described at the end of this section.

Design Types

1. Randomized (RCT)

- Randomized Controlled Trial, or Randomized Clinical Trial: also referred to as Experimental or Type 1 study. RCTs also encompass other different methods, such as cross-over designs.
- The essential feature of an RCT is a set of clients/subjects are identified and then randomly allocated (assigned) to two or more different treatment "groups." One group of clients receives the treatment of interest (often a new treatment) and the other group is the "control" group, which usually receives no treatment or standard practice. Random allocation to different treatment groups allows comparison of the client groups in terms of the outcomes of interest because randomization strongly increases the likelihood of similarity of clients in each group. Thus the chance of another factor (known as a confounding variable or issue) influencing the outcomes is greatly reduced.
- The main disadvantage of RCTs is the expense involved, and in some situations it is not ethical to have "control" groups of clients who do not receive treatment. For example, if you were to study the effectiveness of a multidisciplinary inpatient program for post-surgical patients with chronic low back pain, it may be unethical to withhold treatment in order to have a "control" group.
- RCTs are often chosen when testing the effectiveness of a treatment, or to compare several different forms of treatment.

Participants	→	Stratification	→	Randomization	↗ Experimental Group	→ OUTCOME
					↘ Control Group	

Example: The effects of two different O.T. interventions, functional rehabilitation and reactivation, were evaluated using a randomized controlled trial. 44 patients of a long-term care centre were randomly allocated to one of the two types of intervention. Outcomes were measured using a variety of psychometric tests at 3 different points in time. (Bach et al., 1995).

2. Cohort Design

- A cohort is a group of people (clients) who have been exposed to a similar situation, for example a program, or a diagnosis/disease. Whatever the topic/issue of interest, the groups of clients is identified and followed/observed over time to see what happens.

- Cohort designs are "prospective," meaning that the direction of time is always forwards. Time flows forwards from the point at which the clients are identified. They are sometimes referred to as prospective studies.
- Cohort studies often have a comparison ("control") group of clients/people who have not been exposed to the situation of interest (e.g., they have not received any treatment). One of the main differences between an RCT and a Cohort study is that the allocation of people (clients) to the treatment and control groups is not under the control of the investigator in a Cohort study - the investigator must work with the group of people who have been identified as "exposed" and then find another group of people who are similar in terms of age, gender and other important factors.
- It is difficult to know if the groups are similar in terms of all the important (confounding) factors, and therefore the authors cannot be certain that the treatment (exposure) itself is responsible for the outcomes.
- Advantages of Cohort studies are they are often less expensive and less time-consuming than RCT's.

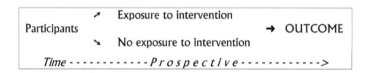

Example: Evaluation of a mental stimulation program used a cohort design to measure changes in mental status in 30 patients over a 2-month time period. The first 15 patients who were admitted to a day care centre received treatment and composed the "exposed" group. The remaining 15 admissions did not receive treatment immediately, and served as a "control" group.(Koh et al., 1994).

3. Single Case Design

- Single subject/case research involves one client, or a number of clients, followed over time, or evaluated on outcomes of interest.
- There are different types of methods used in single case designs, with different terms used such "n of 1" studies, "before-after trial in the same subject"; or single case "series" involving more than one subject/client.
- The basic feature of any single subject design is the evaluation of clients for the outcome(s) of interest both before (baseline) and after the intervention. This design allows an individual to serve as their own "control." However, it is difficult to conclude that the treatment alone resulted in any differences as other factors may change over time, for example the disease severity may change.
- It is useful when only a few clients have a particular diagnosis or are involved in a treatment that you want to evaluate. This type of study is easily replicated with more than one client. Its flexible approach makes it particularly appropriate for conducting research in clinical settings.

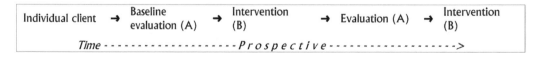

Example: A study examining the effects of environmental changes during an O.T. intervention on a psychiatric ward used a single case design to observe changes in behaviour in 10 individual patients. Observations of each patient's behaviour were made before, during, and after the intevention. (Burton, 1980).

4. Before-After Design

- Before-after design is usually used to evaluate a group of clients involved in a treatment (although as mentioned above, it is a method also used to study single cases/individuals).
- The evaluator collects information about the initial status of a group of clients in terms of the outcomes of interest and then collects information again about the outcomes after treatment is received.
- This is a useful design when you do not wish to withhold treatment from any clients. However, with no "control" group, it is impossible to judge if the treatment alone was responsible for any changes in the outcomes. Changes could be due to other factors such as disease progression, medication use, lifestyle or environmental changes.

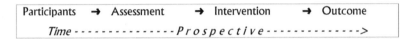

Example: The level of caregiver strain following placement of an elderly family member with dementia in adult cay care was evaluated using a before-after design. Outcomes of caregiver strain and burden of care were measured in 15 subjects before and after the day care placement. (Graham, 1989).

5. Case Control Design

- Case control studies explore what make a group of individuals different. Other terms used are case-comparison study or retrospective study. Retrospective is the term used to describe how the methods look at an issue after it has happened. The essential feature of a case control study is looking backwards.
- A set of clients/subjects with a defining characteristic or situation, for example a specific diagnosis or involvement in a treatment, are identified. The characteristic or situation of interest is compared with a "control" group of people who are similar in age, gender and background but who do not have the characteristic or are not involved in the situation of interest. The purpose is to determine differences between these groups.
- It is a relatively inexpensive way to explore an issue, but there are many potential problems (flaws) that make it very difficult to conclude what factor(s) are responsible for the outcomes.

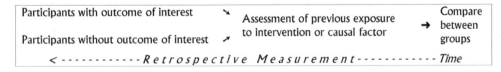

Example: If an occupational therapist wanted to understand why some clients of a day care programme attended a daily activity programme (which was optional) on a regular basis, while other clients did not attend, a case control design could be used to explore differences between the two groups of clients in relation to age, gender, interests, background and current living situation.

6. Cross-Sectional Design

- Involves one group of people, and all the evaluation of the whole group is carried out at the same time.
- This design is often used to explore what factors may have influenced a particular outcome in a group of people. It is useful when relatively little is known about an issue/outcome.
- Surveys, questionnaires, and interviews are common methods used in cross-sectional studies. They are relatively inexpensive and easy, as evaluation takes place at one point in time.
- It is impossible to know if all factors have been included in the evaluation, so it is difficult to draw cause-effect conclusions from the results beyond the group of people being studied.

> Participants → Measurement of outcomes and other factors at the same time
> ▴ *Time: All done at one point in time* ▴

Example: Clients and their families who have been involved in a new activity programme for seniors with dementia can be surveyed or interviewed upon discharge to evaluate the impact of the programme on their quality of life, activity participation and level of satisfaction.

7. Case Study Design

- A case study is carried out in order to provide descriptive information (data) about the relationship between a particular treatment (exposure) and an outcome of interest. It is also called a descriptive study, as that is the primary purpose. There is no control group.
- It is often used to explore a new topic or treatment, when there is little knowledge. However, the results can only be considered in terms of describing a particular situation. It may generate information to support further study of the topic of interest.

> Participants with condition of interest → Information about clinical outcome

Example: Twelve patients on a long-stay geriatric ward were observed over a period of time to determine the effectiveness of providing individual and group activities on the ward. Engagement levels were observed and recorded at 10-minute intervals to determine any differences between no intervention, individual activities and group activities (McCormack & Whitehead, 1981).

Appropriateness of Study Design

- Some of the important issues to consider in determining if the study design is the most appropriate include:
  - Knowledge of the topic/issue: If little is known about an issue, a more exploratory method is appropriate, for example a case study or a cross-sectional design. As our level of knowledge increases, study designs become more rigorous, where most variables that could influence the outcome are understood and can be controlled by the researcher. The most rigorous design is the RCT.
  - Outcomes: If the outcome under study is easily quantified and has well-developed standardized assessment tools available to measure it, a more rigorous design (e.g., An RCT) is appropriate. If outcomes are not fully understood yet, such as quality of life, then a design that explores different factors that may involved in the outcomes is appropriate, such as a case control design.

- **Ethical issues**: It is appropriate to use a research design that uses control groups of people receiving no treatment if there are no ethical issues surrounding the withholding of treatment.
- **Study purpose/question**: Some designs are well-suited to studying the effectiveness of treatment, including RCTs, before-after designs, and single-case studies. Other designs (e.g., case control and cross sectional) are more appropriate if the purpose of the study is to learn more about an issue, or is a pilot study to determine if further treatment and research is warranted.

Biases |

- There are many different types of biases described in the research literature. The most common ones that you should check for are described below under 3 main areas:
  1. Sample (subject selection) biases, which may result in the subjects in the sample being unrepresentative of the population which you are interested in;
  2. Measurement (detection) biases, which include issues related to how the outcome of interest was measured; and
  3. Intervention (performance) biases, which involve how the treatment itself was carried out.
- The reader is directed to the bibliography if more detailed information is needed about biases.
- A bias affects the results of a study in one direction—it either "favors" the treatment group or the control group. It is important to be aware of which direction a bias may influence the results.

| *1. Sample/Selection Biases*

- *a.* Volunteer or referral bias:
  - People who volunteer to participate in a study, or who are referred to a study by someone are often different than non-volunteers/non-referrals.
  - This bias usually, but not always, favors the treatment group, as volunteers tend to be more motivated and concerned about their health.
- *b.* Seasonal bias:
  - If all subjects are recruited and thus are evaluated and receive treatment at one time, the results may be influenced by the timing of the subject selection and intervention. For example, seniors tend to be healthier in the summer than the winter, so the results may be more positive if the study takes place only in the summer.
  - This bias could work in either direction, depending on the time of year.
- *c.* Attention bias:
  - People who are evaluated as part of a study are usually aware of the purpose of the study, and as a result of the attention, give more favorable responses or perform better than people who are unaware of the study's intent. This bias is why some studies use an "attention control" group, where the people in the control group receive the same amount of attention as those people in the treatment group, although it is not the same treatment.

| *2. Measurement/Detection Biases*

- *a.* Number of outcome measures used:
  - If only one outcome measure is used, there can be a bias in the way that the measure itself evaluated the outcome. For example, one ADL measure considers dressing, eating, and toiletting but does not include personal hygiene and grooming or meal preparation.

- This bias can influence the results in either direction; e.g., it can favor the control group if important elements of the outcome that would have responded to the treatment were missed.
- Bias can also be introduced if there are too many outcome measures for the sample size. This is an issue involving statistics, which usually favors the control group because the large number of statistical calculations reduces the ability to find a significant difference between the treatment and control groups.
  - *b.* Lack of "masked" or "independent" evaluation:
    - If the evaluators are aware of which group a subject was allocated to, or which treatment a person received, it is possible for the evaluator to influence the results by giving the person, or group of people, a more or less favorable evaluation. It is usually the treatment group that is favored. This should be considered when the evaluator is part of the research or treatment team.
  - *c.* Recall or memory bias:
    - This can be a problem if outcomes are measured using self-report tools, surveys or interviews that are requiring the person to recall past events. Often a person recalls fond or positive memories more than negative ones, and this can favor the results of the study for those people being questioned about an issue or receiving treatment.

3. Intervention/Performance Biases

- *a.* Contamination:
  - This occurs when members of the control group inadvertently receive treatment, thus the difference in outcomes between the two groups may be reduced. This favors the control group.
- *b.* Co-intervention:
  - If clients receive another form of treatment at the same time as the study treatment, this can influence the results in either direction. For example, taking medication while receiving or not treatment could favor the results for people in either group. The reader must consider if the other, or additional, treatment could have a positive or negative influence on the results.
- *c.* Timing of intervention:
  - Different issues related to the timing of intervention can introduce a bias.
  - If treatment is provided over an extended period of time to children, maturation alone could be a factor in improvements seen.
  - If treatment is very short in duration, there may not have been sufficient time for a noticeable effect in the outcomes of interest. This would favor the control group.
- *d.* Site of treatment:
  - Where treatment takes place can influence the results—for example, if a treatment programme is carried out in a person's home, this may result in a higher level of satisfaction that favors the treatment group. The site of treatment should be consistent among all groups.
- *e.* Different therapists:
  - If different therapists are involved in providing the treatment(s) under study to the different groups of clients, the results could be influenced in one direction—for example, one therapist could be more motivating or positive than another, and hence the group that

she worked with could demonstrate more favorable outcomes. Therapist involvement should be equal and consistent between all treatment groups.

Sample

- $N = ?$ The number of subjects/clients involved in the study should be clear.
- Was the sample described in detail? The description of the sample should be detailed enough for you to have a clear picture of who was involved.
- Important characteristics related to the topic of interest should be reported, in order for you to conclude that the study population is similar to your own and that bias was minimized. Important characteristics include:
  - who makes up the sample—are the subjects appropriate for the study question and described in terms of age, gender, duration of a disability/disease and functional status (if applicable)?;
  - how many subjects were involved, and if there are different groups, were the groups relatively equal in size?;
  - how the sampling was done—was it voluntary, by referral? Were inclusion and exclusion criteria described?
  - if there was more than 1 group, was there similarity between the groups on important (confounding) factors?
- Was the sample size justified? The authors should state how they arrived at the sample size, to justify why the number was chosen. Often, justification is based on the population available for study. Some authors provide statistical justification for the sample size, but this is rare.
- Ethics procedures should be described, although they are often left out. At the very least, authors should report if informed consent was obtained at the beginning of the study.

Outcomes

- Outcomes are the variables or issues of interest to the researcher—they represent the product or results of the treatment or exposure.
- Outcomes need to be clearly described in order for you to determine if they were relevant and useful to your situation. Furthermore, the method (the how) of outcome measurement should be described sufficiently for you to be confident that it was conducted in an objective and unbiased manner.
- Determine the frequency of outcome measurement. It is important to note if outcomes were measured pre- and post-treatment, and whether short-term and/or long-term effects were considered.
- Review the outcome measures to determine how they are relevant to occupational therapy practice, i.e., they include areas of occupational performance, performance components ,and/or environmental components.
- List the measures used and any important information about them for your future reference. Consider if they are well-known measures, or ones developed by the researchers for the specific study being reported. It may be more difficult to replicate the study in the latter situation.
- The authors should report if the outcome measures used had sound (well-established and tested) psychometric properties—most importantly, reliability, and validity. This ensures confidence in the measurement of the outcomes of interest.

- Were the outcome measures reliable? Reliability refers to whether a measure is giving the same information over different situations. The 2 most common forms of reliability are: test-retest reliability—the same observer gets the same information on two occasions separated by a short time interval; and inter-rater reliability—different observers get the same information at the same time.
- Were the outcome measures valid? Asks whether the measure is assessing what it is intended to measure. Consider if the measure includes all of the relevant concepts and elements of the outcome (content validity), and if the authors report that the measure has been tested in relationship to other measures to determine any relationship (criterion validity). For example, a "valid" ADL measure will include all relevant elements of self-care, and will have been tested with other measures of daily living activities and self-care functioning to determine that the relationship between the measures is as expected.

Intervention

- Intervention described in detail? There should be sufficient information about the information for you to be able to replicate it.
- In reviewing the intervention, consider important elements such as:
  - The focus of the intervention—is it relevant to occupational therapy practice and your situation;
  - Who delivered it—was it one person or different people, were they trained?;
  - How often the treatment was received—was it sufficient in your opinion to have an impact? Was the frequency the same if there were different groups involved?;
  - The setting—was treatment received at home or in an institution? Was it the same for different groups of subjects if there was more than one treatment group?
- These elements need to be addressed if you want to be able to replicate the treatment in your practice.
- Contamination, co-intervention avoided? These two factors were described under Biases (see Design section). Were they addressed? If not, consider what possible issues could influence the results of the study, for example, what could happen if some of the clients in the control group received some treatment inadvertently (contamination) or if some subjects were taking medication during the study (co-intervention)? Make note of any potential influences. If there was only one group under study, mark "not applicable (n/a)" on the form.

Results

- Results were reported in terms of statistical significance? Most authors report the results of quantitative research studies in terms of statistical significance, to prove that they are worthy of attention. It is difficult to determine if change in outcomes or differences between groups of people are important or significant if only averages, means, or percentages are reported.
- Refer to the bibliography if you wish to review specific statistical methods.
- Outline the results briefly in this section, focusing on those that were statistically significant. If the results were not significant statistically, examine the reasons: was the sample size not large enough to show an important, or significant, difference; or were too many outcome measures used for the number of subjects involved.
- Were the analysis method(s) appropriate? Do the authors justify/explain their choice of analysis methods? Do they appear to be appropriate for the study and the outcomes. You need to consider the following:

- The purpose of the study—is it comparing 2 or more interventions, or examining the correlation between different variables of interest. Different statistical tests are used for comparison and correlation.
- The outcomes—if there is only one outcome measured to compare 2 different treatments, a simple statistical test such as a t-test will probably be sufficient. However, with a larger number of outcomes, involving different types of variables, more complex statistical methods, such as analysis of variance (ANOVA), are usually required.
- Clinical importance was reported? Numbers are often not enough to determine if the results of a study are important clinically. The authors should discuss the relevance of the results to clinical practice and/or to the lives of the people involved. If significant differences were found between treatment groups, are they meaningful in the clinical world? If differences were not statistically significant, are there any clinically important or meaningful issues that you can consider for your practice?

Drop-outs

- Drop-outs were reported? The number of subjects/participants who drop out of a study should be reported, as it can influence the results. Reasons for the drop-outs and how the analysis of the findings were handled with the drop-outs taken into account should be reported, to increase your confidence in the results. If there were no drop-outs, consider that as "reported" and indicate no drop-outs in the Comments section.

Conclusions and Clinical Implications

- The discussion section of the article should outline clear conclusions from the results. These should be relevant and appropriate given the study methods and results. For example, the investigators of a well-designed RCT study using sound outcome measures could state that the results are conclusive that treatment A is more effective than treatment B for the study population. Other study designs cannot make such strong conclusions, as they likely had methodological limitations or biases, such as a lack of a control group or unreliable measures, that make it difficult to "prove" or conclude that it was the treatment alone that influenced the outcome(s). In these situations, the authors may only conclude that the results demonstrated a difference in the specific outcomes measured in this study for the clients involved. The results may not be generalizable to other populations, including yours. Further study or research should therefore be recommended.
- The discussion should include how the results may influence clinical practice—do they offer useful and relevant information about a client population, or an outcome of interest? Do they warrant further study? Consider the implications of the results, as a whole or in part, for your particular practice and for occupational therapy in general.

Bibliography

Crombie, I.K. (1996). The pocket guide to critical appraisal: A handbook for health care professionals. London: BMJ Publishing Group.

Department of Clinical Epidemiology and Biostatistics, McMaster University Health Sciences Centre (1981). How to read clinical journals: V: To distinguish useful from useless or even harmful therapy. Canadian Medical Association Journal, 124, 1156-1162.

Law, M. (1987). Measurement in occupational therapy: Scientific criteria for evaluation. Canadian Journal of Occupational Therapy, 58, 171-179.

Law, M., King, G., & Pollock, N. (1994). Single Subject Research Design. Research Report #94-2. Hamilton, ON: Neurodevelopmental Clinical Research Unit.

Mulrow, C. D., & Oxman, A. D. (Eds.). (1996). Cochrane Collaboration Handbook. Available in The Cochrane Library [Database on disk and CD-ROM]. The Cochrane Collaboration: Issue 2. Oxford: Updated Software; 1998.

Norman, G. R., & Streiner, D.L. (1986). PDQ Statistics. Burlington, ON: B.C. Decker Inc.

Sackett, D. L. (1979). Bias in analytic research. Journal of Chronic Disability, 32, 51-63.

Sackett, D.L., Haynes, R.B., Guyatt, G.H. & Tugwell, P. (1991). Clinical epidemiology. A basic science for clinical medicine (2nd ed.). Toronto, ON: Little, Brown and Co.

Streiner, D.L., Norman, G.R. & Blum, H.M. (1989). PDQ epidemiology. Toronto, ON: B.C. Decker Inc.

Articles of activity programmes for seniors with dementia (referred to in examples of study designs):

Bach, D., Bach, M., Bohmer, G., Gruhwalk, T., & Grik, B. (1995). Reactivating occupational therapy: a method to improve cognitive performance in geriatric patients. Age and Aging, 24, 222-226.

Burton, M. (1980). Evaluation and change in a psychogeriatric ward through direct observation and feedback. British Journal of Psychiatry, 137, 566-571.

Graham, R.W. (1989). Adult day care: How families of the dementia patient respond. Journal of Gerontological Nursing, 15(3), 27-31, 40-41.

Koh, K., Ray, R., Lee, J., Nair, T., Ho, T., & Ang, P.C. (1994). Dementia in elderly patients: Can the 3R mental stimulation programme improve mental status? Age and Aging, 23, 195-199.

McCormack, D., & Whitehead, A. (1981). The effect of providing recreational activities on the engagement level of long-stay geriatric patients. Age and Aging, 10, 287-291.

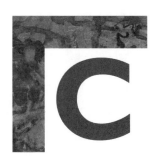

Appendix C:
Critical Review Form
Qualitative Studies (Version 2.0)

© Letts, L., Wilkins, S. Law, M., Stewart, D., Bosch, J., & Westmorland, M., 2007.
McMaster University

CITATION:

	Comments
STUDY PURPOSE: Was the purpose and/or research question stated clearly? ○ yes ○ no	Outline the purpose of the study and/or research question.
LITERATURE: Was relevant background literature reviewed? ○ yes ○ no	Describe the justification of the need for this study. Was it clear and compelling?
	How does the study apply to your practice and/or to your research question? Is it worth continuing this review?[1]
STUDY DESIGN: What was the design? ○ phenomenology ○ ethnography ○ grounded theory ○ participatory action research ○ other _____	Was the design appropriate for the study question? (i.e., rationale) Explain.

1 When doing critical reviews, there are strategic points in the process at which you may decide the research is not applicable to your practice and question. You may decide then that it is not worthwhile to continue with the review.

Was a theoretical perspective identified? O yes O no	Describe the theoretical or philosophical perspective for this study e.g., researcher's perspective.
Method(s) used: O participant observation O interviews O document review O focus groups O other _____	Describe the method(s) used to answer the research question. Are the methods congruent with the philosophical underpinnings and purpose?
SAMPLING: Was the process of purposeful selection described? O yes O no	Describe sampling methods used. Was the sampling method appropriate to the study purpose or research question?
Was sampling done until redundancy in data was reached?[2] O yes O no O not addressed	Are the participants described in adequate detail? How is the sample applicable to your practice or research question? Is it worth continuing?
Was informed consent obtained? O yes O no O not addressed	

DATA COLLECTION:
 	
Descriptive Clarity
Clear & complete description of
site: O yes O no
participants: O yes O no
 	
Role of researcher & relationship with participants:
          O yes O no
 	
Identification of assumptions and biases of researcher:
          O yes O no
	Describe the context of the study. Was it sufficient for understanding of the "whole" picture?
	
	What was missing and how does that influence your understanding of the research?

---

2 Throughout the form, "no" means the authors explicitly state reasons for not doing it; "not addressed" should be ticked if there is no mention of the issue.

Procedural Rigour Procedural rigor was used in data collection strategies? ○ yes ○ no ○ not addressed	Do the researchers provide adequate information about data collection procedures e.g., gaining access to the site, field notes, training data gatherers? Describe any flexibility in the design & data collection methods.
DATA ANALYSES: **Analytical Rigour** Data analyses were inductive? ○ yes ○ no ○ not addressed Findings were consistent with & reflective of data? ○ yes ○ no	Describe method(s) of data analysis. Were the methods appropriate? What were the findings?
Auditability Decision trail developed? ○ yes ○ no ○ not addressed Process of analyzing the data was described adequately? ○ yes ○ no ○ not addressed	Describe the decisions of the researcher re: transformation of data to codes/themes. Outline the rationale given for development of themes.
Theoretical Connections Did a meaningful picture of the phenomenon under study emerge? ○ yes ○ no	How were concepts under study clarified & refined, and relationships made clear? Describe any conceptual frameworks that emerged.

OVERALL RIGOUR Was there evidence of the four components of trustworthiness? Credibility ○ yes ○ no Transferability ○ yes ○ no Dependability ○ yes ○ no Comfirmability ○ yes ○ no	For each of the components of trustworthiness, identify what the researcher used to ensure each. What meaning and relevance does this study have for your practice or research question?

CONCLUSIONS & IMPLICATIONS
 	
Conclusions were appropriate given the study findings?
  ○ yes ○ no
 	
The findings contributed to theory development & future OT practice/ research?
  ○ yes ○ no
	What did the study conclude? What were the implications of the findings for occupational therapy (practice & research)? What were the main limitations in the study?

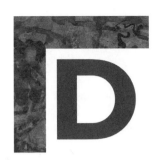

Appendix D:
Guidelines for
Critical Review Form

Qualitative Studies (Version 2.0)

Introduction

- These guidelines accompany the Critical Review Form: Qualitative Studies originally developed by the McMaster University Occupational Therapy Evidence-Based Practice Research Group and revised by Letts et al., 2007. They are written in basic terms that can be understood by researchers as well as clinicians and students interested in conducting critical reviews of the literature.
- Guidelines are provided for the questions in the left hand column of the form and the instructions/questions in the Comments column of each component.
- Examples relate to occupational therapy research as much as possible.
- These guidelines assist readers to complete critical appraisal of qualitative research articles. In recent years, there has been an increase in the number of meta-syntheses i.e., articles that examine more than one qualitative study and synthesize the data from these studies together. The approaches to conducting meta-syntheses are still emerging, and criteria for critical appraisal of meta-syntheses are not yet well-established. Over time, we anticipate that we may either revise this review form to incorporate meta-syntheses or develop another review form.

Critical Review Components

Citation

- Include full title, all authors (last name, initials), full journal title, year, volume number, and page numbers.
- This ensures that another person could easily retrieve the same article.

Study Purpose

- <u>Was the purpose and/or research question stated clearly</u>? - The purpose is usually stated briefly in the abstract of the article, and again in more detail in the introduction. It may be phrased as a research question.
- A clear statement of purpose or research questions helps you determine if the topic is important, relevant, and of interest to you.
- For future reference, it is useful to provide a summary of the purpose or research question in the comments section, so that you or someone else can quickly get a sense of the article.

Literature

- <u>Was relevant background literature reviewed</u>? A review of the literature should be included in an article describing research to provide some background to the study. It should provide a synthesis of relevant information such as previous work/research, and discussion of the clinical importance of the topic.
- The review of the literature could include both qualitative and quantitative evidence related to the study purpose.
- It identifies gaps in current knowledge and research about the topic of interest, and thus justifies the need for the study being reported. The justification for the study should be clear and compelling. Readers should be able to understand the researchers' thinking in conducting the study.
- Consider how the study can be applied to occupational therapy practice and/or your own situation before you continue with your review of the article. If it is not useful or applicable, go on to the next article.

Study Design

- <u>What was the study design?</u> There are many different types of research designs. These guidelines focus on the most common types of qualitative designs in rehabilitation research.
- The essential features of the different types of study designs are outlined to assist in determining which was used in the study you are reviewing.
- Some researchers will not describe their study using these design descriptions; they may simply refer to the research as a 'qualitative design'. In most cases, you should expect the authors to link their research to a specific research tradition, or justify why they have not done so. When reviewing articles in which the design is described only as qualitative, it can be useful to consider which of these traditions best matches the study you are reading; this will help you make a judgement about the appropriateness of the design, sampling, data collection and analyses.
- Numerous issues can be considered in determining the appropriateness of the design chosen. Some of the key issues are listed in the Comments section, and are discussed below.

Design Types

1. Phenomenology

- Phenomenology answers the question: "What is it like to have a certain experience?". It seeks to understand the phenomenon of a lived experience - this may be related to an emotion, such as loneliness or depression, to a relationship, or to being part of an organization or group. The assumption behind phenomenology is that there is an essence to shared experience. It comes from the social sciences and requires a researcher to enter into an individual's life world and use the self to interpret the individual's (or group's) experience. Phenomenology's application to occupational therapy research is discussed in detail by Wilding & Whiteford (2005).

Example: A phenomenological approach was chosen to explore the experiences of people with arthritis who were participants in two different types of arthritis education groups. Data were collected through observations of the groups, individual interviews with group participants, followed by focus groups after initial analyses were completed. Three themes are discussed by the authors: validation through connection; restructuring illness identity; and perceptions of self and disease symptoms. The themes provided insights into notions underlying transformative learning theory (Ashe, Taylor, & Dubouloz, 2005).

2. Ethnography

- Ethnography is a well-known form of qualitative research in anthropology, and focuses on the question: "What is the culture of a group of people, or people in a particular setting?". The goal of ethnographic research is to tell the whole story of a group's daily life, to identify the cultural meanings, beliefs and social patterns of the group, and can include the description of material culture (buildings, tools, and other objects that have cultural meaning). Culture is not limited to ethnic groups, and ethnographers study the culture of organizations, programs and groups of people with common social problems such as smoking and drug addiction. In the area of health care, Krefting (1989) described a disability ethnography, which is a strategic research approach focusing on a particular human problem and those aspects of group life that impact on the problem.

Example: An ethnographic study was conducted to explore the process and outcomes of a program of occupation for seniors with dementia within a day hospital setting, which was the culture being examined. Data from observations, interviews with patients and staff, and field notes were analyzed to discover the opportunities and barriers to conducting an occupational program in a day hospital unit (Borell, Gustavsson, Sandman & Kielhofner, 1994). Jung, Tryssenaar, & Wilkins (2005), in their ethnographic study, interviewed novice tutors and their tutor guides or mentors in order to understand the entry phase of "becoming a tutor" within the culture of problem based learning. The overarching theme was of story telling or an oral tradition within which novice tutors learned from their tutor mentors based on direct modeling and vicarious sharing of stories.

3. Grounded Theory

- Grounded theory focuses on the task of theory construction. The inductive nature of qualitative research is considered essential for generating a theory. The focus is on searching to identify the core social processes within a given social situation. Glaser and Strauss (1967) developed a research process that takes the researcher into and close to the real world to ensure that the results are "grounded" in the social world of the people being studied. More recently, Charmaz (2003, 2006) has argued that the ongoing work of Glaser (1978) and Strauss and Corbin (1990) has resulted in grounded theory becoming more objectivist (positivistic) and suggested that a more constructivist (interpretive) approach allows researchers to focus more on human agency, social and subjective meaning, and problem-solving practices and action. A grounded theory method is an emergent design dependent on continuous data analysis. The theory is seen as a developmental process and therefore is able to capture the nature of social interaction and its structural content.

Example: Grounded theory was used to explore the concept of playfulness in adults (Guitard, Ferland, & Dutil, 2005). Through interviews with a heterogeneous group of fifteen adults, and inductive analyses, the following components of playfulness were identified: creativity, curiosity, sense of humour, pleasure, and spontaneity. The analyses also resulted in the development of a visual model demonstrating the relationships among the components of the model.

4. Participatory Action Research (PAR)

- PAR is an approach to research and social change that can be considered a type of qualitative research. PAR involves individuals and groups researching their own personal beings, socio-cultural settings and experiences. They reflect on their values, shared realities, collective meanings, needs and goals. Knowledge is generated and power is regained through deliberate actions that nurture, empower and liberate persons and groups. The researcher works in partnership with participants throughout the research process. PAR can be time consuming because sometimes delays can occur when researchers from outside the community and community members need to negotiate phases in the research. Research describing PAR should ideally discuss the negotiation processes used in the research.

Example: Cockburn and Trentham (2002) share two examples of participatory action research projects in which they were involved. One project involved adults with mental illness working to create meaningful work experiences. The other involved older adults in a community capacity-building process related to identifying and addressing issues in their housing complex. Letts (2003) also shared a number of examples of participatory research projects that involved occupational therapists.

5. Other Designs

- These are many other qualitative research designs described in the literature. They come from different theoretical traditions and disciplines, and some are extensions of the more popular ethnographic and phenomenological designs. Some of the most frequently described designs in qualitative literature include: heuristics, ethnomethodology, institutional ethnography, hermeneutics, ecological psychology, feminism, and social interactionism. Readers interested in further inquiry of qualitative research designs are directed to the bibliography at the end of this document.

Appropriateness of Study Design

- The choice of qualitative research designs should be congruent with the following:
  - The beliefs and worldviews of the researcher i.e., the qualitative researcher usually expresses an interest in understanding the social world from the point of view of the participants in it, and emphasizes the context in which events occur and have meaning;
  - The nature of the end results desired i.e., the qualitative research is seeking meaning and understanding, which is best described in narrative form;
  - The depth of understanding and description required from participants i.e., qualitative research usually involves the exploration of a topic or issue in depth, with emphasis on seeking information from the people who are experiencing or are involved in the issue;
  - The type of reasoning involved: qualitative research is oriented towards theory construction, and the reasoning behind data analysis is inductive i.e., the findings emerge from the data.

- Crabtree and Miller (1992) suggest that the best way to determine if the choice of a particular qualitative research design is appropriate is to ask how the particular topic of interest is usually shared in the group or culture of interest. For example, if information about how clients responded to occupational therapy treatment is usually shared through discussion and story-telling among individual therapists, then a phenomenological approach may be the most appropriate way to study this experience.

- <u>Was a theoretical perspective identified</u>? The thinking and theoretical perspective of the researcher(s) can influence the study. The researcher should know something conceptually of the phenomenon of interest, and should state the theoretical perspective up front. For example, Ashe et al. (2005) presented findings from an earlier grounded theory study to explain the context of their project, and also discussed the link to adult learning theory.

Qualitative Methods

- A variety of different methods are used by qualitative researchers to answer the research question. The most common ones are described here, including the advantages and disadvantages of each.

1. Participant Observation

- A participant observer uses observation to research a culture or situation from within. There is a difference between the researcher as simply an onlooker and one who is actually participating while observing (i.e., doing what the people are doing). The observer usually spends an extended period of time within the setting to be studied and records 'fieldnotes' of his/her observations. This type of research may be called 'fieldwork', which comes from its roots in social and cultural anthropology.
- Participant observation is useful when the focus of interest is how activities and interactions within a setting give meaning to beliefs or behaviours. It fits with the assumption that everyone in a group or organization is influenced by assumptions and beliefs that they take for granted. It is therefore considered the qualitative method of choice when the situation or issue of interest is obscured or hidden from public knowledge and there are differences between what people say and what they do.
- Participant observation can be time-consuming and costly, as it can take a long time to uncover the hidden meanings of the situation/context. However, if a researcher is expecting to commit to a particular topic as part of an ongoing program of research the investment of this time can prove very valuable. The researcher should allow enough time to get at the complexity of the situation being observed.

2. Interviews

- An interview implies some form of verbal discourse. The participant provides the researcher with information through verbal interchange or conversation. Non-verbal behaviours and the interview context are noted by the researcher and become part of the data.
- Another term used frequently in qualitative research is 'key informant interviews' which refers to the special nature of the participant being interviewed - he or she is chosen by the researcher because of an important or different viewpoint, status in a culture or organization, and/or knowledge of the issue being studied. However, the method of data collection remains an interview.
- Qualitative interviews place an emphasis on listening and following the direction of the participant/informant. A variety of open-ended questions are chosen to elicit the most information possible in the time available. Frequently, the interview protocol provides opportunities for the interviewer to probe following participant responses to open-ended questions.

- Interviews can be done relatively quickly, with little expense, and are useful when a particular issue needs to be explored in depth. However, the drawback to interviewing is related to the constraints imposed by language. The types of questions asked will frame the participants' responses, and this should be taken into account by the researcher.

3. Document Review

- Document review is often used in historical research, which involves the study and analysis of data about past events. The specific methods used are flexible and open because the purpose is to learn how past intentions and events were related due to their meaning and value. Documents are reviewed considering the context within which they were created. The historian learns about particular persons at particular times and places that present unique opportunities to learn about the topic of interest.
- It is a research method that requires the researcher to enter into an in-depth learning process, to become a critical editor of texts, such as diaries, media reports, or blogs. The researcher should explain the method used and readers should feel comfortable that the method involved adequate depth and a critical approach.

4. Focus Groups

- Focus groups are a formal method of interviewing a group of people/participants on a topic of interest.
- The same principles used for individual interviews apply with focus group interviews e.g., the use of open-ended questions, the focus on listening and learning from the participants.
- Focus groups are useful when multiple viewpoints or responses are needed on a specific topic/issue. Group members can build on one another's ideas to result in more in-depth discussions of the topic. Multiple responses can be obtained through focus groups in a shorter period of time than individual interviews. A researcher can also observe the interactions that occur among group members.
- The disadvantages of focus groups relate to the potential constraints that a group setting can place on individuals' responses. A common challenge in focus groups is to ensure that both reticent and gregarious participants have an opportunity to be heard. The facilitator of the focus group must be skilled in group process and interviewing techniques to ensure the success of the group.

5. Other

- Other forms of qualitative research methods include mapping cultural settings and events; recording, using either audio or visual techniques such as photography; life histories (biographies); and genograms.
- Some researchers consider surveys and questionnaires which are open-ended in nature to be qualitative methods if the primary intent is to 'listen' to or learn from the participants/clients themselves about the topic of interest. However, these tend to be limited, and often constrain the participants in ways that other qualitative methods do not. Answering one open-ended question at the end of a survey is not the same as participating in an in-depth interview. It is difficult to ensure that the richness of participants' experiences is really conveyed.

Researchers need to be clear about the intent of such questions, and how the results are analysed and interpreted.

Sampling

- The process of purposeful selection was described? - Sampling in qualitative research is purposeful and the process used to select participants should be clearly described.
- The sampling method needs to fit the study purpose or research question being explored.
- Purposeful sampling selects participants for a specific reason e.g., age, culture, experience, not randomly.
- There are numerous sampling methods in qualitative research: the sampling strategies used by the researcher should be explained and should relate to the purpose of the study. For example, if the purpose of the study is to learn about the impact of a new treatment program from the perspective of all clients involved in the program and their families, the purposeful sampling method should be broad to include maximum variation in perspectives and views. On the other hand, if the purpose is to explore an issue in-depth, such as the numerous factors and interactions that are involved in a family deciding when and where to place an elderly member in a nursing home, an individual, 'key informant' approach may be appropriate.
- Sampling was done until redundancy in data was reached? - The main indicator of sample size in qualitative research is often the point at which redundancy, or theoretical saturation of the data, is achieved. The researcher should indicate how and when the decision was reached that there was sufficient depth of information and redundancy of data to meet the purposes of the study.
- The sampling process should be flexible, evolving as the study progresses, until the point of redundancy in emerging themes is reached.
- The sample should be described in such a way that the reader understands the key characteristics of the participants involved. As a reader, you should then be able to consider the sample in comparison to the purpose of your critical review. You may decide at this point that the sample is different enough from your own population of interest that further appraisal of the study is not warranted.
- Informed consent was obtained? - The authors should describe ethics procedures, including review by a research ethics board and describing how informed consent was obtained and recorded.

Data Collection

Descriptive Clarity

- Clear and complete descriptions? - In qualitative research, the reader should have a sense of personally experiencing the event/phenomenon being studied. This requires a clear and vivid description of the important elements of the study that are connected with the data, namely the participants, and the site or setting.
- The researcher includes relevant information about the participants, often in the form of background demographic data. The unique characteristics of key informants help to explain why they were selected. The credibility of the informants should be explored. Particular to qualitative research, the types and levels of participation of the participants should also be described, so it is clear what contribution each participant made to the data gathering, analysis, and interpretation of the findings.

- It is often useful to consider what information is missing. This sheds light on how the research can be understood.
- Role of the researcher and relationship with participants: Qualitative research involves the 'researcher as instrument', wherein the researcher's use of self is a primary tool for data collection. Documentation of the researcher's credentials and previous experience in observation, interviewing and communicating should be provided to increase the confidence of the reader in the process. The researcher's role(s), level of participation and relationship with participants also needs to be described, as they can influence the findings.
- Identification of assumptions and biases of researcher: The researcher should declare his/her assumptions and biases about the topic under study to make the researcher's views about the phenomenon explicit.
- A vivid but concise description of the participants, site and researcher should provide the reader with an understanding of the 'whole picture' of the topic or phenomenon of interest.

▌Procedural Rigour

- Procedural rigour was used in data collection strategies? The researcher should clearly describe the procedures used to ensure that the reader can understand the tasks undertaken to collect the data. All source(s) of information used by the researcher should be described.
- The reader should be able to describe the data-gathering process including issues of gaining access to the site, data collection methods, training data gatherers, the length of time spent gathering data, and the amount of data collected.

▌Data Analyses

▌Analytical Rigour

- Data analyses were inductive? - The researcher(s) should describe how the findings emerged from the data.
- Different methods are used to analyze qualitative data - the reader should be able to identify and describe the methods used in the study of interest, and make a judgement as to whether the methods are appropriate given the purpose of the study.
- Qualitative analyses are typically inductive i.e., starting with data and organizing them into "chunks" which are typically referred to as codes, categories and themes.
- You should be able to summarize the major findings of the analyses in this section.
- Findings were consistent with and reflective of data? The codes, categories and/or themes developed by the researcher(s) should be logically consistent and reflective of the data. There should be an indication that the themes are inclusive of all data that exists, and data should be appropriately assigned to codes, categories, and themes.

▌Auditability

- Decision trail developed? - The process used to identify codes, categories, patterns, themes and relationships from the data is important to understand as it is complex. This process is best articulated through the use of a decision or 'audit' trail, which tracks decisions made during the process including the development of rules for transforming the data into codes, themes etc. Researchers often confront space limitations in publishing their research, so frequently state that they used a decision trail, but may not provide all of the details. You will need to judge whether you have adequate information about the analyses, and the rationale used to describe the interpretation of the data.

- Process of analyzing the data was described adequately? - The researchers should report on how data was transformed into codes and themes and interrelationships that provide a picture of the phenomenon under study. Often a qualitative researcher will use a specific analysis method, such as an editing style or a template approach (Crabtree & Miller, 1999). The methods used should be described.
- The rationale for the development of the themes should be described.
- These steps in auditing the analysis process provide evidence that the findings are representative of the data as a whole.

Theoretical Connections

- Did a meaningful picture of the phenomenon under study emerge? The findings or discussion section should clearly describe theoretical concepts, relationships between concepts, and integration of relationships among meanings that emerged from the data in order to yield a meaningful picture of the phenomenon under study. The reader should be able to understand concepts and relationships, including any conceptual frameworks that the researchers propose.

Overall Rigour

- Rigour in qualitative studies is critical. While in quantitative research one discusses concepts such as reliability and validity, qualitative researchers argue for the use of different terminology when determining the rigour of a qualitative study (Guba & Lincoln, 1989; Krefting, 1991; Taylor, 2000). The overarching concept when considering rigour is trustworthiness.
- Was there evidence of the four components of trustworthiness? Trustworthiness ensures the quality of the findings and increases the reader's confidence in the findings. This requires that there be logical connections among the various steps in the research process from the purpose of the study through to the analyses and interpretation.

- The four components of trustworthiness are:
  - Credibility which is related to the "true" picture of the phenomenon. Are descriptions and interpretations of the participants' experiences recognizable? Ways of ensuring credibility might include:
    - collection of data over a prolonged period and from a range of participants;
    - use of a variety of methods to gather data;
    - use of reflective approach through keeping a journal of reflections, biases or preconceptions and ideas;
    - triangulation, a strategy used to enhance trustworthiness through the use of multiple sources and perspectives to reduce systematic bias. Main types of triangulation are by sources (people, resources); by methods (interviews, observation, focus groups); by researchers (team of researchers versus single researcher) or by theories (team may bring different perspectives to research question for example a rehabilitation therapist and a sociologist); and
    - the involvement of participants through member checking. Member checking may consist of the involvement of participants in a range of activities to verify data and interpretation such as returning transcriptions to participants for review of accuracy of the interview content or returning to participants at various stages during collection and analysis of data to ensure that the researcher reflects or presents the experience of the phenomenon as it is understood by the participants.

- <u>Transferability</u> which is related to whether the findings can be transferred to other situations. Has the researcher described participants and the setting in enough detail to allow for comparisons with your population of interest? Are there concepts developed that might apply to your clients and their contexts? Transferability is ensured through adequate descriptions of sample and setting.

- <u>Dependability</u> which relates to the consistency between the data and the findings. There should be a clear explanation of the process of research including methods of data collection, analyses and interpretation often indicated by evidence of an audit trail or peer review. The audit trail describes the decision points made throughout the research process.

- <u>Confirmability</u> which involves the strategies used to limit bias in the research, specifically the neutrality of the data not the researcher. This can be enhanced through the researcher being reflective and keeping a journal, peer review such as asking a colleague to audit the decision points throughout the process and checking with expert colleagues about ideas and interpretation of data, checking with participants about ideas and interpretation of data, and having a team of researchers.

Conclusions & Implications

- <u>Conclusions were appropriate given the study findings</u>? - Conclusions should be consistent and congruent with the findings as reported by the researchers. All of the data and findings should be discussed and synthesized.
- <u>The findings contributed to theory development and future OT practice</u>? - The conclusions of the study should be meaningful to the reader, and should help the reader understand the theories developed. It should provide insight into important professional issues facing occupational therapists. The authors should relate the findings back to the existing literature and theoretical knowledge in occupational therapy. Implications and recommendations should be explicitly linked to occupational therapy practice situations and research directions.

▌References:

Ashe, B., Taylor, M., & Dubouloz, C. J. (2005). The process of change: Listening to transformation in meaning perspectives of adults in arthritis health education groups. *Canadian Journal of Occupational Therapy, 72,* 280-288.

Borell, L., Gustavsson, A., Sandman, P., & Kielhofner, G. (1994). Occupational programming in a day hospital for patients with dementia. *Occupational Therapy Journal of Research, 14,* 219-243.

Charmaz, K. (2003). Grounded theory: Objectivist and constructivist methods. In N. K. Denzin & Y. S. Lincoln (Eds.), *Strategies of qualitative inquiry* (2nd ed., pp. 249-291). Thousand Oaks, CA: Sage.

Charmaz, K. (2006). *Constructing grounded theory: A practical guide through qualitative analysis.* Thousand Oaks, CA: Sage.

Cockburn, L., & Trentham, B. (2002). Participatory action research: Integrating community occupational therapy practice and research. *Canadian Journal of Occupational Therapy, 69,* 20-30.

Crabtree, B. F., & Miller, W. L. (1992). *Doing qualitative research: Research methods for primary care.* Newbury Park CA: Sage.

Crabtree, B. F., & Miller, W. L. (1999). *Doing qualitative research* (2nd ed.). Thousand Oaks, CA: Sage.

Glaser, B. G. (1978). *Theoretical sensitivity: Advances in the methodology of grounded theory.* Mill Valley, CA: The Sociology Press.

Glaser, B. G., & Strauss, A. L. (1967). *The discovery of grounded theory: Strategies for qualitative research.* New York: Aldine de Gruyter.

Guba, E. G., & Lincoln, Y. S. (1989). *Fourth generation evaluation.* Newbury Park, CA: Sage.

Guitard, P., Ferland, F., & Dutil, E. (2005). Toward a better understanding of playfulness in adults. *OTJR: Occupation, Participation and Health, 25,* 9-22.

Jung, B., Tryssenaar, J., & Wilkins, S. (2005). Becoming a tutor: Exploring the learning experiences and needs of novice tutors in a PBL programme. *Medical Teacher, 27,* 606-612.

Krefting, L. (1989). Disability ethnography: A methodological approach for occupational therapy research. *Canadian Journal of Occupational Therapy, 56,* 61-66.

Krefting, L. (1991). Rigor in qualitative research: The assessment of trustworthiness. *American Journal of Occupational Therapy, 45,* 214-222.

Letts, L. (2003). Occupational therapy and participatory research: A partnership worth pursuing. *American Journal of Occupational Therapy, 57,* 77-87.

Strauss, A. L., & Corbin, J. M. (1990). *Basics of qualitative research: Grounded theory procedures and techniques.* Newbury Park, CA: SAGE.

Taylor, M. C. (2000). *Evidence-based practice for occupational therapists.* Oxford, UK: Blackwell Science Inc.

Wilding, C., & Whiteford, G. (2005). Phenomenological research: An exploration of conceptual, theoretical, and practical issues. *OTJR: Occupation, Participation and Health, 25,* 98-104.

Bibliography:

Bentz, V. M., & Shapiro, J. J. (1998). *Mindful inquiry in social research.* Thousand Oaks, CA: Sage.

Burns, N. (1989). Standards for qualitative research. *Nursing Science Quarterly, 2*(1), 44-52.

Creswell, J. W. (2006). *Qualitative inquiry and research design: Choosing among five approaches* (2nd ed.). Thousand Oaks, CA: Sage.

Denzin, N. K., & Lincoln, Y.S. (Eds.). (2005). *The SAGE Handbook of qualitative research* (3rd ed.). Thousand Oaks, CA: SAGE.

de Laine, M. (1997). *Ethnography: Theory and application in health research.* Sydney, Australia: MacLennan & Petty.

Farmer, T., Robinson, K., Elliott, S. J., & Eyles, J. (2006). Developing and implementing a triangulation protocol for qualitative health research. *Qualitative Health Research, 16,* 377-394.

Patton, M. Q. (1990). *Qualitative evaluation and research methods* (2nd ed.). Newbury Park, CA: Sage.

Smith, S. E., Willms D. G., & Johnson, N. A. (Eds.). (1997). *Nurtured by knowledge: Learning to do participatory action-research.* Ottawa ON: The Apex Press.

van Manen, M. (1997). *Researching lived experience: Human science for an action sensitive pedagogy* (2nd ed.). London, ON: The Althouse Press.

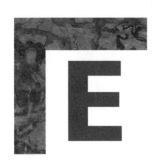

Appendix E:
Outcome Measures
Rating Form

CANCHILD CENTRE FOR DISABILITY RESEARCH
INSTITUTE OF APPLIED HEALTH SCIENCES, MCMASTER UNIVERSITY
1400 MAIN STREET WEST, ROOM 408
HAMILTON, ONTARIO,CANADA L8S 1C7
Fax (905) 522-6095
lawm@mcmaster.ca

To be used with: Outcome Measures Rating Form Guidelines (CanChild,2004)

Name and initials of measure: _____

_____

Author(s): _____

_____

Source and year published: _____

_____

Date of review: _____

Name of Reviewer: _____

---

1. FOCUS

a. Focus of measurement – Using the ICF framework
   ☐ Body Functions.................. are the physiological functions of body systems(includes psychological functions)

   ☐ Body Structures................... are anatomical parts of the body such as organs, limbs, and their components

   ☐ Activities and Participation.... Activity is the execution of a task or action by an individual. Participation is involvement in a life situation.

   ☐ Environmental Factors......... make up the physical, social and attitudinal environment in which people live and conduct their lives.

b. Attribute(s) being measured – Check as many as apply.
   This list is based on attributes cited in the ICF, 2001: WHO.

Body Functions

Global Mental Functions

□ consciousness
□ orientation
□ sleep

□ intellectual
□ global psychosocial

□ temperament and personality
□ energy and drive

Specific Mental Functions

□ attention
□ memory
□ psychomotor
□ calculation

□ thought
□ higher level cognitive
□ perceptual

□ mental functions of language
□ experience of self and time
□ mental function of sequencing
   complex measurements

Sensory Functions and Pain

□ seeing and related

□ hearing and vestibular

Voice and Speech Functions

□ voice
□ articulation

□ fluency and rhythm of speech
□ alternative vocalization

Functions of the Cardiovascular, Hematological, Immunological, and Respiratory Systems

□ cardiovascular
□ haematological and
   immunological systems

□ respiratory system
□ additional functions and sensations of the
   cardiovascular and respiratory systems

Functions of the Digestive, Metabolic, and Endocrine Systems

□ related to the digestive
   system

□ related to metabolism and the endocrine system

Genitourinary and Reproductive Functions

□ urinary

□ genital and reproductive

Neuromuscular and Movement-Related Functions

Joints and Bones

□ mobility of joint
□ stability of joint

□ mobility of bone

Muscle

□ muscle power
□ muscle tone

□ muscle endurance

Movement

□ motor reflex
□ involuntary movement
   reaction
□ control of voluntary
   movement

□ involuntary movement
□ sensations related to
   muscle and movement
□ gait patterns

Functions of the Skin and Related Structures

Skin
- □ protection
- □ repair

- □ other functions
- □ sensations

Hair
- □ function of the hair

Nails
- □ function of nails

Body Structures

Structures of the Nervous System
- □ brain
- □ meninges
- □ parasympathetic nervous system

- □ spinal cord and related structures
- □ sympathetic nervous system

The Eye, Ear and Related Structures
- □ eye socket
- □ eyeball

- □ around eye
- □ external ear

- □ middle ear
- □ inner ear

Structures Involved in Voice and Speech
- □ nose
- □ mouth

- □ pharynx
- □ larynx

Structures of the Cardiovascular, Immunological, and Respiratory Systems

Cardiovascular System
- □ heart
- □ arteries

- □ veins
- □ capillaries

Immune System
- □ lymphatic vessels
- □ thymus
- □ bone marrow

- □ lymphatic nodes
- □ spleen

Respiratory System
- □ trachea
- □ thoracic cage

- □ lungs
- □ muscles of respiration

Structures Related to the Digestive, Metabolic, and Endocrine Systems
- □ salivary glands
- □ oesophagus
- □ stomach

- □ pancreas
- □ liver
- □ gall bladder

- □ intestines
- □ endocrine glands

Structures Related to the Genitourinary and Reproductive Systems
- □ urinary system
- □ pelvic floor
- □ reproductive system

Structures Related to Movement

- □ head and neck
- □ upper extremity
- □ additional musculoskeletal structures related to movement
- □ shoulder region
- □ trunk
- □ lower extremity
- □ pelvic region

Skin and Related Structures

- □ skin
- □ nails
- □ skin and glands
- □ hair

Activities and Participation

Learning and Applying Knowledge

Purposeful Sensory Experiences
- □ watching
- □ listening
- □ other purposeful sensing

Basic Learning
- □ copying
- □ learning to read
- □ learning to calculate
- □ rehearsing
- □ learning to write
- □ acquiring skills

Applying Knowledge
- □ focusing attention
- □ thinking
- □ reading
- □ writing
- □ calculating
- □ solving problems
- □ making decisions

General Tasks and Demand

- □ undertaking a single task
- □ carrying out daily routine
- □ undertaking multiple tasks
- □ handling stress and other psychological demands

Communication

- □ receiving (verbal, nonverbal, written, formal sign language)
- □ producing (verbal, nonverbal, written, formal sign language)
- □ conversation and use of communication devices and techniques

Mobility

- □ changing and maintaining body position
- □ walking and moving
- □ carrying, moving, and handling objects
- □ moving around using transportation

Self-Care

- □ washing oneself
- □ caring for body parts
- □ toileting
- □ dressing
- □ eating
- □ drinking

Looking after one's health
- □ ensuring oneself physical comfort
- □ managing diet and fitness
- □ maintaining one's health

Domestic Life

Acquisition of Necessities
☐ acquiring a place to live
☐ acquisition of goods and services

Household Tasks
☐ preparing meals
☐ caring for household objects and assisting others
☐ doing housework

Interpersonal Interactions and Relationships

General
☐ general interpersonal interactions (basic and complex)

Particular Interpersonal Relationships
☐ informal social realtionships
☐ formal relationships
☐ relating with strangers
☐ family relatonships
☐ intimate relationships

Major Life Areas

Education
☐ informal
☐ preschool
☐ school

Work and Employment
☐ apprenticeship
☐ acquiring, keeping, and terminating a job
☐ renumerative employment
☐ non-renumerative employment

Economic Life
☐ basic economic transactions
☐ complex economic transactions
☐ economic self-sufficiency

Community, Social, and Civic Life

Community
☐ community life

Recreation and Leisure
☐ play
☐ sports
☐ arts and culture
☐ crafts
☐ hobbies
☐ soicalizing

Civic
☐ religion and spirituality
☐ human rights
☐ political life and citizenship

Environmental Factors

Products and Technology
☐ communication
☐ culture, recreation, and sport
☐ design, construction, and buildings for public use
☐ religion and spirituality
☐ education
☐ products or substances for personal consumption
☐ design, construction, and buildings for private use
☐ land development
☐ employment
☐ products and technology for personal use in daily living
☐ for personal indoor and outdoor mobility and transportation
☐ assets

Natural Environment and Human-Made Changes to Environment

- □ physical geography
- □ flora and fauna
- □ natural events
- □ light

- □ sound
- □ air quality
- □ population
- □ climate

- □ human events
- □ time-related changes
- □ vibration

Support and Relationships

- □ immediate family
- □ health professionals
- □ people in positions of authority
- □ acquaintances, peers, colleagues, neighbors, and community members

- □ extended family
- □ other professionals
- □ people in subordinate positions
- □ domesticated animals

- □ friends
- □ strangers
- □ personal care providers and personal assistants

Attitudes

- □ of immediate family
- □ of strangers
- □ of people in positions of authority
- □ of acquaintances, peers, colleagues, neighbors, and community members

- □ of extended family
- □ of health professionals
- □ of people in subordinate positions
- □ societal attitudes

- □ of friends
- □ of health-related professionals
- □ of personal care providers and personal assistants
- □ social norms, practices, and idealogies

Services, Systems and Policies

- □ production of consumer goods
- □ open space planning
- □ utilities
- □ transportation
- □ legal
- □ media

- □ architecture and construction
- □ social security
- □ health
- □ labour and employment
- □ housing
- □ communication

- □ associations and organizations
- □ civil protection
- □ economic
- □ general social support
- □ education and training
- □ political

c. Does this measure assess a single attribute or multiple attributes?

□ Single
□ Multiple

d. Check purposes that apply and indicate (*) primary purpose of the measure

□ To describe or discriminate   □ To predict   □ To evaluative

Comments:_____
_____
_____

e. Perspective - Indicate possible respondents:
    □ Client   □ Other professional
    □ Caregiver/parent   □ Other
    □ Service provider

f. Population measure designed for:
    Age: Please specify all applicable ages if stated in the manual
    □ Infant (birth - < 1 year)   □ Adult (> 18 years - <65 years)
    □ Child (1 year - < 13 years)   □ Senior (> 65 years)
    □ Adolescent (13 - < 18 years)   □ Age not specified

    Diagnosis:
    List the diagnostic group(s) for which this measure is designed to be used:

    _____
    _____
    _____
    _____

g. Evaluation context—Indicate suggested/possible environments for this assessment
    □ Home   □ Education setting   □ Community
    □ Workplace   □ Community agency   □ Rehabilitation centre/
                                              health care setting

    □ Other_____

2. CLINICAL UTILITY

a. Clarity of Instructions: (check one of the ratings)
    □ Excellent: clear, comprehensive, concise, and available
    □ Adequate: clear, concise, but lacks some information
    □ Poor: not clear and concise or not available
    Comments:_____
    _____

b. Format (check applicable items)
    □ Interview   Questionnaire: □ Self completed
    □ Task performance   □ Interview administered
    □ Naturalistic observation   □ Caregiver completed

    □ Other_____

    Physically invasive: □ Yes   □ No
    Active participation of client: □ Yes   □ No
    Special Equipment Required: □ Yes   □ No

c. Time to complete assessment: _____ minutes
        Administration: □ Easy   □ More complex   *(Consider time,*
        Scoring: □ Easy   □ More complex   *amount of training,*
        Interpretation: □ Easy   □ More complex   *and ease)*

d. Examiner Qualifications: Is formal training required for administering and/or interpreting?

　☐ Required　　☐ Recommended　　☐ Not required　　☐ Not addressed

e. Cost (Cdn. Funds)
　manual: $_____
　score sheets: $_____ for_____Sheets
　Indicate year of cost information:_____
　Source of cost information:_____

---

3. SCALE CONSTRUCTION

a. Item Selection (check one of the ratings)

　☐ Excellent:　　included all relevant characteristics of attribute based on comprehensive literature review and survey of experts

　☐ Adequate:　　included most relevant characteristics of attribute

　☐ Poor:　　· convenient sample of characteristics of attribute

　Comments:_____
　_____
　_____

b. Weighting
　Are the items weighted in the calculation of total score? ☐ Yes　☐ No
　　　　If yes, are the items weighted: ☐ Implicitly　☐ Explicitly

c. Level of Measurement　　☐ Nominal　　☐ Ordinal　☐ Interval　　☐ Ratio

　　Scaling method (Likert, Guttman, etc.):_____

　　Number of items:_____

　　Indicate if subscale scores are obtained:　☐ Yes　　☐ No

　　If yes, can the subscale scores be used alone:　Administered: ☐Yes ☐ No
　　　　　　　　　　　　　　　　　　　　　　Interpreted:　☐ Yes ☐ No

List subscales:	Number of Items:

4. STANDARDIZATION

a. Manual (check one of the ratings)

    □ Excellent: published manual which outlines specific procedures for administration; scoring and interpretation; evidence of reliability and validity

    □ Adequate: manual available and generally complete but some information is lacking or unclear regarding administration; scoring and interpretation; evidence of reliability and validity

    □ Poor: no manual available or manual with unclear administration; scoring and interpretaion; no evidence of reliability and validity

b. Norms available (N/A for instrument whose purpose is only evaluative)

    □ Yes   □ No   □ N/A

Age: Please specify all applicable ages for which norms are available

□ Infant (birth - < 1 year)   □ Adult (> 18 years - <65 years)
□ Child (1 year - < 13 years)   □ Senior (> 65 years)
□ Adolescent (13 - < 18 years)

Populations for which it is normed:

_____
_____

Size of sample: n = _____

5. RELIABILITY

a. Rigor of standardization studies for reliability (check one of the ratings)

    □ Excellent: more than 2 well-designed reliability studies completed with adequate to excellent reliability values

    □ Adequate: 1 to 2 well-designed reliability studies completed with adequate to excellent reliability values

    □ Poor: reliability studies poorly completed, or reliability studies showing poor levels of reliability

    □ No evidence available

Comments:_____
_____
_____
_____

b. Reliability Information

Type of Reliability	Statistic Used	Value	Rating (excellent, adequate or poor)

* guidelines for levels of reliability coefficient (see instructions)
Excellent: >.80   Adequate: .60 - .79   Poor: <.60

---

6. VALIDITY

a. Rigor of standardization studies for validity (check one of the ratings)
  □ Excellent: more than 2 well-designed validity studies supporting the measure's validity
  □ Adequate: 1 to 2 well-designed validity studies supporting the measure's validity
  □ Poor: validity studies poorly completed or did not support the measure's validity
  □ No evidence available

Comments:
_____
_____
_____
_____

b. Content Validity (check one of the ratings)
  □ Excellent: judgmental or statistical method (e.g. factor analysis) was used and the measure is comprehensive and includes items suited to the measurement purpose
  Method: □ judgmental   □ statistical
  □ Adequate: has content validity but no specific method was used
  □ Poor: instrument is not comprehensive
  □ No evidence available

c. Construct Validity (check one of the ratings)
  □ Excellent: more than 2 well-designed studies have shown that the instrument conforms to prior theoretical relationships among characteristics or individuals
  □ Adequate: 1 to 2 studies demonstrate confirmation of theoretical formulations
  □ Poor: construct validation poorly completed, or did not support measure's construct validity
  □ No evidence available

Strength of Association:_____
_____
_____
_____
_____

d. Criterion Validity (check ratings that apply)
            □ Concurrent   □ Predictive

□ Excellent: more than 2 well-designed studies have shown adequate agreement with a criterion or gold standard

□ Adequate: 1 to 2 studies demonstrate adequate agreement with a criterion or gold standard measure

□ Poor: criterion validation poorly completed or did not support measure's criterion validity

□ No evidence available

Criterion Measure(s) used: _____

_____

Strength of Association:_____

_____

e. Responsiveness (check one of the ratings)
□ Excellent: more that 2 well-designed studies showing strong hypothesized relationships between changes on the measure and other measures of change on the same attribute.

□ Adequate: 1 to 2 studies of responsiveness

□ Poor: studies of responsiveness poorly completed or did not support the measure's responsiveness

□ N/A

□ No evidence available

Comments:

_____
_____

---

7. OVERALL UTILITY (based on an overall assessment of the quality of this measure)

□ Excellent: adequate to excellent clinical utility, easily available, excellent reliability, and validity

□ Adequate: adequate to excellent clinical utility, easily available, adequate to excellent reliability, and adequate to excellent validity

□ Poor: poor clinical utility, not easily available, poor reliability, and validity

Comments/Notes/Explanations:

_____
_____
_____
_____
_____
_____
_____
_____

MATERIALS USED FOR REVIEW/RATING

Please indicate the sources of information used for this review/rating:
□ Manual
□ Journal articles: (attach or indicate location)
    □ by author of measure
    □ by other authors
List sources:

_____
_____
_____
_____
_____
_____

□ Books—provide reference

□ Correspondence with author—attach

□ Other sources:

_____
_____
_____

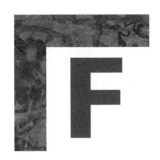

Appendix F:
Outcome Measures
Rating Form Guidelines

OUTCOME MEASURES RATING FORM GUIDELINES

FROM: CanChild Centre for Childhood Disability Research
Institute of Applied Health Sciences, McMaster University
1400 Main Street West. Room 408
Hamilton, Canada L8S 1C7
fax (905) 522-6095
lawm@mcmaster.ca

PREPARED BY: Mary Law, Ph.D. O.T.(C)

FOR FURTHER DISCUSSION OF ISSUES: Law, M. (1987). Measurement in occupational therapy: Scientific criteria for evaluation. *Canadian Journal of Occupational Therapy, 54*, 133-138.

GENERAL INFORMATION: Name of Measure, Authors, Source and Year.

---

1. FOCUS

---

a. FOCUS OF MEASUREMENT. Use the ICF framework to indicate the focus of the measurement instrument that is being reviewed. The definitions are as follows: BODY FUNCTIONS: are the physiological functions of body systems (including psychological functions). BODY STRUCTURES: are anatomical parts of the body such as organs, limbs and their components. ACTIVITIES AND PARTICIPATION: activity is the execution of a task or action by an individual. Participation is involvement in a life situation. ENVIRONMENTAL FACTORS: make up the physical, social and attitudinal environment in which people live and conduct their lives.

b. ATTRIBUTE(S) BEING MEASURED. The rating form lists attributes organized using the ICF framework. Check as many attributes as apply to indicate what is being measured by this instrument.

c. SINGLE OR MULTIPLE ATTRIBUTE. Check the appropriate box to indicate whether this measure assesses a single attribute only or multiple attributes.

d. List the PRIMARY PURPOSE for which the scale has been designed. Secondary purposes can also be listed but the instrument should be evaluated according to its primary purpose (i.e., discriminative, predictive, evaluative).

DISCRIMINATIVE: A discriminative index is used to distinguish between individuals or groups on an underlying dimension when no external criterion or gold standard is available for validating these measures.

PREDICTIVE: A predictive index is used to classify individuals into a set of predefined measurement categories... either concurrently or prospectively, to determine whether individuals have been classified correctly.

EVALUATIVE: An evaluative index is used to measure the magnitude of longitudinal change in an individual or group on the dimension of interest.
(Kirshner, B. & Guyatt G. (1985). A methodological framework for assessing health indices. *Journal of Chronic Diseases, 38,* 27-36.)

e. PERSPECTIVE. Indicate the possible respondents.

f. POPULATION for which it is designed (AGE). If no age is stated, mark as age unspecified. List the diagnostic groups for which the measure is used.

g. EVALUATION CONTEXT refers to the environment in which the assessment is completed. Check all possible environments in which this assessment can be completed.

---

2. CLINICAL UTILITY

a. CLARITY OF INSTRUCTIONS. Check one of the ratings. Excellent: clear, comprehensive, concise and available; Adequate: clear, concise but lacks some information; Poor: not clear and concise or not available.

b. FORMAT. Check all applicable items to indicate the format of data collection for the instrument. Possible items include naturalistic observation, interview, a questionnaire (self-completed, interview administered or caregiver-completed), and task performance.

PHYSICALLY INVASIVE indicates whether administration of the measure requires procedures which may be perceived as invasive by the client. Examples of invasiveness include any procedure which requires insertion of needles or taping of electrodes, or procedures which require clients to take clothing on or off.

ACTIVE PARTICIPATION OF CLIENT. Indicate whether completion of the measure requires the client to participate verbally or physically.

SPECIAL EQUIPMENT REQUIRED. Indicate whether the measurement process requires objects which are not part of the test kit and are not everyday objects. Examples of this include stopwatches, a balance board or other special equipment.

c. TIME TO COMPLETE THE ASSESSMENT. Record in minutes. For ADMINISTRATION, SCORING and INTERPRETATION, consider the time and the amount of training and the ease with which a test is administered, scored, and interpreted, and indicate whether these issues are easy or more complex. For ADMINISTRATION, SCORING, and INTERPRETATION to be rated as easy, each part of the task should be completed in under one hour with minimal amount of training and is easy for the average service provider to complete.

d. EXAMINER QUALIFICATIONS. Indicate if formal training is required for administering and interpreting this measure.

e. COST. In Canadian funds, indicate the cost of the measurement manual and score sheets. For SCORE SHEETS, indicate the number of sheets obtainable for that cost. List the SOURCE and the YEAR of the cost information so readers will know if the information is up to date.

---

3. SCALE CONSTRUCTION

---

a. ITEM SELECTION. Check one of the ratings. Excellent: included all relevant characteristics of the attribute based on comprehensive literature review and survey of experts—a comprehensive review of the literature only is enough for an excellent rating, but a survey of experts alone is not enough; Adequate: included most relevant characteristics of the attribute; Poor: convenient sample of characteristics of the attribute.

b. WEIGHTING. Indicate whether the items in the tool are weighted in the calculation of the total score. If items are weighted, indicate whether the authors have weighted these items implicitly or explicitly. Implicit weighting occurs when there are a number of scales and each have a different number of items and the score is obtained by simply adding the scores for each item together. Explicit weighting occurs when each item or score is multiplied by a factor to weight its importance.

c. LEVEL OF MEASUREMENT. State whether the scale used is NOMINAL (descriptive categories), ORDINAL (ordered categories), or INTERVAL or RATIO (numerical) for single and for summary scores. Indicate the SCALING METHOD that was used and the NUMBER OF ITEMS in the measure. Indicate if SUBSCALE SCORES are obtained. Indicate whether the subscales can be administered alone and the scores interpreted alone. In some cases, the scores can be interpreted alone, but the whole measure must be administered first. List the subscales with the number of items and indicate if there is evidence of reliability and validity for the subscales so that the scores can be used on their own. *Standardization* is the process of administering a test under uniform conditions.

---

4. STANDARDIZATION

---

a. MANUAL. Check one of the ratings. Excellent: published manual which outlines specific procedures for administration; scoring and interpretation; evidence of reliability and validity. Adequate: manual available and generally complete but some information is lacking or unclear regarding administration; scoring and interpretation; evidence of reliability and validity. Poor: no manual available or manual with unclear administration; scoring and interpretation; no evidence of reliability and validity.

b. NORMS. Indicate whether norms are available for the instrument. Please note that instruments which are only meant to be evaluative do not require norms. Indicate all AGES for which norms are available, the POPULATIONS for which the measure has been normed (e.g., children with cerebral palsy, people with spinal cord injuries), and indicate the SIZE OF THE SAMPLE which was used in the normative studies.

5. RELIABILITY

Reliability is the process of determining that the test or measure is measuring something in a reproducible and consistent fashion.

a. RIGOUR OF STANDARDIZATION STUDIES FOR RELIABILITY. Excellent: More than 2 well-designed reliability studies completed with adequate to excellent reliability values; Adequate: 1 to 2 well-designed reliability studies completed with adequate to excellent reliability values; Poor: No reliability studies or poorly completed, or reliability studies showing poor levels of reliability.

b. RELIABILITY INFORMATION. *Internal Consistency*: the degree of homogeneity of test items to the attribute being measured. Measured at one point in time.

Observer: i) *intra-observer* - measures variation which occurs within an observer as a result of multiple exposures to the same stimulus. ii) *inter-observer*—measures variation between two or more observers. *Test-Retest*: measures variation in the test over a period of time. Complete the table and reliability information by filling in the TYPE OF RELIABILITY which was tested (internal consistency, observer, test-retest); the STATISTIC that was used (e.g., Cronbach's coefficient alpha, kappa coefficient, Pearson correlation, intra-class correlation); the VALUE of the statistic that was found in the study; and the RATING of the reliability. Guidelines for levels of the reliability coefficient indicate that it will be rated excellent if the coefficient is greater than .80, adequate if it is from .60 to .79, and poor if the coefficient is less than .60.

6. VALIDITY

a. RIGOUR OF STANDARDIZATION STUDIES FOR VALIDITY. Excellent: More than 2 well-designed validity studies supporting the measure's validity; Adequate: 1 to 2 well designed validity studies supporting the measure's validity; Poor: No validity studies completed, studies were poorly completed or did not support the measure's validity.

b. CONTENT VALIDITY. Check one of the ratings. *Content Validity*: the instrument is comprehensive and fully represents the domain of the characteristics it claims to measure (Nunnally, J. C. [1978]. *Psychometric theory*. New York: McGraw-Hill). Excellent: judgmental or statistical method (e.g. factor analysis) was used and the measure is comprehensive and includes items suited to the measurement purpose; Adequate: has content validity but no specific method was used; Poor: instrument is not comprehensive. METHOD. Note whether a judgmental (e.g., consensus methods) or statistical method (e.g., factor analysis) of establishing content validity was used.

c. CONSTRUCT VALIDITY. *Construct Validity*: the measurements of the attribute conform to prior theoretical formulations or relationships among characteristics or individuals (Nunnally, J. C. [1978]. *Psychometric theory*. New York: McGraw-Hill). Excellent: More than 2 well-designed studies have shown that the instrument conforms to prior theoretical relationships among characteristics or individuals; Adequate: 1 to 2 studies demonstrate confirmation of theoretical formulations; Poor: No construct validation completed.

Indicate the STRENGTH OF ASSOCIATION of the findings for construct validity by listing the value of the correlation coefficients found.

d. CRITERION VALIDITY. Check one of the ratings.

Criterion Validity: the measurements obtained by the instrument agree with another more accurate measure of the same characteristic, that is, a criterion or gold standard measure (Nunnally, J. C. [1978]. *Psychometric theory*. New York: McGraw-Hill).

Indicate whether the type of criterion validity which was investigated is CONCURRENT, PREDICTIVE, or both. Excellent: More than 2 well-designed studies have shown adequate agreement with a criterion or gold standard; Adequate: 1 to 2 studies demonstrate adequate agreement with a criterion or gold standard measure; Poor: No criterion validation completed. Indicate the STRENGTH OF ASSOCIATION of the evidence for criterion validity by listing the values of the correlation coefficients which were found in the criterion validity studies. Using the information from the assessment that has been completed on this measure, check the appropriate rating to give an overall assessment of the quality of the measure.

e. RESPONSIVENESS. Check one of the ratings (applicable only to evaluative measures). *Responsiveness*: the ability of the measure to detect minimal clinically important change over time (Guyatt, G., Walter, S. D., & Norman, G. R. [1987]. Measuring change over time: Assessing the usefulness of evaluative instruments. *Journal of Chronic Diseases*, *40*, 171-178). Excellent: More that 2 well-designed studies showing strong hypothesized relationships between changes on the measure and other measures of change on the same attribute; Adequate: 1 to 2 studies of responsiveness; Poor: No studies of responsiveness; N/A: Check if the measure is not designed to evaluate change over time.

7. OVERALL UTILITY

Excellent: Adequate to excellent clinical utility, easily available, excellent reliability and validity. Adequate: Adequate to excellent clinical utility, easily available, adequate to excellent reliability and adequate to excellent validity. Poor: Poor clinical utility, not easily available, poor reliability and validity.

8. MATERIALS USED

Please indicate and list the sources of information which were used for this review. By listing sources of information and attaching appropriate journal articles or correspondence with authors, it will be easier to find further information about this measure if it is required.

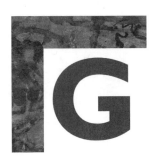

Appendix G:
Critical Appraisal of
Study Quality for
Psychometric Articles

Evaluation Form

Critical Appraisal Of Study Design For Psychometric Articles
Evaluation Form

Authors: _____ Year: _____ Rater: ____

Use this form to rate the quality of a psychometric study. To decide which score to provide for each item on your quality checklist pick the descriptor that sounds <u>most</u> like the study you were evaluating with respect to a given item. Items ranks are described in the guide. (Forms and guides to extract the actual psychometric information available from developer at macderj@mcmaster.ca)

Evaluation criteria	Score		
Study question	2	1	0
1. Was the relevant background work cited to define what is currently known about the psychometric properties of measures under study, and the potential contributions of the current research question?			
Study Design			
2. Were appropriate inclusion/exclusion criteria defined?			
3. Were specific psychometric hypotheses identified?			
4. Was an appropriate scope of psychometric properties considered?			
5. Was an appropriate sample size used?			
6. Was appropriate retention/follow-up obtained? (Studies involving retesting or follow-up only)			
Measurements			
7. Were specific descriptions provided of the techniques used to collect measurements reported?			
8. Did measurement procedures use standardized techniques (and other methods required) to minimize potential sources of error/misinterpretation in the individual measures taken within the study?			
Analyses			
9. Were analyses conducted for each specific hypothesis or purpose?			
10. Were appropriate statistical tests conducted to obtain point estimates of the psychometric property?			
11. Were appropriate ancillary analyses done to describe properties beyond the point estimates? (Confidence intervals, benchmark comparisons, SEM/MID)			
Recommendations			
12. Were the conclusions/clinical recommendations supported by the study objectives, analysis, and results?			
Subtotals (of columns 1 and 2)			
Total score (sum of subtotals/24*100); if for a specific paper or topic an item is deemed inappropriate then you can sum of items/2*number of items *100			

© MacDermid 2007

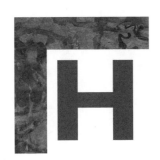

Appendix H:
Critical Appraisal of
Study Quality for
Psychometric Articles
Interpretation Guide

Critical Appraisal Of Study Quality For Psychometric Articles
Interpretation Guide

To decide which score to provide for each item on your quality checklist, read the following descriptors. Pick the descriptor that sounds most like the study you were evaluating with respect to a given item.

		Descriptors
Study question		
Score		
1	2	The authors: - performed a thorough literature review indicating what is currently known about the psychometric properties of the instruments or tests under study - presented a critical and unbiased view of the current state of knowledge - indicated how the current research question evolves from a current knowledge base - Established a research question based on the above.
	1	All of these above criteria were not fulfilled, but a clear rationale was provided for the research question.
	0	A foundation for the current research question was not clear or was not founded on previous literature.
Study design		
2	2	Specific inclusion/exclusion criteria for the study were defined, the practice setting was described and appropriate demographic information was presented yielding a study group generalizable to a clinical situation.
	1	Some information on person and place is provided (NOT ALL). For example, age/sex/diagnosis and the name of the practice (clinic name) without additional information. Information on the type of patients is briefly defined, but it is insufficient to allow the reader to generalize the study to a specific population.
	0	No information on type of clinical settings or study participants is provided.
3	2	Authors identified specific hypotheses that included the specific type of reliability (intra/inter-rater or test-retest) or validity (construct/ criterion/ content; longitudinal/concurrent; convergent/divergent) being tested. For validity, expected relationships or constructs were defined.
	1	Types of reliability and validity being tested were stated, but not clearly defined in terms of specific hypotheses.
	0	Specific types of reliability or validity under evaluation were not clearly defined nor were specific hypotheses on reliability and validity stated. ("*The purpose of this study was to investigate the reliability and validity of...*" can be rated it is zero if no further detail on the types of reliability and validity or the nature of specific hypotheses is stated.)

4	2	An appropriate scope of psychometric properties would be indicated by 1. A detailed focus on reliability that included multiple forms of reliability (at least two of intra-rater, inter-rater, test-retest) where both relative and absolute reliability were addressed (e.g., ICCs and SEM/MID). 2. A detailed focus on validity that included multiple forms of validity (content-judgmental; structured e.g. expert review/survey or qualitative interviews) or statistical (e.g. factor analyses), construct (known group differences; convergent/divergent associations), criterion (concurrent/predictive), responsiveness; predictive, evaluative or discriminative properties were established 3. Some aspects of both reliability and validity were examined concurrently using multiple approaches/analyses.
	1	Two psychometric properties were evaluated, however, the scope of both was superficial or narrow (e.g. point estimates used for one type of reliability and only a single unidimensional validity hypotheses tested)
	0	The scope of psychometric properties was very narrow as indicated by only one form of reliability or validity hypothesis estimated/tested.
5	2	Authors performed a sample size calculation and obtained their recruitment targets. Post-doc power analyses and/or confidence intervals confirm that the sample size was sufficient to define relatively precise estimates of reliability or validity.
	1	The authors provide a rationale for the number of subjects included in the study, but did not present specific sample size calculations or post-doc power analyses.
	0	Size of the sample was not rationalized or is clearly underpowered.
6	2	90% or more of the patients enrolled for study were re-evaluated.
	1	More than 70% of the eligible patients were re-evaluated.
	0	Less than 70% of the patients eligible for study were re-evaluated
Measurements		
7	2	The authors provided or referenced a published manual/article that outlines specific procedures for administration, scoring (including scoring algorithms handling of missing data), and interpretation that included any necessary information about positioning/active participation of the client, any special equipment required, calibration of equipment if necessary, training required, cost, examiner procedures/actions. Text describes key details of procedures.
	1	Procedures are referenced without any details or a limited description of procedures is included within text.
	0	Minimal description of procedures without appropriate references
8	2	All of the measurement techniques, including administration and scoring of the measurements were performed in a standardized way. This would include calibration of any equipment; use of consistent measurement tools and scoring, a priori exclusion of any participants likely to give invalid results/unable to complete testing (no exclusion of after enrollment participants); use of standardized procedures.
	1	No obvious sources of bias, but minimal attention or description to ascertain the extent to which the above standards were maintained.
	0	No description of the extent to which the above standards were maintained or an obvious source of bias in data collection methods.

Analyses		
9	2	Authors clearly defined which specific analyses were conducted for the stated specific hypotheses of the study. This may be accomplished through organization of the results under specific subheadings or by demarcating which analyses addressed specific psychometric properties. Data was presented for each hypothesis.
	1	Data was presented for each hypothesis, but authors did not clearly link analyses to hypotheses.
	0	Data was not presented for each hypothesis or psychometric property outlined in the purposes or methods
10	2	Appropriate statistical tests were conducted: 1. Reliability (e.g. Relative=ICCs for quantitative, Kappa for nominal data); absolute (SEM)) 2. Clinical relevance—e.g., minimal detectable change, minimally important difference, number needed to treat 3. Validity a. Validity associations—e.g., Pearson correlations for normally distributed data, Spearman rank correlations for ordinal data; or other correlations if appropriate b. Validity tests of significant difference—e.g., an appropriate global test like analysis of variance was used where indicated, with post-hoc tests that adjusted for multiple testing 4. Responsiveness—e.g., standardized response means or effect sizes or other recognized responsiveness indices were used.
	1	Appropriate statistical tests were used in some instances but suboptimal choices were made in other analyses.
	0	Inappropriate use of statistical tests
11	2	For key indicators like reliability coefficients indices at least 2 of the following were presented: 1. appropriate confidence intervals, 2. Comparison to appropriate benchmarks or standards, or 3. SEM. Correlation matrices for validity analysis may not require that each individual correlation be presented with its associated confidence intervals; however, confidence intervals and benchmarks should be used according to standards for that type of analysis.
	1	Either confidence intervals or appropriate benchmarks were used—not both.
	0	Inappropriate use of benchmarks or confidence intervals or neither included.
Recommendations		
12	2	Authors made specific conclusions and clinical recommendations that were clearly related to specific hypotheses stated at the beginning of the study and supported by the data presented.
	1	Authors made conclusions and clinical recommendations that were general but basically supported by the study data; OR authors made conclusions and clinical recommendations for only some of the study hypotheses.
	0	Authors made vague conclusions without any clinical recommendations; conclusions or recommendations were in contradiction to the actual data presented.

© MacDermid 2007

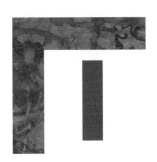

Appendix I:
Worksheet for
Evaluating and Using
Articles About
Diagnostic Tests

Title	
Authors	
Citation	
Test(s) evaluated	
Reference Standard	☐ blinded/independent ☐ gold standard /reasonable alternative ☐ applied to all
Test methods	
Setting	

Subjects		Cases	Non- cases
	n		
	Included (Criteria/ Description)		
	Excluded (Criteria/ Description)		

Test Results	Sensitivity Specificity (see calculation appendix) Other

Evaluation	Y	N
*1. Was there an independent, blind comparison with a reference standard test ?		
* 2. Was the reference standard/ true diagnosis selected a gold standard or reasonable alternative?		
* 3. Was the reference standard applied to all patients?		
4. Did the actual cases include an appropriate spectrum of severity?		
*5. Were the non-cases patients who might reasonably present for differential diagnosis?		
6. Did the non-cases include an appropriate spectrum of patients with alternate diagnoses?		
7. Did the study have an adequate sample size?		
8. Was the description of the test maneuver described insufficient detail to permit replication?		
9. Were exact criteria for interpreting the test results provided?		
10. Was the reliability of the test procedures documented?		
11. Were the number of positive and negative results reported for both cases and non-cases?		
12. Were appropriate statistics (sensitivity, specificity, likelihood ratios) presented?		
13. If the test required an element of examiner interpretation were the qualifications and skills of the examiner described (if n/a leave blank)		
14. Were the training, skills and experience of the examiner appropriate to the test conducted? (if n/a leave blank)		

Application criteria	Y	N
1. Will I be able to accurately apply and interpreting the test in my practice setting? (Instrumentation, training, personnel)		
2. Are the results applicable to my patients? i.e., Are my patients similar in terms of the distribution of disease severity and comorbidities		
3. Will the test results influence my clinical decision-making?		
4. Will my patient benefit from the test result?		
5. Is there any potential for harm to my patient from the test or its result?		

A significant problem with any of these criteria make one question the validity and/or applicability of the study results, although the items with * are particularly important. The final decision must be made by the clinician, based on a preponderance of the information.

This form was designed by JC MacDermid based on principles of evidence-based practice described by D Sackett (1)

DIAGNOSTIC TESTS CALCULATIONS

		Target disorder		Totals
		Present	Absent	
Diagnostic test result	Positive	a	b	a+b
	Negative	c	d	c+d
	Totals	a+c	b+d	a+b+c+d

Sensitivity = a/(a+c) =
Specificity = d/(b+d) =
Likelihood ratio for a positive test result = LR+ = sens/(1-spec) =
Likelihood ratio for a negative test result = LR - = (1-sens)/spec =
Positive Predictive Value = a/(a+b) =
Negative Predictive Value = d/(c+d) =
Pre-test probability (prevalence) = (a+c)/(a+b+c+d) =
Pre-test odds = prevalence/(1-prevalence) =
Post-test odds = pre-test odds × LR
Post-test probability = post-test odds/(post-test odds +1)

For further explanation of these calculations and how to apply them in evidence-based decision making consult texts or websites that describe evidence-based practice methods

Interpretation Guidelines

A "yes" response indicates that the criterion was fulfilled. A "no" indicates that it was not fulfilled or that no documentation of the criteria being fulfilled was provided.

1. The independence of the reference standard test or gold standard diagnosis is critical to study validity and should be documented within the methods. The reference standard test should be obtained without knowledge of other test results or clinical history (blinded) .

2. The reference standard should either be a recognized gold standard or where a gold standard does not exist, a suitable best alternative. Where a gold standard does not exist, suitable justification for the alternative should be provided.

3. The same reference standard should be applied to all patients in the study (patients and controls) . Results of the test under evaluation should not influence the application of the reference standard. Nor should specific pretests be done which would affect either the application or interpretation of the reference standard.

4. The patients with the target disorder should include mild, moderate and severe cases. A description of the spectrum of disease severity should be provided.

5. Patients without the target disorder should be those for whom the test might reasonably be applied in a clinical situation - as a component of differential diagnosis. Asymptomatic controls are not appropriate. Patients with the same disorder in a different location, patients with different disorders in the same location, are examples of types of appropriate non-cases. Where the reference standard is truly a gold standard i.e. accepted to be almost perfectly accurate, then a negative test should be taken as establishing the absence of the condition; where the reference standard is known to be flawed, the actual diagnosis of the non-cases should be defined to minimize the likelihood that they are not false negatives from the reference standard testing.

6. Patients without the target disorder should include *a spectrum* of patients who might conceivably be exposed to this test in a clinical situation, i.e. a variety of appropriate alternative diagnoses or locations. The severity of illness/disability should include mild, moderate and severe cases of other competing diagnoses. The specific diagnosis determined for the controls should be documented.

7. Sample size should be justified and/or not be less than 40.

8. The test maneuver should be described in sufficient detail that it could be implemented by another clinician. This may include test instruments, calibration procedures, training procedures, patient set-up and test application as dictated by the type of test involved.

9. The specific outcome or observation required in order for test to be interpreted as positive should be described. This may include elements of appearance, symptoms, timing or numerical cutoffs - as appropriate to the test.

10. The author should documented the reliability of the test procedures either by conducting reliability analyses themselves or referencing previous work which has done so.

11.   When reporting results, the number of positive and negative cases should be reported for both cases and non-cases regardless of how these numbers are used in decision-making. Where sensitivity and specificity are reported or likelihood ratios are reported, this criterion has been fulfilled. Where raw numbers are provided that could be used in a 2 by two table to compute these values, this criterion has been fulfilled.

12.   If the appropriate analyses were conducted one would expect to see sensitivity, specificity, positive/ negative predictive values and/or likelihood ratios.

13.   For any test where the examiner interprets whether a score was normal or abnormal based on interpretation of a patient's response, observation or physical assessment (other than automated tests),   the training and experience of the examiner is relevant to the accuracy of the test. Therefore, it it should be described so that the reader will be able to determine whether the examiners have similar training and experience to those who would be applying the test in future clinical situations. If this information is provided (regardless of whether the reader agrees that the examiner was appropriate) the item is scored as "yes". If this information is not provided, the score is "no".

14. Certain physical assessments or test interpretations are known to be reliable only with more experienced examiners or those with specific training. If this information is provided and is consistent with the training and experience required for competency in performing the test, the item is scored as a "yes". If the information is not provided or if the training and experience is inadequate, then this item is scored as a "no"

Reference List

1.   Sackett DL; Straus SE; Richardson WS; Rosenberg W; Haynes RB. Evidence-based Medicine. How to practice and teach EBM. 2nd. 2000. Toronto,ON, Churchill Livingstone.

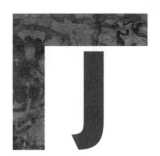

Appendix J:
Occupational Therapy
in the ICU

Title

"Does the provision of splints for people with stroke or burn injuries decrease contractures and improve upper limb functioning in acute care settings?"

Reviewer

Laura Bradley, MSc OT (prepared in April 2006 while a candidate for her MSc OT at McMaster University)

Dilemma

Often occupational therapists in hospital settings are requested to perform interventions in units to which they are not assigned. This can lead to dilemmas surrounding quality of patient care if the requests are not honoured, and therapist burnout if they are. As there is little literature surrounding the effectiveness of occupational therapy in hospital intensive care units (ICUs), a different approach to address this dilemma needed to be found.

The number one reason that OTs are called into the adult ICU is for the provision of splints for people who have sustained strokes or severe burn injuries. By looking more in depth at these two populations with regards to splinting, we can hopefully see the importance of OT services in the ICU, thereby potentially directing more service coverage and funding to these units.

Search

Database	Keywords	Yield	Hits	Obtained
Cochrane Central Register of Controlled Trials	Splint$ (limit RCT) + Function	31	1	1*
CINAHL (1992-2005)	Splint$+ Acute care	5	1	0
	Splint$ + ICU	2	0	0
	Splint$ + Function (limit clinical trial)	8	1	1*
	Burn$ + Acute Care	70	5	0
Medline (1996-2005)	Splint$ + Contracture	32	3	1*
	Splint$ + Burns	16	2	1 ®
	Splint$ + Function (limit RCT)	31	1	1 ®
	Splint$ + ICU	5	1	1®
	Splint$ + Burns (mp)	42	4	4 (1*,1®)
EMBASE (1996-2005)	Splint$ + Burns	32	3	2 ®
	Splint$ + Contractures + Burn$	17	2	0
OT Seeker	Burn	12	0	0
	Splint	37	2	2 ®

Legend: *=critically reviewed; ®=repeat articles

Date

Date of search: September/October, 2005
Proposed date for re-evaluation: September/October 2007

Citations

Lannin, N.A., Horsely, S., Herbert, R., McCluskey, A., & Cusick, A. (2003). Splinting the hand in the functional position after brain impairment: A randomized controlled trial. *Archives of Physical Medicine and Rehabilitation, 84*(2), 297-302.

Lannin, N., & Herbert, R.D. (2003). Is splinting effective for adults following stroke? A systematic review and methodological critique of published research. *Clinical Rehabilitation, 17,* 807-816.

Richard, R., Miller, S., Stanley, M., & Johnson, M. (2000). Multimodal versus progressive treatment techniques to correct burn scar contractures. *Journal of Burn Care and Rehabilitation, 18,* 64-71.

Summary and Appraisal of Studies

Author: Lannin & Herbert (2003) :Systematic Review			
Research design	*Strengths*	*Limitations*	*Conclusions*
Purpose To assess the effectiveness of hand splinting on the hemiplegic upper extremity following stroke	-systematic search -research question focused to a specific population and area of the body -homogeneous studies examined	-81% of studies were excluded due to 'poor quality', indicating some clinically important results may have been lost to methodological weaknesses -studies accepted or rejected by a single reviewer -varied outcome measures	-insufficient evidence to support or refute the effectiveness -although there was no sig. differences in many of the studies, ROM was showing positive trends (95%CI) -clinically important results may have been lost due to high number of outcome measures

Author: Lannin, Horsely, Herbert, McCluskey & Cusick (2003): Randomized Controlled Trial			
Research Design	*Strengths*	*Limitations*	*Conclusions*
Purpose: To evaluate the effects of 4 weeks of hand splinting on the length of finger and wrist flexors, hand function and pain in people with acquired brain impairment	-Outcome measures taken at days 1,30,38 -showed trial profile with dropouts included -appropriate statistical analysis -intention to treat analysis -assessor blinded	-@50% of referred patients excluded from study due to cognitive impairments associated with stroke. -both intervention and control group were given a stretching and exercise program.	-Splinting increased ROM 1° after intervention (-3.7° to 6.1°), and ROM was reduced 2V at 1 week follow up post intervention (-7.2° to 3.2°). Not statistically significant, however showing trends towards effectiveness -if patients are already receiving a motor program with stretching, splinting may not increase their ROM, decrease pain or improve hand skills.

Author: Richard, Miller, Stanley & Johnson (2000): Cohort study			
Research Design	*Strengths*	*Limitations*	*Conclusions*
Purpose: To investigate successful outcomes of scar contracture resolution with physical rehabilitation alone in order to determine best treatment practice	-looked at best clinical outcome for non-surgical interventions -population and pathology very clearly defined	-only examined populations who were successfully treated for contractures. Those who were not corrected were not included -little information as to statistical method analysis -sample of convenience can create difficulties with generalizability	-The greater the total burn surface area (TBSA), the greater the likelihood of splint provision -In order to increase the possibility of contracture revision, splints must be given while scar tissue is still immature -The provision of splints corrected contractures more quickly (35 days as opposed to 76 days, p≤.05)

Conclusions

Although Lannin and Herbert (2003) found insufficient to either support or refute the effectiveness of splinting in the stroke population, the ROM scores after treatment showed a positive trend towards effectiveness. In the population of adults with severe burns, splinting was seen to be effective to restore functional movement (Sheridan et al., 1995), as well as correct contractures up to two times more quickly in those who can potentially be corrected (Richard et al., 2000)

What does this mean for therapists working in the ICU? Splinting to prevent deformities and correct contractures can be effective if the following is kept in mind. Splinting, accompanied with a stretching or exercise program has shown beneficial results (Lannin et al., 2003; Sheridan et al., 1995). Also, the faster splints are given to appropriate populations, the more likely there is to be a favourable outcome (Lannin et al., 2003; Richard et al., 2000). It is apparent that further research must be done to provide us with stronger evidence to justify broader OT services in the adult ICU. However, the narrower scope of splinting in the population of those with stroke or burn injury can be seen to be beneficial, or show trends towards effectiveness.

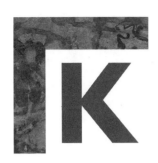

Appendix K:
Recognizing and Referring Children With Developmental Coordination Disorder

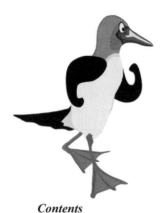

Recognizing and Referring Children with Developmental Coordination Disorder

Role of the Physical Therapist

Physical therapists assess young children with motor difficulties and/or delays by observing movement skills and asking critical key questions about their motor abilities and development. They do so in order to differentiate between patterns of motor behaviour that are characteristic of different conditions, a differentiation that guides the therapist in selecting a course of intervention.

Recently, increased attention is being given to the motor difficulties of children who used to be labeled "clumsy" or "physically awkward" but who would now be recognized as having Developmental Coordination Disorder (DCD: APA, 2000). In the past, these children received little attention from physical therapists because many believed that they would overcome their difficulties with time. It is now being realized that their motor in-coordination significantly impacts their physical, social and emotional well-being.

It is important for physical therapists to learn to differentiate the motor behaviour of children with DCD from other movement disorders in order to enable early identification and appropriate intervention. Children referred in the early years with motor difficulties or delays may have disorders such as cerebral palsy, muscular dystrophy, global developmental delay or developmental coordination disorder. Some key questions may help you focus on differentiating between each of these patterns of motor behaviour.

In a young child, you might ask: Is there evidence of increased or fluctuating tone? Observed alterations in muscle tone might be suggestive of a condition such as cerebral palsy. Are the delays global rather than just a motor delay, a situation in which global developmental delay might be suspected? With a preschool or schoolaged child, questions might centre around the history of the in-coordination. Have the difficulties been present from an early age? Are the motor concerns appearing to worsen over time? Has there been a loss of previously acquired skills? If so, this might be suggestive of a condition like muscular dystrophy.

If a child does not show the above signs but demonstrates uncoordinated movements and motor abilities below those expected for their age, they may have Developmental Coordination Disorder (DCD). This paper will help you recognize children at risk for DCD and recognize the need to intervene and to refer the child to other service providers for further evaluation.

Contents

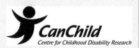

CanChild
Centre for Childhood Disability Research

Visit our web site and check for new information at
www.canchild.ca
or call (905) 525-9140 ext 27850

Recognizing Children with Developmental Coordination Disorder (DCD)

Described by those around them as being clumsy, children presenting with the characteristics of DCD are often referred to as "motor delayed." You might hear or observe that these children have difficulty with *skipping, hopping, jumping, and balancing. Handwriting, printing, copying, cutting* and other fine motor tasks also present challenges. Children with DCD usually also have difficulty with *zippers, snaps, buttons, tying shoelaces, throwing and catching balls, learning to ride a bicycle. Organizational skills* might be less well developed than their peers. *Motor skills require effort* so children with DCD are often slow to complete tasks at school and may appear inattentive. Children with DCD usually begin to withdraw from and avoid motor and sports activities at an early age. They often seem verbally advanced but immature socially and might have behavioural or emotional problems.

Definition:

Developmental Coordination Disorder is a "marked impairment in the development of motor coordination... only if this impairment significantly interferes with academic achievement or activities of daily living." Developmental Coordination Disorder may exist in isolation OR may co-occur with other conditions such as learning disabilities or attention deficit disorder.

Diagnostic Criteria:

A) Performance in daily activities that require motor coordination is substantially below that expected, given the person's chronological age and measured intelligence. This may be manifested by marked delays in achieving motor milestones (e.g., walking, crawling, sitting), dropping things, "clumsiness", poor performance in sports, or poor handwriting.

B) The disturbance in Criterion A significantly interferes with academic achievement or activities of daily living.

(APA Diagnostic and Statistical Manual, 2000; pp. 56-58)

C) The disturbance is not due to a general medical condition (e.g., cerebral palsy, hemiplegia, or muscular dystrophy) and does not meet criteria for Pervasive Developmental Disorder.

D) If mental retardation is present, motor difficulties are in excess of those usually associated with it.

> *Note: Criteria C and D require the involvement of a family practitioner or developmental pediatrician to rule out other explanations for the clumsiness. In the province of Ontario, only a medical doctor or a psychologist is permitted to make this diagnosis.*

Prevalence: 5-6% of the school-aged population, more commonly identified in boys

For more information on this topic:
Missiuna, C., Rivard, L. & Bartlett, D. (2003). Early identification and risk management of children with developmental coordination disorder. *Pediatric Physical Therapy, 15,* 32-38.

**Characteristic Features of Children with Developmental
Coordination Disorder:**

- Clumsiness and/or incoordination
- Handwriting / printing / copying difficulties
- Difficulty finishing academic tasks on time
- Requires extra effort and attention when tasks have a motor component
- Difficulty with activities of daily living (e.g., dressing, feeding, grooming)
- Difficulty with sports and on the playground (last to "get picked" for teams)
- Difficulty learning new motor skills
- Difficulty with, or reduced interest in, physical activities

If you suspect that a child is demonstrating the characteristics of DCD, you might want to ask parents about other developmental concerns (fine motor, self-care, leisure). It will be important to inquire whether or not there are difficulties at home or at school. Is your child having trouble with buttons, using eating utensils or tying shoelaces? Are fine motor activities such as printing and cutting difficult for your child? Does your child have to exert a lot of effort to complete motor tasks? Does your child participate in organized sports or other physical activity?

A child with DCD is usually seen by a physical therapist due to low tone or gross motor concerns: you will want to conduct further assessment and might provide intervention for these difficulties. It is probable, however, that a child with DCD will also experience delays in fine motor and/or self-care skill acquisition that may not have been identified. If your observations and parental report are consistent with the characteristics outlined above, you might consider making a referral to an occupational therapist (see page 4 for parent information).

You should also consider encouraging the family to have the child seen by their physician. It is important that a medical practitioner rule out other conditions that might explain the motor in-coordination. Also, since DCD often coexists with other developmental conditions (expressive and receptive language difficulties, attention deficit disorder), the primary care physician should be investigating these further and making appropriate referrals to other service providers.

**For more information, access the *CanChild* website
(www.canchild.ca)**
or contact:

Cheryl Missiuna, PhD, OTReg(Ont)	**Lisa Rivard, B.Sc. , M.Sc., PT**
Associate Professor and Investigator	Project Coordinator
missiuna@mcmaster.ca	lrivard@mcmaster.ca

**School of Rehabilitation Science and *CanChild*
McMaster University, Hamilton, Ontario**

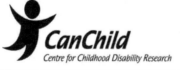
CanChild
Centre for Childhood Disability Research

canchild@mcmaster.ca
(905) 525-9140, ext. 27850

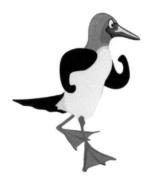

When Your Child is Having Motor Difficulties.......

Children can have motor difficulties in the early years for a number of reasons. Some children have trouble coordinating their movements to run, skip or jump. They might experience frustration at learning to ride a tricycle or to catch a ball. Others might have difficulty managing stairs and might avoid playing on playground equipment or participating in childhood motor games.

You may have some concerns about your child's ability to participate in motor activities. Your child has now been seen by a physical therapist and his/her motor skills have been assessed. Your physical therapist thinks that there is a reason for your child to also be seen by an occupational therapist. Occupational therapists, like physical therapists work with children who have coordination problems or organizational difficulties that can impact on their ability to perform well at school, at home and on the playground. Some children who have these types of problems have developmental coordination disorder and may also benefit from working with an occupational therapist on self-care or early academic tasks.

What can an occupational therapist do?
An occupational therapist will:
- Provide a thorough assessment of your child's developmental skills
- Determine how different aspects of your child's daily life are affected
- Teach your child ways of thinking his/her way through learning new tasks
- Provide adapted equipment and materials to improve task performance
- Help you and your child to set appropriate expectations
- Modify environmental factors to maximize participation
- Guide you in your selection of leisure activities for success
- Help you, your child and others to maximize his/her strengths

How do I find an occupational therapist in my area?
Your child's physical therapist can help you find and make a referral to an occupational therapist.
It may also be a good idea for your child to be seen by your family physician. Your doctor will be able to assist the physical and occupational therapists in determining the possible reasons for your child's motor difficulties. You can find more information about developmental coordination disorder at:

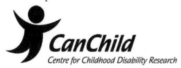

CanChild
Centre for Childhood Disability Research

www.canchild.ca
(905) 525-9140, ext. 27850

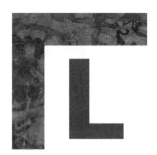

Appendix L:
Do You Know a
Child Who Is Clumsy?

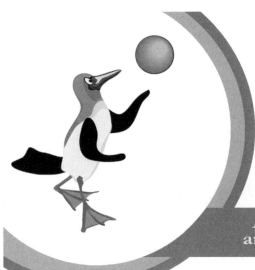

Do You Know A Child Who Is Clumsy?

A flyer for coaches and sports instructors

Do you know a child who is motivated to participate in sports activities at first, but they experience significant frustration when they just can't seem to "get the hang of it"? While other children learn and progress with good instruction, this child may seem to learn slowly and may show very little improvement from one practice session to another.

Children with these types of difficulties may have *Developmental Coordination Disorder* (DCD). Even though many people have never heard of it, DCD affects about 5% of school-aged children in North America. Children with DCD have trouble learning to coordinate their movements and may appear to be awkward or clumsy. These children often struggle with participation in organized sports and leisure activities. Activities that are hardest for them are those that require new learning and those that require coordination of their bodies in response to things that move (like balls, pucks and other children).

Repeated failure experiences cause children with DCD to eventually withdraw from physical activities altogether. They often cannot overcome the physical challenges, and they begin to feel isolated from their peers.

If children with movement difficulties avoid or drop out of physical games and activities then, over time, they will develop poor overall fitness and low self-esteem. With encouragement and individualized instruction, children with DCD can receive enjoyment from the activities they participate in and be healthy throughout their lives.

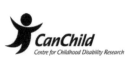

CanChild
Centre for Childhood Disability Research

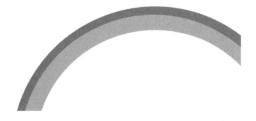

What might you see in a child with movement difficulties?

➢ Appears clumsy or uncoordinated

➢ Is slow to learn new motor skills

➢ Requires more instruction than other children

➢ Works hard but is often unsuccessful; becomes frustrated easily

➢ Has difficulty with ball skills (catching, throwing, kicking) and activities that require good balance (running, hopping, jumping, skipping, climbing stairs)

   ➢ May demonstrate distracting or disruptive behaviour

     ➢ Demonstrates decreased interest or motivation, poor self-esteem

     ➢ May withdraw or avoid coming to practices and games

How can you help a child with movement difficulties?

   ➢ REWARD EFFORT!

   ➢ Encourage participation and fun rather than competition

   ➢ If possible, provide one-to-one instruction for new skills

➢ Break down skills into smaller, meaningful parts

➢ Use different teaching methods to demonstrate the skill (show the movement while using words to describe it)

➢ When giving feedback, use clear and specific language (raise your arm up higher when you throw)

➢ Provide hand over hand instruction (e.g., have child demonstrate a new skill to a group with the instructor guiding the movement)

➢ Keep the environment as predictable as possible when teaching a new skill

➢ Review rules of game play when the child is not concentrating on the movements

➢ Modify or adapt equipment to ensure safety

➢ Provide frequent verbal instruction and encouragement

➢ Ask questions to ensure that the child understands the game rules or movements required

For more information, please go to www.fhs.mcmaster.ca/canchild.

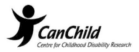

Download our free booklet called, *"Children with Developmental Coordination Disorder: At home and in the classroom."* To order a hard copy of this booklet, or for more information, please call (905) 525-9140, ext. 27850

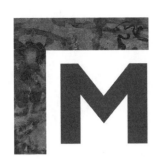

Appendix M:
Effectiveness Study
Quality Checklist

Evaluation of Quality of an Intervention Study

This form is used to extract relevant data on effectiveness from your study and to rate the quality of the published study (for item interpretation see guide)

Citation: _____

Authors: _____

Title: _____

Reviewer: _____   Date: _____

Patient Characteristics (age, sex, disorder, co-morbidity/important co-variates)
1._____
2._____

Sample Size _____

Interventions   (Describe type, timing, frequency, equipment, provider, progression etc.)
1._____

2._____

Outcome Measures   (Type and when evaluated)
1E_____
2E_____

Results:
Outcomes (absolute change, significance)
         1E_____
         2E_____

Time to Return to work/function _____

Describe any risk factors for non-response indicated in this study ?

_____

Describe any complications indicated by this study ?

_____

Evaluation of Study Design

Evaluation Criteria	Score		
Study question	2	1	0
1. Was the relevant background work cited to establish a foundation for the research question?			
Study design			
2. Was a comparison group used?			
3. Was patient status at more than 1 time point considered?			
4. Was data collection performed prospectively?			
5. Were patients randomized to groups?			
6. Were patients blinded to the extent possible?			
7. Were treatment providers blinded to the extent possible?			
8. Was an independent evaluator used to administer outcome measures?			
Subjects			
9. Did sampling procedures minimize sample/selection biases?			
10. Were inclusion/exclusion criteria defined?			
11. Was an appropriate enrollment obtained?			
12. Was appropriate retention/follow-up obtained?			
Intervention			
13. Was the intervention applied according to established principles?			
14. Were biases due to the treatment provider minimized (i.e. attention, training)?			
15. Was the intervention compared to an appropriate comparator?			
Outcomes			
16. Was an appropriate primary outcome defined?			
17. Were appropriate secondary outcomes considered?			
18. Was an appropriate follow-up period incorporated?			
Analysis			
19. Was an appropriate statistical test(s) performed to indicate differences related to the intervention?			

20. Was it established that the study had significant power to identify treatment effects?			
21. Was the size and significance of the effects reported?			
22. Were missing data accounted for and considered in analyses?			
23. Were clinical and practical significance considered in interpreting results?			
Recommendations			
24. Were the conclusions/clinical recommendations supported by the study objectives, analysis and results?			
Total Quality Score (Sum of above) =			
Level of Evidence (Sackett) 1 □ 2 □ 3□ 4□ 5□			

© Joy MacDermid 2003

Notes:

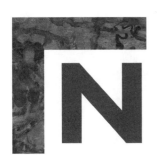

Appendix N:
Effectiveness Study
Quality Checklist
Interpretation Guidelines

Evaluation Guidelines for Rating the Quality of an Intervention Study

This guide helps you interpret the correct score for each critical appraisal item on your checklist. To decide which score to choose read the following descriptors for each item. Pick the descriptor that sounds <u>most</u> like what was described in the study you were evaluating with respect to that item.

Question		Descriptors
#	Score	
1	2	The authors -performed a thorough literature review indicating what is currently known about the problem and the intervention at present - presented a critical, but unbiased, view of the current state of knowledge - indicated how the current research question evolves from the current knowledge base - established a clear research question(s) based on the above.
	1	All of these above were not fulfilled, but a clear rationale was provided for the research question
	0	A foundation for the current research question was not developed.
		Study design
2.	2	Two or more contemporary (same point in time) groups of similar patients were compared. Crossover trials which include randomization/blinding of intervention order and complete wash-out of effects can be considered equivalent.
	1	A comparator group was present, but did not fulfill the above criteria.
	0	No comparator group was included.
3.	2	Patients were evaluated prior to the intervention, and at one or more clinically relevant time points, following the intervention using the same evaluation criteria.
	1	Patients were evaluated at more than one point in time (including case control studies); but the above criteria were not fulfilled
	0	Patients were evaluated at only one point in time.
4.	2	A standardized set of (prospective) data were collected at specific pre-set intervals according to a preplanned study protocol.
	1	A core set of prospective data were collected from patients or obtained from database retrieval. This data was collected across multiple intervals, but the actual data collection strategy was not determined specifically for this study
	0	Data were based on retrospective records/interpretations or recall of past events.
5.	2	An appropriate randomization strategy was used to allocate patients to interventions and the specifics of randomization were described.

	1	Randomization was used, but information describing the randomization process was not included or did not confirm a truly random process.
	0	Randomization was not used
6.	2	Patients were blinded as to the intervention that was provided and either a post- hoc analyses indicated that blinding procedures were effective or it was evident that patients would be unable to distinguish which intervention they received.
	1	Blinding patients was not possible or it was unclear whether an effective blinding strategy was used.
	0	Blinding was possible, but not utilized (includes all studies without comparison groups).
7.	2	Treatment providers were blinded to the intervention they were administering and this blinding was substantiated either through audits or other post-hoc analyses indicated that the blinding procedure was effective.
	1	Blinding was not possible or it was unclear whether an effective blinding strategy was used
	0	Blinding was possible, but was not utilized
8.	2	Outcome measures were administered by an evaluator who was blind to the treatment provided and/or the purpose of the study. Self-report can be considered as equivalent if provided by an independent person
	1	Evaluators were not blinded, but were not involved in treatment of patients (were independent) or Self-report administered by treatment provider.
	0	Outcome measures were obtained by unblinded treatment providers
	Subjects	
9.	2	The authors documented a specific recruitment strategy that was intended to maximize the representation of subjects in relation to specific target population and sampling procedures were applied equally across comparison groups.
	1	The study sample appears representative of the population of clinical interest, but adequate information on sampling procedures or description of the reference population is not provided.
	0	Sampling biases are evident; systematic differences occurred between the comparison groups; and/or selection procedures used make it impossible to determine what types of patients were included.
10.	2	Specific inclusion and exclusion criteria for the study were defined and designed to yield a study group generalizable to clinical situation.
	1	Some information on the type of patients included in the study and excluded are defined, but the information is insufficient to allow the reader to generalize the study results to a specific clinical population.
	0	No information on inclusion and exclusion criteria and limited patients descriptors are provided.

11.	2	Authors performed a sample size calculation upon which their recruitment targets were defined, described the target population from which subjects were drawn, and the response from the target population in terms of participation in the study
	1	The authors performed a sample size calculation and/or provided a satisfactory rationale for the number of subjects included in the study.
	0	The size of the sample or its relationship to target population were not rationalized.
12.	2	90% or more of the patients enrolled or eligible for study were evaluated for outcomes.
	1	More than 70% of the patients eligible for study or enrolled were evaluated for outcomes.
	0	Less than 70 percent of patients eligible for study or enrolled were evaluated.
		Intervention
13.	2	The parameters of the treatment (provider/equipment, frequency, duration, application process, progression and other technical components) and compliance/monitoring were sufficiently described that they could be replicated. The specific parameters used were based on published basic science or clinical evidence documenting that the specific treatment effects intended are achievable given the treatment parameters used.
	1	A sound rationale OR adequate description was provided for the treatment intervention, but the above level of documentation was not cited.
	0	A rationale for the treatment intervention was not provided AND an adequate description of the intervention was not included OR the application of the intervention did not conform to present knowledge on potentially effective parameters.
14.	2	The study was designed to minimize biases due to the treatment provider. Treatment provider biases can be minimized if the treatment provider is blinded to which treatment they provide. In cases where this is impossible, methods such as equalize attention to groups, selecting treatment providers without vested interests in a specific intervention, training treatment providers according to a standardized process or assuring a specific level of training when recruiting providers can be used to assure sufficient equipoise.
	1	Minimal attention was directed either in methods or discussion to the potential for treatment provider biases, but no inherent opportunity for bias was apparent.
	0	No attention was directed at the potential for treatment provider biases and the opportunity for bias is evident, given the nature in which interventions were applied.
15.	2	A rationale was provided for the comparison group selected. Where no specific intervention has previously been demonstrated to be effective, placebo is an appropriate comparator. A comparator group that has previously been shown to be effective or is commonly considered as acceptable standard of care is also appropriate.
	1	A rationale for the comparison group was not established.
	0	No comparison group was included.
		Outcome

16.	2	A primary outcome measure which represented important clinical outcomes was selected and supported by evidence of appropriate psychometric properties (reliability, validity, responsiveness).
	1	A relevant primary outcome measure was evident, but was insufficient in either its clinical relevance or its psychometric properties.
	0	A primary outcome was not evident or was inappropriate, because it was irrelevant or methodologically unsupported.
17.	2	Appropriate secondary outcome measures were identified that augmented the perspective provided by the primary outcome measure, ensuring a comprehensive view of outcomes was obtained; and these secondary outcome measures had sound psychometric properties.
	1	Secondary outcomes were considered, but were not identified as being secondary or were deficient either in terms of their relevance or methodological properties.
	0	Appropriate secondary outcomes were not considered.
18.	2	Patients were followed at important time points that provided an indication as to the early response and longer-term outcomes achieved. These time points were sufficient to support a clear definition of the relative value of the intervention, over a clinically meaningful time period. A rationale and/or discussion of the appropriateness of these follow-up periods was included.
	1	At least one relevant follow-up evaluation was incorporated, but the study did include other important clinical time points or a rationale for the specific follow-up time.
	0	The follow-up period was insufficient to establish the true outcome of the intervention.
	Analysis	
19.	2	The statistical tests utilized to determine whether differences existed due to the intervention were appropriate and specifically related to their stated research objectives. The authors documented important elements on the statistical tests (software used, that statistical assumptions underlying tests were met, Alpha levels).
	1	Test(s) of statistical difference was used, but were insufficient to describe whether statistical differences occurred because of treatment; there was insufficient documentation of the specifics of the analyses performed
	0	Statistical tests were not performed or those selected were not appropriate to the research question or data collected.
20.	2	Power was established. A justified sample with significant statistical difference are one indication of this. If statistical differences were not obtained, a post-hoc power analysis was conducted and identified that the study was appropriately powered.
	1	The sample size was substantial, but post-hoc power analyses were not conducted in response to nonsignificant results.
	0	The sample size was small and post-hoc power analyses were not conducted in response to nonsignificant results.

21.	2	The authors appropriately conveyed both the statistical significance and size of the treatment effect when reporting the results. This could be indicated by the inclusion of p-values and the associated confidence intervals; effect sizes, number-needed-to-treat; or other similar statistical methods.
	1	Statistical significance of the outcomes achieved by the intervention group were described (means and p-values), but no quantitative description of the confidence intervals/effect sizes of these differences was presented
	0	Descriptive, statistical information on the size of the treatment effects was not reported.
22.	2	1) complete data collection was achieved on all subjects or 2) a specific described strategy for handling missing data was documented and where missing data occurred in more than 10 percent of cases a specific analysis was conducted to determine the impact of missing data management.
	1	Missing data was not an apparent issue, but the exact protocol for handling missing data was not adequately described.
	0	Missing data may have been an issue and the protocol for handling missing data was not adequately described.
23.	2	The authors fully addressed clinical significance by relating the observed differences to that required for clinically important change (or minimally important significant differences) and described practical issues such as specific training or equipment required to achieve the effects described in the study.
	1	The relevant issues on the clinical and practical significance were addressed in the discussion of the study results, but not documented in relation to specifically established criteria (certifications of treatment provider's or established minimally/clinically important differences.)
	0	Clinical and practical significance were not considered when interpreting the results.
		Recommendations
24.	2	Specific conclusions and clinical recommendations made by the authors directly related to the objectives of the study, the specific analyses conducted and results of those analyses. Recommendations neither 1. ignored observed results 2. overstated their generalizability/clinical application or 3. stated that the treatment is ineffective when there was insufficient power to establish this was the case.
	1	Conclusions and clinical recommendations are either incomplete, or generalize beyond the domain of the study or the results actually obtained.
	0	Conclusions and or clinical recommendations were not founded on the results of the study or contradict findings of the study.

Guidelines for Multiple Reviewers

1. Use the accompanying data collection sheets to extract content information from the study and your ratings of research design rigor on the 24 items above
2. Suggested Consensus Process Policy for Design Rigor Items:
    - Reviewers will review their scores for all 24 items
    - Differences of 2 points on the score for any item must be adjudicated so that they are minimized by consensus to a difference of 1 point or less for any given item. If the primary reviewers cannot agree to within 1 point, secondary reviewers will be used.
- Differences of 1 point will be adjudicated and an attempt made for reviewers to assign a score by consensus; if a consensus cannot be reached, then the lower score will be assigned.

Index

WAIT

...There's More!

Please visit

www.slackbooks.com
to order any of these titles!
24 Hours a Day...7 Days a Week!

Attention Industry Partners!
Whether you are interested in buying multiple copies of a book, chapter reprints, or looking for something new and different — we are able to accommodate your needs.

Multiple Copies
At attractive discounts starting for purchases as low as 25 copies for a single title, SLACK Incorporated will be able to meet all of your needs.

Chapter Reprints
SLACK Incorporated is able to offer the chapters you want in a format that will lead to success. Bound with an attractive cover, use the chapters that are a fit specifically for your company. Available for quantities of 100 or more.

Customize
SLACK Incorporated is able to create a specialized custom version of any of our products specifically for your company.

Please contact the Marketing Communications Director of the Health Care Books and Journals for further details on multiple copy purchases, chapter reprints or custom printing at 1-800-257-8290 or 1-856-848-1000.

*Please note all conditions are subject to change.

CODE: 328

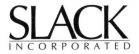

SLACK Incorporated • Health Care Books and Journals
6900 Grove Road • Thorofare, NJ 08086

1-800-257-8290 or 1-856-848-1000
Fax: 1-856-848-6091 • E-mail: orders@slackinc.com • Visit: www.slackbooks.com